Selected Papers from XVI MaNaPro and XI ECMNP

Selected Papers from XVI MaNaPro and XI ECMNP

Editors

Susana P. Gaudêncio
Rui Pedrosa
Vitor Vasconcelos

MDPI • Basel • Beijing • Wuhan • Barcelona • Belgrade • Manchester • Tokyo • Cluj • Tianjin

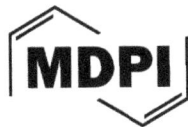

Editors
Susana P. Gaudêncio
UCIBIO, NOVA School of
Science and Technology,
NOVA University of Lisbon
Portugal

Rui Pedrosa
MARE—Marine and
Environmental Sciences Centre,
Polytechnic of Leiria
Portugal

Vitor Vasconcelos
CIIMAR/CIMAR,
University of Porto
Portugal

Editorial Office
MDPI
St. Alban-Anlage 66
4052 Basel, Switzerland

This is a reprint of articles from the Special Issue published online in the open access journal *Marine Drugs* (ISSN 1660-3397) (available at: https://www.mdpi.com/journal/marinedrugs/special_issues/MaNaPro-ECMNP-2019).

For citation purposes, cite each article independently as indicated on the article page online and as indicated below:

LastName, A.A.; LastName, B.B.; LastName, C.C. Article Title. *Journal Name* **Year**, *Volume Number*, Page Range.

ISBN 978-3-0365-0642-5 (Hbk)
ISBN 978-3-0365-0643-2 (PDF)

© 2021 by the authors. Articles in this book are Open Access and distributed under the Creative Commons Attribution (CC BY) license, which allows users to download, copy and build upon published articles, as long as the author and publisher are properly credited, which ensures maximum dissemination and a wider impact of our publications.

The book as a whole is distributed by MDPI under the terms and conditions of the Creative Commons license CC BY-NC-ND.

Contents

About the Editors vii

Preface to "Selected Papers from XVI MaNaPro and XI ECMNP" ix

Matthias Köck, Michael Reggelin and Stefan Immel
The Advanced Floating Chirality Distance Geometry Approach—How Anisotropic NMR Parameters Can Support the Determination of the Relative Configuration of Natural Products
Reprinted from: *Mar. Drugs* **2020**, *18*, 330, doi:10.3390/md18060330 1

Yan Xie, Yunjiang Feng, Angela Di Capua, Tin Mak, Garry W. Buchko, Peter J. Myler, Miaomiao Liu and Ronald J. Quinn
A Phenotarget Approach for Identifying an Alkaloid Interacting with the Tuberculosis Protein Rv1466
Reprinted from: *Mar. Drugs* **2020**, *18*, 149, doi:10.3390/md18030149 23

Chia-Chi Peng, Chiung-Yao Huang, Atallah F. Ahmed, Tsong-Long Hwang and Jyh-Horng Sheu
Anti-Inflammatory Cembranoids from a Formosa Soft Coral *Sarcophyton cherbonnieri*
Reprinted from: *Mar. Drugs* **2020**, *18*, 573, doi:10.3390/md18110573 37

Anton N. Yurchenko, Phan Thi Hoai Trinh, Elena V. Girich (Ivanets), Olga F. Smetanina, Anton B. Rasin, Roman S. Popov, Sergey A. Dyshlovoy, Gunhild von Amsberg, Ekaterina S. Menchinskaya, Tran Thi Thanh Van and Shamil Sh. Afiyatullov
Biologically Active Metabolites from the Marine Sediment-Derived Fungus *Aspergillus flocculosus*
Reprinted from: *Mar. Drugs* **2019**, *17*, 579, doi:10.3390/md17100579 51

Che-Yen Chiu, Xue-Hua Ling, Shang-Kwei Wang and Chang-Yih Duh
Ubiquitin-Proteasome Modulating Dolabellanes and Secosteroids from Soft Coral *Clavularia flava*
Reprinted from: *Mar. Drugs* **2020**, *18*, 39, doi:10.3390/md18010039 63

Concetta Imperatore, Roberto Gimmelli, Marco Persico, Marcello Casertano, Alessandra Guidi, Fulvio Saccoccia, Giovina Ruberti, Paolo Luciano, Anna Aiello, Silvia Parapini, Sibel Avunduk, Nicoletta Basilico, Caterina Fattorusso and Marialuisa Menna
Investigating the Antiparasitic Potential of the Marine Sesquiterpene Avarone, Its Reduced Form Avarol, and the Novel Semisynthetic Thiazinoquinone Analogue Thiazoavarone
Reprinted from: *Mar. Drugs* **2020**, *18*, 112, doi:10.3390/md18020112 73

Florbela Pereira, Joana R. Almeida, Marisa Paulino, Inês R. Grilo, Helena Macedo, Isabel Cunha, Rita G. Sobral, Vitor Vasconcelos and Susana P. Gaudêncio
Antifouling Napyradiomycins from Marine-Derived Actinomycetes *Streptomyces aculeolatus* [†]
Reprinted from: *Mar. Drugs* **2020**, *18*, 63, doi:10.3390/md18010063 95

Nuna Araújo, Carla S. B. Viegas, Eva Zubía, Joana Magalhães, Acácio Ramos, Maria M. Carvalho, Henrique Cruz, João Paulo Sousa, Francisco J. Blanco, Cees Vermeer and Dina C. Simes
Amentadione from the Alga *Cystoseira usneoides* as a Novel Osteoarthritis Protective Agent in an Ex Vivo Co-Culture OA Model
Reprinted from: *Mar. Drugs* **2020**, *18*, 624, doi:10.3390/md18120624 115

Elham Kamyab, Norman Goebeler, Matthias Y. Kellermann, Sven Rohde, Miriam Reverter, Maren Striebel and Peter J. Schupp
Anti-Fouling Effects of Saponin-Containing Crude Extracts from Tropical Indo-Pacific Sea Cucumbers
Reprinted from: *Mar. Drugs* **2020**, *18*, 181, doi:10.3390/md18040181 . . . . **131**

Sébastien Duperron, Mehdi A. Beniddir, Sylvain Durand, Arlette Longeon, Charlotte Duval, Olivier Gros, Cécile Bernard and Marie-Lise Bourguet-Kondracki
New Benthic Cyanobacteria from Guadeloupe Mangroves as Producers of Antimicrobials
Reprinted from: *Mar. Drugs* **2020**, *18*, 16, doi:10.3390/md18010016 . . . . **151**

Alison E. Murray, Nicole E. Avalon, Lucas Bishop, Karen W. Davenport, Erwan Delage, Armand E.K. Dichosa, Damien Eveillard, Mary L. Higham, Sofia Kokkaliari, Chien-Chi Lo, Christian S. Riesenfeld, Ryan M. Young, Patrick S.G. Chain and Bill J. Baker
Uncovering the Core Microbiome and Distribution of Palmerolide in *Synoicum adareanum* Across the Anvers Island Archipelago, Antarctica
Reprinted from: *Mar. Drugs* **2020**, *18*, 298, doi:10.3390/md18060298 . . . . **165**

Mariaelena D'Ambrosio, Ana Catarina Santos, Alfonso Alejo-Armijo, A. Jorge Parola and Pedro M. Costa
Light-Mediated Toxicity of Porphyrin-Like Pigments from a Marine Polychaeta
Reprinted from: *Mar. Drugs* **2020**, *18*, 302, doi:10.3390/md18060302 . . . . **189**

About the Editors

Susana P. Gaudêncio PhD in Organic Chemistry, is the Head of the Blue Biotechnology & Biomedicine Lab at UCIBIO—Applied Molecular Biosciences Unit, Department of Chemistry, Faculty of Sciences and Technology, NOVA University of Lisbon (FCT-NOVA) (https://www.requimte.pt/ucibio/research-groups/lab/blue-biotechnology-biomedicine).
Her research interests focus on marine-derived actinobacteria from Portugal and the Macaronesia Archipelagos for the discovery of bioactive natural products as lead-like agents for drug discovery and biotechnological applications. She is responsible for a collection of over 1000 actinobacteria obtained from ocean sediments. SPG has published over 30 papers on marine natural product chemistry and marine biotechnology.

Rui Pedrosa PhD in Human Biology, is Coordinator Professor at the School of Tourism and Maritime Technology (ESTM) from the Polytechnic Institute of Leiria and President of the same institute. His research is focused on algae for the discovery of natural products and their biotechnological applications. RP has published over 60 papers on marine biotechnology and cellular pharmacology and biology.

Vitor Vasconcelos PhD in Biology, is Full Professor at the Faculty of Sciences of Porto University and Director of CIIMAR—Interdisciplinary Center of Marine and Environmental Research. He is the Head of the Blue Biotechnology and Ecotoxicology Group (LEGE lab). His main research focus is on cyanobacteria secondary metabolites and their uses: toxins and molecules with biotechnological applications. He is responsible for the LEGE culture collection comprising over 400 cyanobacteria strains. VV has published over 400 papers on toxicology and biotechnology.

Preface to "Selected Papers from XVI MaNaPro and XI ECMNP"

The International Symposium on Marine Natural Products (MaNaPro) and the European Conference on Marine Natural Products (ECMNP) are two of the top three most prestigious conferences on marine natural products. MaNaPro started in 1975 and ECMNP began in 1997, and they are conducted in triennial and biennial frequencies, respectively. Both conferences focus on studies related to marine chemistry. The MaNaPro symposia are the world's most noteworthy events in marine natural products. The ECMNP mission is to promote the participation of younger researchers in high-quality scientific meetings in this field and encourage collaborations worldwide.

In 2019, the 2nd joint XVI MaNaPro and XI ECMNP meeting (http://wmnp2019.ipleiria.pt/) was held in Peniche, Portugal, from the 1st to the 5th of September. A Special Issue dedicated to this symposium entitled "Selected Papers from the XVI MaNaPro and XI ECMNP" was developed to maximize the impact of this conference in the marine natural products community. The conference Special Issue resulted in 1 conference report and 12 articles published in *Marine Drugs* (https://www.mdpi.com/journal/marinedrugs/special_issues/MaNaPro-ECMNP-2019).

The 12 articles are included in this volume and provide a good representation of the richness of the joint XVI MaNaPro and XI ECMNP conference topics: (1) the development of an advanced floating chirality distance geometry approach that uses anisotropic NMR parameters to support the determination of the relative configuration of natural products; (2) the use of a phenotarget approach for identifying an alkaloid that interacts with the tuberculosis protein; (3) the discovery of anti-inflammatory cembranoids from the soft coral *Sarcophyton cherbonnieri*; (4) the finding of anticancer metabolites from the marine sediment-derived fungus *Aspergillus flocculosus*; (5) the discovery of dolabellanes and secosteroids that potentiate proteasome inhibition from the soft coral *Clavularia flava*; (6) the investigation of avarone, avarol, and the novel semisynthetic thiazinoquinone analog thiazoavarone as antiparasitic agents; (7) the assessment of napyradiomycins from the marine-derived actinomycetes *Streptomyces aculeolatus* as antifouling agents; (8) the evaluation of amentadione from the alga *Cystoseira usneoides* as an osteoarthritis protective agent; (9) the study of the antifouling properties of saponin-containing crude extracts from sea cucumbers; (10) the discovery of new benthic cyanobacteria from Guadeloupe Mangroves as producers of antimicrobials; (11) the uncovering of the core microbiome and distribution of palmerolide in *Synoicum adareanum* across the Anvers Island, Antarctica; and (12) the light-mediated toxicity of porphyrin-like pigments from a marine polychaeta.

This collection of selected scientific publications provides a comprehensive overview of the wide diversity of marine bioresources, the relentless search for new tools for advancing structure elucidation and configuration assignment and for the rapid discovery of bioactive natural products, and the interdisciplinary nature of the research of marine natural products and their extensive medical and biotechnological potential.

Susana P. Gaudêncio, Rui Pedrosa, Vitor Vasconcelos

Editors

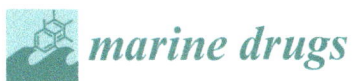

Article

The Advanced Floating Chirality Distance Geometry Approach—How Anisotropic NMR Parameters Can Support the Determination of the Relative Configuration of Natural Products

Matthias Köck [1,*], Michael Reggelin [2] and Stefan Immel [2,*]

[1] Alfred-Wegener-Institut für Polar-und Meeresforschung in der Helmholtz-Gemeinschaft, Am Handelshafen 12, 27570 Bremerhaven, Germany
[2] Clemens-Schöpf-Institut für Organische Chemie und Biochemie, Technische Universität Darmstadt, Alarich-Weiss-Straße 4, 64287 Darmstadt, Germany; re@chemie.tu-darmstadt.de
* Correspondence: mkoeck@awi.de (M.K.); lemmi@chemie.tu-darmstadt.de (S.I.)

Received: 4 May 2020; Accepted: 18 June 2020; Published: 24 June 2020

Abstract: The configurational analysis of complex natural products by NMR spectroscopy is still a challenging task. The assignment of the relative configuration is usually carried out by analysis of interproton distances from NOESY or ROESY spectra (qualitative or quantitative) and scalar (J) couplings. About 15 years ago, residual dipolar couplings (RDCs) were introduced as a tool for the configurational determination of small organic molecules. In contrast to NOEs/ROEs which are local parameters (distances up to 400 pm can be detected for small organic molecules), RDCs are global parameters which allow to obtain structural information also from long-range relationships. RDCs have the disadvantage that the sample needs a setup in an alignment medium in order to obtain the required anisotropic environment. Here, we will discuss the configurational analysis of five complex natural products: axinellamine A (**1**), tetrabromostyloguanidine (**2**), 3,7-*epi*-massadine chloride (**3**), tubocurarine (**4**), and vincristine (**5**). Compounds **1**–**3** are marine natural products whereas **4** and **5** are from terrestrial sources. The chosen examples will carefully work out the limitations of NOEs/ROEs in the configurational analysis of natural products and will also provide an outlook on the information obtained from RDCs.

Keywords: chirality; configurational analysis; distance geometry; NMR spectroscopy; NOE data; residual dipolar couplings

---

1. Introduction

The determination of the relative and absolute configuration of natural products is essential to understand their interactions in the biological field and to allow their procurement through total synthesis. The structure determination of natural products by NMR spectroscopy [1–3] is usually divided into two more or less "independent" approaches: (a) constitutional assignment and (b) configurational and conformational assignment (see Figure 1). The constitutional assignment will not be covered in the present manuscript. We will focus on the discussion of the assignment of the relative configuration and conformation only.

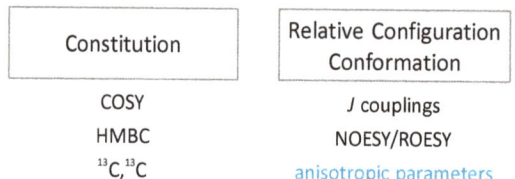

Figure 1. Structure elucidation of natural products by NMR spectroscopy.

1.1. NOEs/ROEs in Structure Elucidation

So far, there is no general NMR method for a secure assignment of the relative configuration of non-crystallizable natural products [4–6]. Valuable information is provided by NOEs or ROEs which allow to derive actual interproton distances by volume integration of the cross-peaks in the NOESY or ROESY spectrum. The H, H distances are obtained by the comparison of the peak volume with a cross-peak of known distance (the so-called calibration or reference peaks). The determination of the relative configuration from NOE- or ROE-derived interproton distances can be accomplished in different ways [3]. In the past, this was mainly carried out in a qualitative way using molecular-mechanics or density functional theory (DFT) derived structure models. In particular, the DFT approach is restricted to relatively small systems because these types of calculation quickly become prohibitively expensive for larger structures or large numbers of diastereomers that need to be considered.

Another possibility would be to run rEM (restrained energy minimization) [7] or rMD (restrained molecular dynamics) [8,9] simulations for all possible relative configurations, and generally, the one with the lowest error with respect to the experimental restraints is chosen as the correct relative configuration of the investigated molecule. The disadvantage of this approach is that it is very time consuming, especially for molecules with many unknown stereogenic centers because for every diastereomer separate simulations need to be run (2^{n-1} calculations), albeit these may be automated in computer-assisted structure elucidation protocols [10,11]. However, MD simulations are biased by the choice of the force-field (for uncommon structural fragments these might even lack appropriate parameters at all) and the user's choice of the initial geometry ("starting configuration and conformation"). Relative conformational energies obtained from DFT calculations may be inaccurate up to ~1–2 kcal/mol^{-1} (amounting to errors in Boltzmann weights of conformers differing by factors of ~0.20–0.03 at 300 K!) depending on the treatment of electron-electron correlation and/or dispersion interactions [12].

One method of choice for small molecules with several stereogenic centers is the combination of distance geometry (DG) [13–16] and distance bounds driven dynamics (DDD) calculations using NOE/ROE-derived distance restraints (r) [3,5,16–19]. The most important aspects of the NOE/ROE-restrained DG/DDD method (rDG/DDD) is the possibility to allow configurations to dynamically change during the simulation (floating chirality, fc) and therefore to determine the conformation and the relative configuration of small organic molecules simultaneously (fc-rDG/DDD). The DG approach (see Figure 2) considers holonomic distance restraints as lower (d_{min}) and upper (d_{max}) bounds of atom-atom distance relations, which are derived from the molecular constitution (which must be known!), as well as 1,2- (bonds), 1,3- (angles), and 1,4-connectivities (torsions) and experimental NOE/ROE-derived restraints can be added to this set of limits. Within these restraints, structure models are generated solely based on distance information, removing the bias to any initial input reference model, and these models are further refined in a simulated annealing approach. Chirality is incorporated in the DG approach using signed chiral volumes, which basically describe the volume enclosed by the substituents on tetrahedral centers, and which simultaneously encode for opposite configurations through sign inversion (see Section 4).

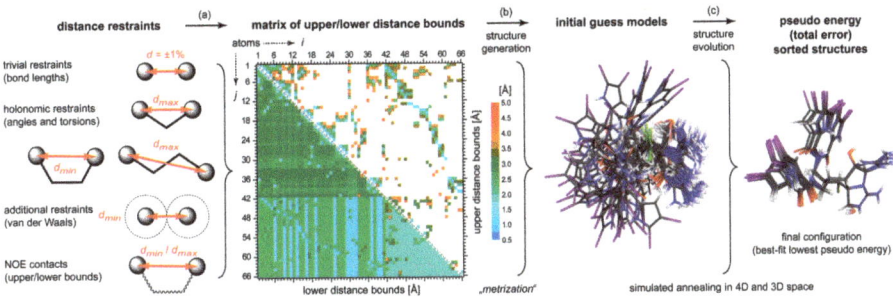

Figure 2. Workflow of rDG/DDD calculations: Based on distance restraints such as bond lengths (1,2-distance), angles and torsions (1,3- and 1,4-distances), excluded van der Waals volumes, and NOE/ROE derived distance limits, a matrix of upper (top right triangle) and lower (bottom left triangle) distance bounds between all atom-atom pairs i, j is constructed (**a**). Based on these distance limits, initial guess structure models of arbitrary configuration and conformation are generated through a "metrization" procedure in 4D space (**b**, for clarity shown as 3D models). These models are subsequently refined through an automated sequence of simulated annealing steps in 4D and 3D space (**c**), by which finally the correct configuration evolves as the best-fit structures of lowest pseudo energy (total error). In particular step (**a**) ensures that the final structures generated are not biased by any input structure, and through step (**b,c**), evolve solely on the basis of experimental data. At no point of a rDG/DDD simulation, neither a conventional parametrized force-field is involved, nor are any presumptions on conformational preferences implied. All relative configurations of stereogenic centers emerge exclusively based on experimental data.

The concept of floating chirality (fc) was introduced for the assignment of diastereotopic protons or methyl groups in proteins. This approach was first applied in 1988 to distance geometry (DG) calculations [20] and in 1989 to rMD simulations [21]. In DG calculations, floating chirality is achieved by not using chiral restraints (chiral volumes) for unknown prochiral and stereogenic centers, whereas in rMD, floating chirality is achieved by reducing or removing the force constants of the angles which define the chiral centers. Even more, DG uses no energy penalty or additional out-of-plane terms to guarantee that the full set of permutations for all stereogenic centers is generated. In general, DG uses a single chiral volume restraint on one selected stereogenic center only in order to avoid enantiomeric configurations (see discussions below). However, in contrast to rMD simulations, DG does not use any physical force-field of any type, and thus removes any intrinsic bias imposed on the results by this choice. DG relies solely on experimental data like distances between atoms or anisotropic data (see below) and all stereogenic centers are allowed to adopt their relative configuration in accordance with the experimental data.

Moreover, the strength of the DG approach is that all structure models are first generated in four-dimensional (4D) space before these are transferred into "real" 3D space. The extra dimension provides additional degrees of freedom to assemble structures of different configurations and conformations within the limits of the distance bounds. Most notably, the sequence of 4D and 3D simulated annealing steps has major benefits for the robustness and quality of configurational sampling, as inversions of 3D objects (e.g., stereogenic centers) become simple rotations in 4D, and thus the "energy" barriers between alternate diastereomers are effectively lowered or even removed altogether (see Figure 2, and in the Section 4, Figure 12).

NMR-derived experimental data such as NOE/ROE distances, scalar couplings, residual dipolar couplings (RDCs), residual quadrupolar couplings (RQCs), and residual chemical shift anisotropies (RCSAs) can be incorporated in this DG approach. Here, all experimental parameters are accounted for as sums of squared violations $\Delta X^2 = (X^{exp} - X^{calc})^2$ of experimental versus back-calculated values, and these deviations are added up in a harmonic approximation as pseudo energy terms $E = 1/2K \sum \Delta X^2$

with empirical force constants K. In total, the sum of these terms based on NMR data, and violations of distance bounds or, if applicable chiral volume restraints, define a dimensionless total penalty or pseudo energy function, which must not be confused with a MD- or DFT-derived "real" molecular energy, and the lower this pseudo energy penalty becomes, the better the restraints based on experimental data are fulfilled. A comprehensive description of all energy terms is given in the Section 4. In this context, these violation energies, and in particular their partial derivatives $\partial E_{total}/\partial r$ with respect 4D and 3D Cartesian atomic coordinates, are considered as forces which drive the structure evolution in a simulated annealing type approach–and thus the structures evolve from the data rather than being evaluated against pre-calculated structures only.

Up till now a general application of the DG approach to all different kind of natural products was hindered by the fact that NOEs/ROEs cover only short-range interactions (up to 400 pm for small molecules) and was hampered or even impossible for proton-deficient structures. This can now be overcome by the use of anisotropic NMR parameters (RDCs, RQCs, and RCSA) in the structure under investigation.

1.2. RDCs in Structure Elucidation

In contrast to NOEs/ROEs, residual dipolar couplings (RDCs) are anisotropic NMR parameters, which are global in nature and independent from the distances between the vectors connecting the coupling nuclei. RDCs, RQCs, and RCSAs are NMR observables that can now be used within the fc-rDG/DDD method using the recently published software ConArch+ [22,23]. Within this investigation, only the usage of RDCs will be discussed here.

Standard NMR investigations are carried out in isotropic solutions, where usually the dipolar couplings are averaged out by isotropic tumbling of the molecules. If this is not the case, either by the presence of paramagnetic metal ions [24] or anisotropic susceptibility of diamagnetic macromolecules [25] or, more general, the presence of an anisotropic medium, the molecules will be partially oriented with respect to the external magnetic field, and residual dipolar couplings (RDCs) can be measured (detailed reviews can be found at [26–31]). An anisotropic environment is generated by an alignment medium (AM), examples for AMs are stretched gels [32–40] or lyotropic liquid crystalline (LLC) phases [41–49].

The size of $^1D_{CH}$ RDCs depends on the time-averaged orientation of the CH-vector and its averaged angle with respect to the external magnetic field B_0 (see Figure 3). The one-bond (CH) dipolar coupling is usually obtained by comparison of HSQC-type experiments run in isotropic and anisotropic environment [50,51]. A very popular variant of these HSQC experiments is the so-called CLIP/CLAP-HSQC [52], which is run without F_2 decoupling in order to observe the one-bond coupling in F_2. The residual dipolar coupling adds to the scalar coupling leading to a total coupling constant ($^1T_{CH}$) from which the residual dipolar coupling ($^1D_{CH}$) can be calculated ($^1T_{CH} = {}^1J_{CH} + 2\,{}^1D_{CH}$).

Analysis of RDC data is less straightforward than the interpretation of isotropic data such as chemical shifts and scalar coupling. However, given a molecular geometry for the compound analyzed, RDCs can be back-calculated from the experimental data and this structural model in a parameter-free fashion using natural constants only, and an alignment tensor can be computed which describes the average orientation of the molecule in relation to the magnetic field [53]. Frequently, alternative relative configurations of analytes imply different relative orientations of CH vectors, and thus RDCs are very sensitive configuration probes even for cases, where stereogenic centers are separated by many bonds. Usually, the configuration which displays the best correlation between experimental and back-calculated RDC data (D^{exp} vs. D^{calc}) is considered as the correct one (see Figure 3). RDC analysis is based on the assumption that the chemical shifts in the isotropic and anisotropic phases do not change or change only slightly. The standard procedure does not include a re-assignment of the molecule under study in the anisotropic phase, but the assignment could be questionable if larger changes in the chemical shifts are observed.

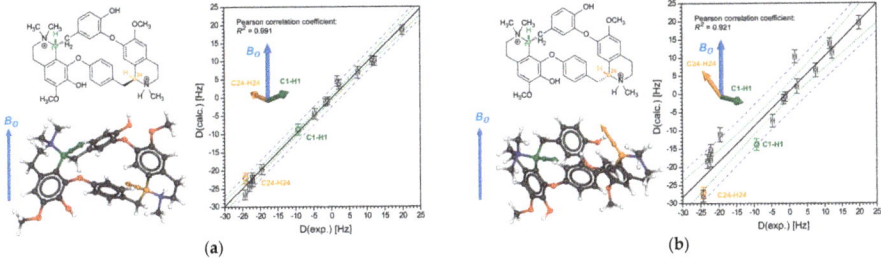

Figure 3. Matching of RDC data against two alternative diastereomers of tubocurarine (**4**), which differ in their configuration at C-24: (**a**) correct, and (**b**) wrong relative configuration of C-1 and C-24. The stereogenic centers C-1 and C-24 are marked in green and orange, respectively, and the directionality of the corresponding methine C-H bonds is indicated by the colored vectors in both structure models. The differing average orientation of each of these C-H bond vectors relative to the external magnetic field (blue vector) of the NMR spectrometer leads to different RDCs back-calculated for both diastereomers (colored values in the plots of D^{exp} vs. D^{calc}), the better correlation between experimental and back-calculated data identifies (**a**) as the correct relative configuration of **4**, whereas (**b**) could be ruled out.

However, crucial for the interpretation of RDC data is the fact that accurate structure proposals must be provided at first hand, which are then evaluated against the experimental NMR data, and a thorough error analysis has to be carried out in order to ascertain configurational assignments [23]. The necessity for pre-evaluation of conformational preferences may become problematic for flexible or larger molecules. Moreover, this type of analysis has to be repeated for all 2^{n-1} diastereomers if the molecule contains n stereogenic elements. In a recent report [22], we have demonstrated on how to include RDC information in DG simulations in both 4D and 3D space, using a pseudo energy penalty function $E_{RDC} = 1/2 K_{RDC} \sum (D^{exp} - D^{calc})^2$ similar as described above. This now provides the advantage that the prerequisite of the beforehand structure generation is dropped altogether. Instead, the correct configuration emerges from these RDC-driven rDG types of simulations as a direct consequence and within the boundaries of these experimental restraints.

Though the mathematical details for the treatment of NOEs/ROEs and RDCs differ vastly, the pseudo energy error function allows to arbitrarily combine these different types of restraints within DG, and structures are generated fulfilling all experimental parameters best. However, there is one additional fundamental difference between NOE and RDC data. For the former, only a single NOE "data set" can be obtained, whereas for the latter RDCs multiple "data sets" can be obtained when measuring the NMR data under different alignment conditions (i.e., different alignment media [23,54–57], multi-component multi-phase AM [46], temperature dependent AM [43,58], etc.). Though this might entail considerable experimental effort, these multi-alignment data sets can also be exploited in the DG implementation of ConArch$^+$ [22]. Under the assumption that the conformational preferences of the analyte do not change significantly for alternate alignment conditions, different sets of RDCs can provide crucial additional and independent structure information, which may contribute significantly to the certainty with which configurational assignments are supported by experimental data [23,54–57].

In the sequel, the application of the fc-rDG/DDD method will be demonstrated on five complex natural products (see Scheme 1). The dimeric cyclic pyrrole-imidazole alkaloid (PIA) axinellamine A (**1**) isolated from the marine sponge *Axinella* sp. in 1999 [59] is the first compound to study. The second example is also a dimeric cyclic PIA from the marine sponge *Stylissa caribica*, tetrabromostyloguanidine (**2**) from 2007 [60], and the synthetic massadine derivative 3,7-*epi*-massadine chloride (**3**) is the last one of the PIA series from 2008 [61]. Finally, the terrestrial plant alkaloids tubocurarine (**4**) from *Chondrodendron tomentosum* [62] and vincristine (**5**) from *Catharanthus roseus* [63] are examples discussed here to illustrate the limitations of configurational analysis based on NOE/ROE data solely, and only the combined approach of using distance as well as RDC data allows to deduce their configurations unequivocally.

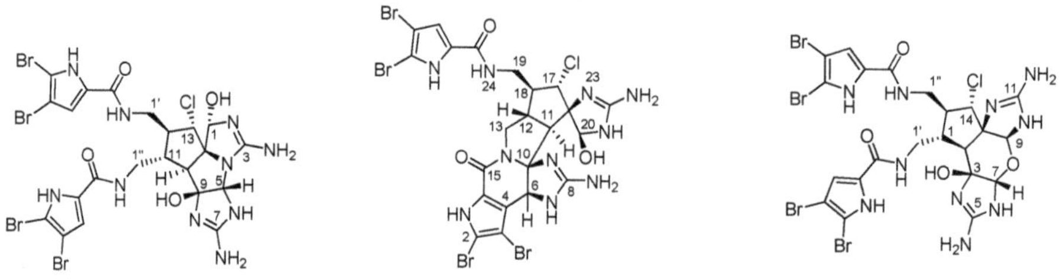

Axinellamine A (**1**) Tetrabromostyloguanidine (**2**) 3,7-*epi*-Massadine chloride (**3**)

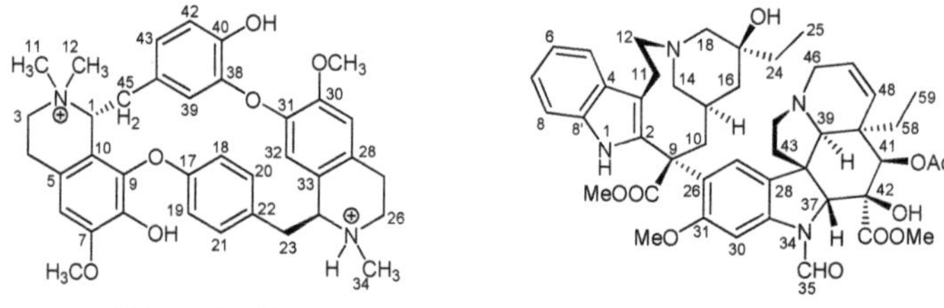

Tubocurarine (**4**) Vincristine (**5**)

Scheme 1. Structural formulae of the investigated molecules with atom numbering: axinellamine A (**1**), tetrabromostyloguanidine (**2**), 3,7-*epi*-massadine chloride (**3**), tubocurarine (**4**), and vincristine (**5**).

2. Results and Discussion

Compounds **1–3** are cyclic dimeric pyrrole-imidazole alkaloids (PIAs) with eight contiguous stereogenic centers each, resulting in 128 possible relative configurations (diastereomers), respectively. Axinellamine A (**1**) and 3,7-*epi*-massadine chloride (**3**) possess tetracyclic cores, whereas tetrabromostyloguanidine (**2**) features an even more complex hexacyclic core. For the PIAs **1–3** only ROE-derived interproton distances were used. The interproton distances were extracted from a ROESY spectrum with a mixing time of 100 ms (in case of **3**: 300 ms). For all compounds the interproton distances ±10% were used as distance restraints in the floating chirality restrained DG/DDD calculations (fc-rDG/DDD), additional details on the calculations on **1–3** are given in the Section 4 and the Supporting Information. As NMR can anyhow determine relative configurations only, in all rDG simulations a single stereogenic center of **1–3** each was fixed by applying a chiral volume restraint in order to avoid enantiomeric structures. The number of the generated structures in the fc-rDG/DDD calculations was set to 1000 to allow for reasonable sampling of the configurational and conformational space. Additional simulations applying different chiral volume restraints and/or sampling lengths, as well as in-depth analyses of the rDG runs are described in the Supporting Information. In the following, we report the application of the fc-rDG/DDD method to assign the relative configuration of all stereogenic centers for compounds **1–3** simultaneously, and based on ROE data alone.

2.1. *Configurational Assignment with ROEs Only*

2.1.1. Axinellamine A (**1**)

For the configurational assignment of axinellamine A (**1**) 35 interproton distances from ROESY spectra were used (the complete list of ROEs of **1** is given in the SI, Table S1). As mentioned above, one stereogenic center of **1** was fixed and set as reference (C-14). In the traditional approach of pre-calculating structures, this would entail the necessity to evaluate a total of 128 diastereomers. Indeed, inspection of the output on the rDG protocol shows that all 128 configurations are actually generated by the "metrization" process in 4D space, but many of these molecular geometries severely violate the restraints imposed by the ROE data even in this higher dimension, and thus do not "survive" even the 4D refinement of simulated annealing. At the end of the 4D sampling phase, 40 alternative configurations were obtained (see Supplementary Figures S2 and S3), out of which even only 37 did emerge finally from the 3D sampling, albeit many of these structures display severe ROE violations.

The over-all exceedingly high efficiency of configurational sampling by rDG, and the results for 1000 generated possible structural candidates of axinellamine A (**1**) are shown in Figure 4a ("best 700") as a graphical representation of the total error (dimensionless) for each structure, ordered according to ascending total errors. The first wrong structure (wrong configuration of **1**) in respect to the eight stereogenic centers is No. #598 (red circle in Figure 4a). This structure differs from structures #1 to #597 by the configuration of C-1. The first "pseudo-configurational" change was already observed at structure No. #365 (orange circle in Figure 4a). This is the alternative assignment of the diastereotopic protons at the methylene group C-1'. Mathematically there is no difference between stereogenic and prochiral centers, which means that for axinellamine A (**1**) altogether ten centers needed to be assigned. Chemically only the stereogenic centers are of importance for the differentiation of the stereoisomers, but the prochiral centers are important to support the configurational assignment. In this example, only C-1' is used, whereas the second prochiral center (C-1'') does not contribute to the results since no ROE to both H's of C-1'' have been observed.

Most notably, the first wrong configuration of **1** (#598) appears rather late in this sequence of energy sorted structures sampled, visualizing the efficiency of sampling (the total number of structures with the correct configuration for axinellamine A (**1**) is even 760/1000). Additionally, the second best (first wrong) alternative configuration is separated from the best-fit global energy minimum structure by significant energy steps and a large pseudo energy difference of the penalty error function ($\Delta E_{total} = 3.15$). Within the rDG approach, both of these characteristics are indicative for an unambiguous configurational assignment of **1** based on the experimental NMR data used, and the plot in Figure 4b shows, that all structures #1 to #597 indeed feature the same relative configuration of all stereogenic centers.

Figure 4a illustrates very well that the correct relative configuration of axinellamine A (**1**) appears in different conformations with respect to the orientation of the side chains. There are already six steps before a different configuration is observed, which originate from alternate local conformational changes that mainly include the orientation of the side chains (see Figure 4b). The inset plot in Figure 4a shows the first "energy" step in detail.

It must be stressed, that this rDG simulation is actually a single, fully automated sequence of calculations–and not 128 individual calculations on alternate diastereomers–by which the correct configuration of axinellamine A (**1**) is quickly and highly reliably identified. At no point of this simulation is a physical force-field involved, and the final assignment emerges based on experimental data only irrespective of the starting configuration.

2.1.2. Tetrabromostyloguanidine (**2**)

For the configurational assignment of tetrabromostyloguanidine (**2**) 27 interproton distances from ROESY spectra were used (the complete list of ROEs of **2** is given in the SI, Table S2). Using the same methodology as in case of axinellamine A (**1**), the results for the 1000 generated possible structures of tetrabromostyloguanidine (**2**) are shown in Figure 5a ("best 400") as a graphical representation of the total error (dimensionless) for each structure, ordered according to ascending total errors. As already discussed for **1**, one stereogenic center of **2** was again set as reference and fixed by the application of a chiral volume restraint (C-10). In order to verify and demonstrate that the results of the fc-rDG/DDD calculations do not depend on the choice of the stereogenic center that is fixed, these calculations were also repeated for all eight centers of **2** and are reported in the Supporting Information (see Supplementary Figures S5–S7).

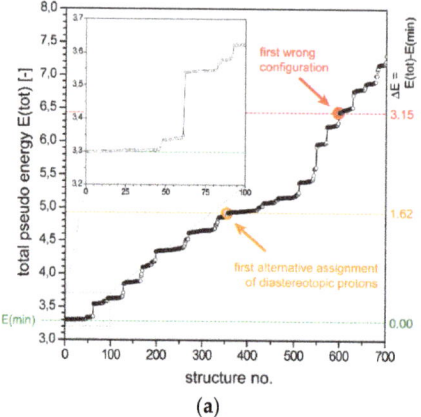
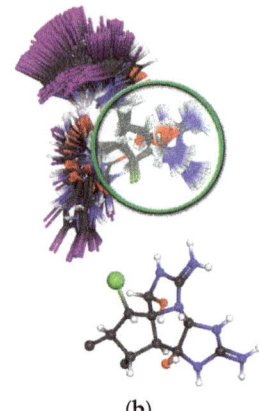

(a) (b)

Figure 4. (a) Plot of the total *"pseudo energy"* of ranked rDG structures of axinellamine A (**1**), showing the first 700 out of 1000 structures generated ($K_{NOE} = 10.0$ Å^{-2}), the minimum energy level is indicated by the green line. The dashed lines at higher energies indicate the differentiability of the best-fit solution with respect to alternate assignments of diastereotopic methylene protons (orange) or wrong (red) configurations, the corresponding ΔE values are given on the right. The inset plot shows the first 100 structures with all-correct assignments and their separation into distinct conformational families by smaller energy steps. (b) Molecular structures of axinellamine A (**1**) showing the superposition of all DG structures identified up to the first wrong configuration (597 structures); the central fragment (green circle) of the DG best-fit (lowest pseudo energy) structure is plotted below, displaying the correct configuration of **1**.

The first wrong structure with respect to the eight stereogenic centers is No. #378 (red circle in Figure 5). This structure differs from structures #1 to #377 by the configuration of C-20, which is actually the same position (different atom numbering, see Scheme 1) for the first change as observed in case of axinellamine A (**1**). The first "pseudo-configurational" change, i.e., an alternative diastereotopic assignment of methylene protons of the exocyclic methylene group C-19, was already observed at structure No. #99 (orange circle in Figure 5) with a very low energy difference of $\Delta E = 0.14$, indicating some ambiguity in the assignment of these CH$_2$-protons. The second and more characteristic "jump" in energy is observed at structure No. #203. This jump in energy includes both either a new conformation of **2** and its side chains, or an alternative assignment of the diastereotopic protons at the endocyclic methylene group C-13, both changes have similar penalties in experimental versus calculated NMR parameters. At structure No. #277 the alternative assignment of the diastereotopic protons at C-13 is observed, and at structure No. #302 both methylene groups are inverted and both changes are manifested in rather small changes in pseudo energy only. The total number of structures with the correct configuration for tetrabromostyloguanidine (**2**) generated is 702/1000. Though all 128 relative configurations of **2** were initially generated by the rDG "metrization" step, only a few "survived" the 4D (36 configuration) and 3D (19 diastereomers) stages of sampling, and of the latter, all 18 wrong configurations appear after structure No. #377, and are ranked in their pseudo energy significantly higher ($\Delta E \geq 5.32$) than the best-fit geometry of **2** with correct configuration (see discussion of **1**).

The diastereotopic assignment of the methylene protons can also be alternatively obtained by a J coupling approach ($^3J_{HH}$ and HMBC intensities). Using this information within the fc-rDG/DDD calculation, the results can still be improved (see Supporting Information, Figures S8 and S9). For this calculation the two methylene groups are used with a fixed chiral volume, changing the number of floating centers from nine to seven (C-10 fixed). The first wrong structure for this calculation in respect to the eight stereogenic centers changes from No. #378 to No. #420, and many of the smaller steps in pseudo energy originating from alternate CH$_2$-assignments vanish altogether.

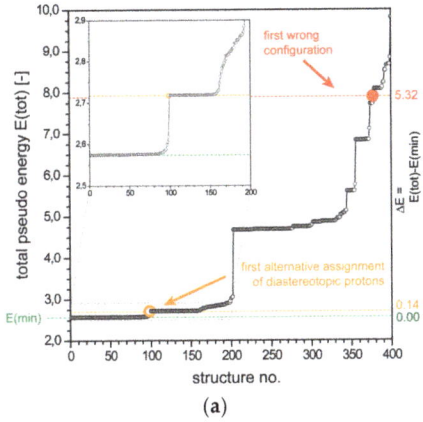 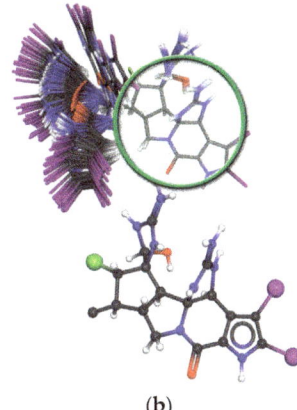

(a) (b)

Figure 5. (a) Plot of the total *"pseudo energy"* of ranked rDG structures of tetrabromostyloguanidine (**2**), showing the first 400 out of 1000 structures generated (K_{NOE} = 10.0 Å^{-2}), the minimum energy level is indicated by the green line. The dashed lines at higher energies indicate the differentiability of the best-fit solution with respect to alternate assignments of diastereotopic methylene protons (orange) or wrong (red) configurations. (b) Molecular structures of tetrabromostyloguanidine (**2**) showing the superposition of all DG structures identified up to the first wrong configuration (377 structures); the central fragment (green circle) of the DG best-fit (lowest pseudo energy) structure is plotted below, displaying the correct configuration of **2**.

In total, the relative configuration of all stereogenic centers in **2** is unequivocally determined by the ROE data used, although some ambiguities remain on the assignment of diastereotopic protons. However, both the unambiguity of the configurational assignment, as well as the ambiguity of the CH$_2$-assignments is again established by a single rDG simulation, without any other assumptions or restraints used rather than experimental NMR data exclusively.

2.1.3. 3,7-*epi*-Massadine chloride (**3**)

For the configurational assignment of 3,7-*epi*-massadine chloride (**3**) 36 interproton distances from ROESY spectra were used (the complete list of ROEs of **3** is given in the SI, Table S3). Results for the 1000 generated structures of 3,7-*epi*-massadine chloride (**3**) are shown in Figure 6a ("best 200") as a graphical representation of the total error for each structure, ordered according to ascending total errors. As already discussed for **1** and **2** one stereogenic center of **3** was set as reference (C-13).

The first wrong structure in respect to the eight stereogenic centers is No. #56 (red circle in Figure 6). This structure differs from the preceding structures by a configurational change of C-3 and C-7, which represents the original massadine configuration. The first "pseudo-configurational" change was again observed earlier at structure No. #25 (orange circle in Figure 6a), which represents the alternative assignment of the diastereotopic protons at the methylene group C-1″. The results of the calculations for **3** can be improved if a diastereotopic assignment of the methylene protons is carried out prior to the DG/DDD calculations (see discussion of compound **2**). In this case, the first wrong structure becomes No. #123 (see Figures S11 and S12). The diastereomeric differentiability in this case is not as pronounced as for compounds **1** and **2**. This becomes obvious just by looking at the occurrence of the first wrong structure (**1**: #597, **2**: #377, and **3**: #56), but it is still an unambiguous result. Another difference to the first two examples is the energy difference between the different configurations, which is much lower for **3**. This indicates that the extent and certainty with which the experimental data does differentiate between the different structures (diastereomers) is not as pronounced as it was observed for **1** and **2**. For 3,7-*epi*-massadine chloride (**3**), the NMR data set was less well defined because of the longer mixing time of the ROESY experiment.

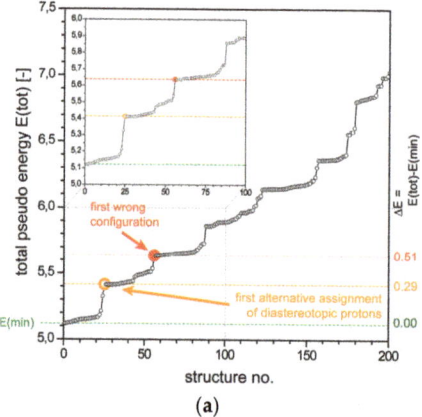
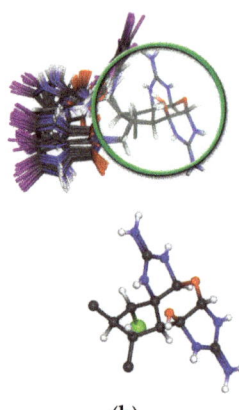

Figure 6. (a) Plot of the total *"pseudo energy"* of ranked rDG structures of 3,7-*epi*-massadine chloride (**3**), showing the first 200 out of 1000 structures generated (K_{NOE} = 10.0 Å^{-2}), the minimum energy level is indicated by the green line. The dashed lines at higher energies indicate the differentiability of the best-fit solution with respect to alternate assignments of diastereotopic methylene protons (orange) or wrong (red) configurations. (b) Molecular structures of 3,7-*epi*-massadine chloride (**3**) showing the superposition of all DG structures identified up to the first wrong configuration (55 structures); the central fragment (green circle) of the DG best-fit (lowest pseudo energy) structure is plotted below, displaying the correct configuration of **3**.

2.2. Configurational Assignment with NOEs and RDCs

The terrestrial alkaloids tubocurarine (**4**) and vincristine (**5**) form the completion of the current investigation. In case of **4** only one stereogenic center relative to a second one needs to be assigned and is therefore a seemingly rather simple model for the described approach, but was chosen for demonstration purposes and its long-range separated stereogenic centers. Vincristine (**5**) is a more complex structure with nine stereogenic centers. In both examples, NOEs involving diastereotopic protons of methylene groups were used as unassigned and averaged restraints only, and in the case of **4**, the *o*/*o*'-protons of the *p*-disubstituted aryl ring were treated similarly (see Supplementary Tables S4 and S5 and Figure S4). As it will be demonstrated later in the manuscript, NOEs are not sufficient for the unambiguous assignment of the relative configuration of compounds **4** and **5**. Further data was necessary for a complete assignment. Due to the lack of experimental RDC data, we have decided to use synthetic RDC data sets for both compounds. Though one might argue that is a general weakness of the method, it is important to know for demonstration purposes that additional NMR parameter may help to solve the structural problem. Where applicable, RDCs involving CH$_2$-groups were also treated as unassigned values, and only the sum of both individual $^1D_{CH}$ methylene RDCs are used as restraining parameters. Though this reduces the quality of the data set that might be experimentally accessible, this method was chosen to reduce the amount of prior information to learn more about the limits of the DG based structure analysis described here. The full data sets of NOEs and RDCs used for **4** and **5** are listed in Supplementary Tables S4–S7. As this data explicitly does not allow to differentiate diastereotopic CH$_2$-protons, we will not get into a debate on the subject of assignments on prochiral centers in this chapter.

2.2.1. Tubocurarine (4)

The toxic alkaloid ("arrow poison") tubocurarine (**4**) was chosen as a model compound with only two stereogenic centers (C-1 and C-24) being nine bonds apart from each other (either counting the orange or the blue pathway in the macrocycle; see Figure 7). Additionally, along either way only three out of the eight atoms in between have a proton attached, and thus **4** represents a prototype example where the relative configuration of the two remote stereogenic centers is expected to be indefinable on the basis of NOE data alone. The question is now: can RDCs contribute significantly to the assignment of the relative configuration of tubocurarine (**4**)?

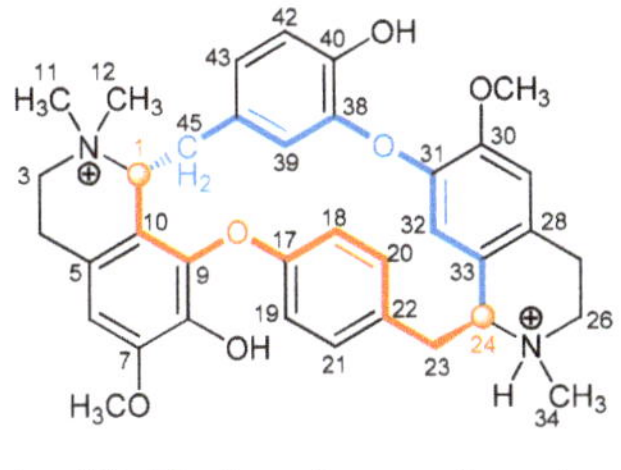

Figure 7. Structure of tubocurarine (**4**). The two stereogenic centers (C-1 and C-24) are represented as orange circles. The nine bonds between the two centers (either way) are printed as bold orange or blue lines.

For the configurational assignment of tubocurarine (**4**), a total of 17 NOE-derived interproton distances and 16 $^1D_{CH}$ RDCs were used for up to three independent alignment media, respectively, the RDC data for **4** was taken from Ref. [22] (see also Supplementary Tables S4 and S5).

Results for 1000 structures of tubocurarine (**4**) are shown in Figure 8a ("best 500") as a graphical representation of the total error for each structure, ordered according to ascending total errors. Following the methodology outlined in the previous chapter for **1** to **3**, one stereogenic center of **4** was set as reference and fixed by a single rDG chiral volume restraint (C-1), and therefore, only one center needed to be assigned in the calculations. Using NOE data exclusively, the first wrong structure is No. #80 (black curve/circle in Figure 8a). The energy difference between the two structures of opposite configuration at C-24 is extremely low ($\Delta E_{total} = 0.04$, see black symbols in Figure 8a). Accordingly, the total number of structures for tubocurarine (**4**) generated by rDG is almost equally distributed between both possibilities (the correct and the wrong configuration), and therefore a differentiation of the two alternative relative configurations of **4** by the NOE data set used here is impossible, as long as no further assumptions are made or additional experimental data is included.

The results can be significantly improved by adding RDC data to the restraints. A single alignment medium RDC data set with 16 individual $^1D_{CH}$ RDCs added to the restraints of the rDG/DDD simulation leads to a clearly recognizable step in pseudo energy separating the first occurrence of a structure with wrong configuration (#334) from the energy minimum family of structures displaying the correct configuration of **4** (blue line and symbols in Figure 8a). This already pronounced diastereomeric differentiability is improved considerably when adding a second (Figure 8a, green line) or even third (Figure 8a, dark red line) RDC data set. Though these data sets require NMR measurements under different alignment conditions (alignment media) and are associated with quite some experimental effort, the resultant additional structural restraints add valuable information to the discrimination of diastereomers. With an increasing number M of alignment data sets used, the rDG/DDD simulations show a significantly increasing step in pseudo energy ($M = 1$: $\Delta E = 0.95$, $M = 2$: $\Delta E = 1.73$, and $M = 3$: $\Delta E = 11.33$, cf. Figure 8a) between both alternate configurational assignments of **4**, and the total number of correctly identified structures increases consistently. The second and third AM RDC data sets remove the last remaining doubts on the configuration of **4** that might prevail after single-AM analysis. The predictive power of AM data sets cannot be estimated in advance of a measurement, but needs to be evaluated thoroughly after the NMR data has been acquired. For the experimentalist, this is of high significance, as adding further data and re-running a rDG/DDD simulation is very straight-forward–it simply requires adding a new RDC table in an additional input file–and within a couple of minutes a clear-cut answer on the decidability of a given structural problem is provided by the DG method presented here.

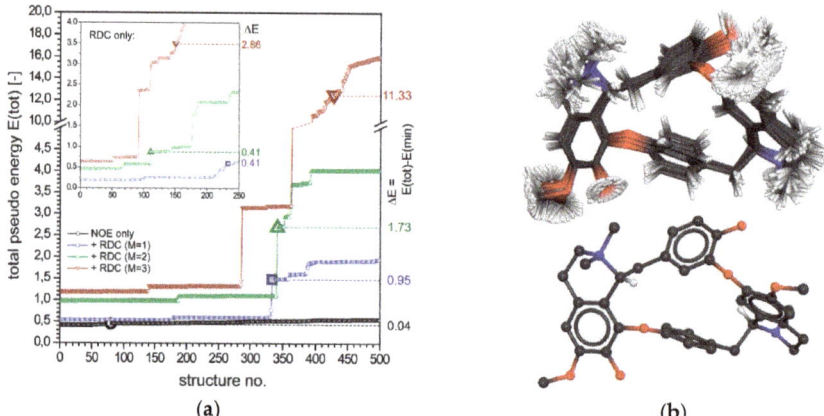

Figure 8. (**a**) Plot of the total "*pseudo energy*" of ranked rDG structures of tubocurarine (**4**), showing the first 500 out of 1000 structures generated ($K_{NOE} = 10.0$ Å^{-2}, $K_{RDC} = 1.5/M$ Hz^{-2}) using only NOE restraints (black symbols) and an increasing number M of additional RDC data sets (blue, green, and dark red with $M = 1$–3 alignment media). The dashed lines and ΔE values on the right indicate the energy levels of the first wrong configuration identified ($M = 1$: #334, $M = 2$: #342, $M = 3$: #429), respectively, and thus the increasing differentiability of the correct configuration when using an increasing number of RDC restraints. The inset plot shows the corresponding data obtained using only RDCs ($M = 1$–3 data sets) without any NOE restraints. (**b**) Superposition of the first 428 DG structures (top plot) of correct configuration ($M = 3$), and backbone representation of the best-fit geometry (lowest pseudo energy, bottom plot, hydrogen atoms not connected to stereogenic centers have been omitted for clarity) of tubocurarine (**4**).

The main plot of Figure 8a shows the combined usage of NOE and RDC data, whereas the inset graph reveals, that the discriminative power for alternate configurations based on RDCs alone is smaller than the combined usage of NOE and RDC data. Though the level of differentiation still increases with the number of alignment media data sets applied, the energy is smaller and less significant ($M = 1$: $\Delta E = 0.41$, $M = 2$: $\Delta E = 0.41$, and $M = 3$: $\Delta E = 2.86$, cf. Figure 8a, inset plot).

2.2.2. Vincristine (5)

The alkaloid vincristine (**5**) from the pink-colored catharanthe (*Catharanthus roseus*) was chosen as very complex natural product. Vincristine (**5**) is an approved drug in cancer therapy. It has nine stereogenic centers, six of which are arranged consecutively in a six-membered ring and three are located in a remote ring fragment connected to the former segment by a single rotatable bond only, and therefore **5** is a challenging goal for a configurational analysis by NMR spectroscopy. For the configurational assignment of vincristine (**5**) altogether 23 NOEs and 24 RDCs in up to three AM, respectively, were used (all restraints were again used without assignments of diastereotopic methylene protons as described for **4**). The RDC data for **5** were taken from Ref. [22] for three independent alignment scenarios, respectively (see also Supplementary Tables S6 and S7). It also must be noted that due to the absence of NOE and RDC associated with the substituents of C-42 (a quaternary carbon carrying a hydroxyl group and a COOMe ester moiety), the configuration of this stereogenic center is not assignable based on the data used here, and thus C-42 was excluded from any further analysis.

Results for 1000 structures of vincristine (**5**) are shown in Figure 9a ("best 100") as a graphical representation of the total error for each structure, ordered according to ascending total errors. Again, a single stereogenic center of **5** was set as reference and fixed (C-9). Using NOE data only, the first wrong structure is already the structure No. #1 ranked best (black curve/circle in Figure 9a), which is a clear indication that NOEs alone are insufficient to accomplish the configurational analysis of vincristine (**5**). In analogy to the methodology employed in the case of **4**, the results can be improved by further adding RDC data to the restraints.

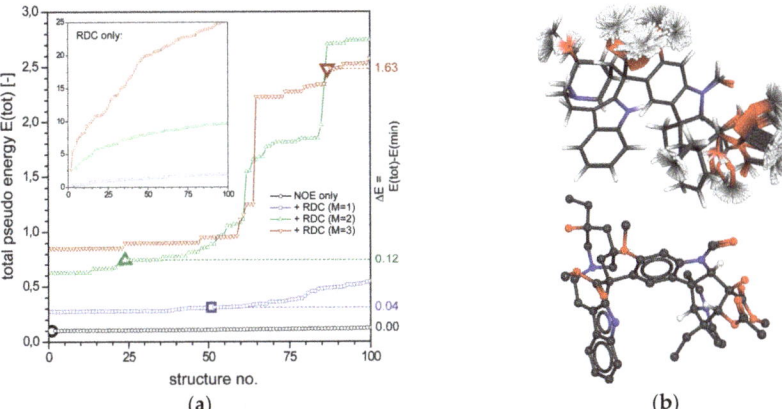

Figure 9. (a) Plot of the total "*pseudo energy*" of ranked rDG structures of vincristine (**5**), showing the first 100 out of 1000 structures generated ($K_{NOE} = 10.0$ Å^{-2}, $K_{RDC} = 1.5$/M Hz^{-2}) using only NOE restraints (black symbols) and an increasing number of additional RDC data sets (blue, green, and dark red with $M = 1$–3 alignment media). The dashed lines and ΔE values on the right indicate the energy levels of the first wrong configuration identified, respectively, and thus the increasing differentiability of the correct configuration when using an increasing number of RDC restraints. The inset plot shows the corresponding data obtained using only RDCs ($M = 1$–3 data sets) without any NOE restraints. (b) Superposition of the first 86 DG structures (top plot, $M = 3$) of correct configuration, and backbone representation of the best-fit geometry (lowest pseudo energy, bottom plot, only hydrogen atoms connected to stereogenic centers are shown) of vincristine (**5**).

Successively adding multiple AM, RDC data sets slowly increases the certainty with which the correct configuration of **5** can be assigned: with $M = 1$ (blue curve), 2 (green), and 3 (dark red) AMs (see Figure 9a). However, the level of differentiability of the correct configuration from alternate wrong diastereomers is at first very low ($M = 1$: $\Delta E = 0.04$, and $M = 2$: $\Delta E = 0.12$), but raises constantly to $\Delta E = 1.63$ when using RDCs from three alignment media ($M = 3$). In the latter case, the first wrong structure is No. #87 (dark red triangle in Figure 9a), and this diastereomer is already separated from the best-fit (pseudo energy minimum) correct diastereomer of **5** by a now significant step in the error function, which is due to a configurational change of the quaternary carbon C-17 (at structure #87). Another step (not shown) follows at structure #245 ($\Delta E = 6.04$) due to a misassignment of C-41. In conclusion, the most problematic stereogenic centers to be determined for vincristine (**5**) are–as discussed above–C-42, C-17, and C-41 (in this order), whereas the reliability with which any of the other six stereogenic centers is differentiated from alternate configurations is high when NOE and RDC data is used in combination (see Figure 10 for a traffic-light type encoded pictorial description of these assignment probabilities). The problems associated with C-17 arise from limited RDC data available for the rotating ethyl side chain, and for C-41, only a single CH RDC and two NOEs indicate some preference for the correct configuration over a wrong assignment. However, Figure 9a and the inset plot therein clearly indicate the importance of using combinations of both NOE and RDC data sets, as neither NOEs nor RDCs alone provide conclusive evidence for the correct configuration of **5**, and in particular calculations relying on RDCs only gave much less conclusive results as compared to the combined approach.

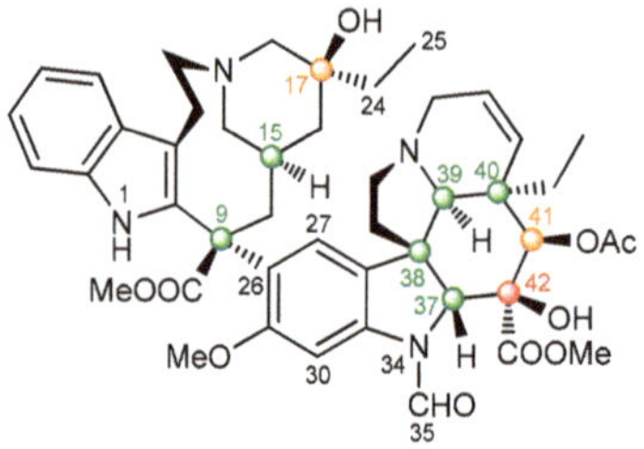

Figure 10. Structure of vincristine (**5**). The color-coded atom markers in the formula of **5** correspond to difficulties in the configurational assignment (for details, see text).

3. Conclusions

In this study, we have shown with the aid of five examples of natural products, that the ROEs or NOEs/RDCs driven floating chirality distance geometry (fc-rDG/DDD) approach represents a valuable method to assign the configuration (and conformation) of complex molecules in just one single calculation. Given the known constitution of a compound, the method produces all configurations that are in accordance with the experimental NMR data, without the necessity to carry out separate configurational and conformational analyses on 2^{n-1} diastereomers for n stereogenic centers. In the case of the marine natural products **1–3**, the relative configuration of eight stereogenic centers is unequivocally derived in just one instead of individual 128 simulations. In addition, it was demonstrated for the terrestrial alkaloids **4** and **5**, that the DG method also clearly reveals remaining ambiguities if NOE data alone is insufficient for configurational assignments–as e.g., for the long-range separated stereogenic centers of **4**–and indicates to the NMR spectroscopist that additional data such as RDCs has to be acquired. Successively adding RDC data obtained for different alignment media as additional restraints to the DG calculations is straight forward, and can be easily repeated until the level of confidence of the assignment is raised beyond any reasonable doubt.

The method discussed here neither requires individual treatment of alternate diastereomers under consideration, nor does it rely on force-field based MM/MD or DFT derived pre-calculated structures. In particular the use of force-field parameters–which may not even be available for uncommon structural fragments of natural products–in the traditional MD approach introduces an implied bias towards low-energy structures (in a thermodynamic sense) that might be misleading as in the case of tetrabromostyloguanidine (**2**). Here, the correct configuration of two *trans*-anellated five-membered rings is about 24 kJ mol^{-1} less favorable than the more stable wrong configuration with *cis*-fused rings (which represents the original palau'amine configuration from 1993 [64–68]; see Figure 11), and any MD approach would have to overcome this pronounced bias in order to identify the correct configuration of **2**.

Most importantly, the methodology outlined here does not depend on pre-calculated structures that are traditionally evaluated against experimental data, but DG represents the opposite approach, which produces structures that evolve from experimental restraints exclusively. The "FF- and DFT-free" types of simulations are unbiased, reliable, and fast (completed within minutes), and the NMR data itself governs the mode with which these structures emerge.

The full methodology outlined here for the interpretation of NOEs/ROEs and RDCs has been implemented in our ConArch$^+$ (Configurational Architect) program, which also produces convenient pseudo energy and configuration sorted lists that were used for all plots presented here. The software can be obtained along with the source code (free of charge for academic institutions) from our web site (https://www.chemie.tu-darmstadt.de/reggelin).

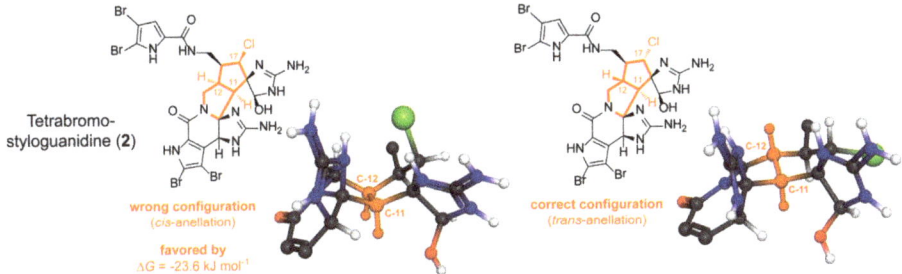

Figure 11. Selected structure plots underpinning the importance of an unbiased rDG/DDD approach compared to the traditional force-field based rMD approach: the left plot of tetrabromostyloguanidine (**2**) features a wrong configuration of two C–11/C–12 *cis*-anellated five-membered ring systems, which is energetically significantly favored over the correct configuration with an *trans*-type anellation of both ring systems (energy difference given based on DFT B3LYP/6-311+G(2d,p) optimized structures including thermal corrections at T = 298.15 K, the lower dibromopyrrole ring and the side chain have been removed for clarity).

4. Methods

4.1. NMR Data

The ROEs for compounds **1–3** were taken from refs [60,69]. For compounds **1** and **2** three ROESY spectra with different mixing times (100, 150 and 200 ms) were measured [60,69]. In the case of **3**, only one ROESY spectrum with a mixing time of 300 ms was recorded [69]. The spectra were integrated with TOPSPIN and SPARKY.

For the compounds **4** and **5**, sets of NOEs were predicted using the corresponding X-ray structures and all proton-proton contacts $\leq$ 3.5 Å. All NOEs involving CH_3- or CH_2- groups were treated as averaged values between unassigned (diastereotopic) protons only, in order to reduce the amount of prior information, thus simulating situations where no diastereotopic assignment was possible. The *ortho*- and *ortho'*-protons of the central benzene ring (C-17 to C-22) were treated equivalently (see Tables S4 and S5). Simulated RDC data for **4** and **5** was taken from Ref. [22] for three independent alignment scenarios, respectively.

4.2. DG/DDD

The ROE-/NOE-interproton distances as well as the RDCs served as input for the distance geometry (DG) and distance bounds driven dynamics (DDD) calculations. The DG pseudo force-field employed for all simulations presented in this study takes the form defined by Equation (1):

$$E_{total} = E_{dist} + E_{chir} + E_{NOE} + E_{RDC} + E_{DBL}, \qquad (1)$$

where the dimensionless total pseudo energy E_{total} is a sum of distance (holonomic bond lengths) errors (E_{dist}), chiral volume violations (E_{chir}), NOE (E_{NOE}), and RDC (E_{RDC}) deviations of experimental data from values back-calculated from structures and a special term denoting the deviations of double bonds from planarity (E_{DBL}). There are no additional or customary atom-type dependent force-field parameters of physical force-fields used. All pseudo energy terms take the form of sums of squared violations $(\Delta X)^2$ as defined by Equation (2):

$$E_X = \frac{1}{2} K_X \sum (\Delta X)^2, \qquad (2)$$

with $\Delta X = X^{exp} - X^{calc}$, and empirically chosen force-constants K_X to appropriately account for the size and allowed ranges of each type of parameter violations ΔX.

E_{dist} and E_{chir} (Equation (1)) represent the violations originating from differences in holonomic distances $\Delta r_{i,j}$ (i.e., bond lengths) and ΔV_i (chiral volumes). The latter are defined by the scalar triple product $V_{chir} = \vec{a} \cdot (\vec{b} \times \vec{c})$ of three vectors spanning planar sp^2-type ($V_{chir} = 0$) or tetrahedral sp^3-type atomic centers (i.e., stereogenic centers with $V_{chir} \neq 0$), thus encoding for the configuration of the latter through opposite signs ($|V_{chir}^{(S)}| = |V_{chir}^{(R)}|$), respectively (see Figure 12a). For reference, holonomic distance bounds (for all atom-atom pairs for which upper and lower bounds of inter-atom distances can be established based on the molecular constitution) and chiral volumes are obtained from an initial guess (input) structure of arbitrary configuration and conformation. As these values depend solely on the constitution (which must be known), the DG approach is completely independent from the structure initially assumed [22]. Here, chiral volume restraints were used only on a single stereogenic center simply to avoid enantiomeric structures, as well as on CH$_3$-groups (to keep them tetrahedral) and all sp^2-centers (to keep them planar, $V_{chir} = 0$). Thus, through the deliberate absence of chiral volume restraints, all stereogenic centers (except one), and all CH$_2$-groups with diastereotopic protons were allowed to "float" and thus their configurations and/or assignments evolve on the basis of experimental NMR data (NOEs and/or RDCs) only.

In Equation (1), E_{NOE} denotes the deviations of back-calculated (and $<r^{-6}>$ averaged where applicable) NOE distances from experimental upper and lower distance bounds with Δr defined as follows:

$$\Delta r = \begin{cases} r_{i,j} - r_{lower} & \text{for} \quad r_{i,j} < r_{lower} \\ 0 & \text{for} \quad r_{lower} \leq r_{i,j} \leq r_{upper} \\ r_{i,j} - r_{upper} & \text{for} \quad r_{i,j} > r_{upper} \end{cases} \quad . \tag{3}$$

In this study, all NOE bounds r_{lower} and r_{upper} were derived from the corresponding NMR volume integrals and used as $r_{mean} \pm 10\%$, with force-constants $K_{NOE} = 10.0$ Å^{-2} unless stated otherwise.

The mathematics of RDC calculations used here has been taken from Glaser et al. [53], and the formalism on how to include RDC data in 4D and 3D DG simulations (see below) has been described in full detail in Ref. [22]. The harmonic RDC "pseudo energy" E_{RDC} is based on violations $\Delta D = D^{exp} - D^{calc}$ between experimental and back-calculated values, and RDC data sets derived from multiple alignment media can be used simultaneously as an increasing number of experimental NMR restraints in our ConArch$^+$/DG approach simply by expanding the corresponding sum in E_{RDC}. Empirically, it proved best to scale the force-constant K_{RDC} used with the number of RDCs, or equivalently, with the number M of alignment media used, and thus we employ $K_{RDC} = 1.5/M$ Hz^{-2} in this study.

In addition to the application of chiral volume restraints on sp^2-type atomic centers ($V_{chir} = 0$), the term E_{DBL} in Equation (1) is used to reasonably restrain double bonds and aryl rings to planarity (restraining $V_{chir} = 0$ on neighboring atomic centers alone is not sufficient). Here, ΔX (used cf. Equation (2)) is defined as $\Delta X = 1 - \cos^2 \phi$, where $\phi_{i,j,k,l}$ are the corresponding torsion angles $i-j-k-l$ with sp^2-sp^2-type central bonds, and ΔX vanishes for $\phi = 0°$ and $\phi = 180°$ only (cis- and trans-configurations). The rather high force-constant $K_{DBL} = 100$ used here efficiently removes local energy minima which originate from slight bending of C=C-double bonds and aromatic rings, revealing more distinctive energy steps separating alternate conformational families. In general, the final best-fit energy-minimum structures have very low distortional energy terms of $E_{DBL} \leq 5 \times 10^{-3}$, and the efficiency with which different configurations and conformations are sampled on the basis of experimental NMR data is largely unhampered by these types of restraints.

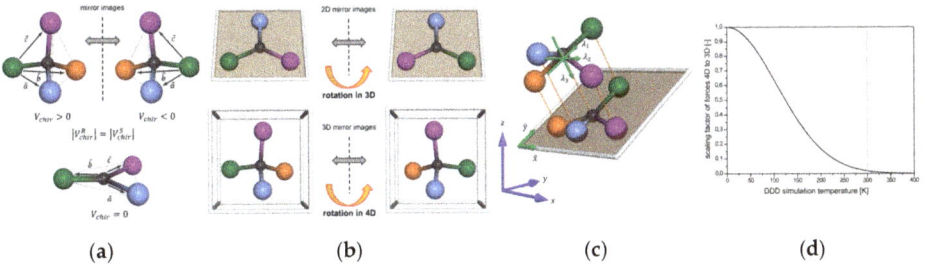

Figure 12. (a) Definition of chiral volumes as scalar triple products $V_{chir} = \vec{a} \cdot (\vec{b} \times \vec{c})$ for sp^3- and sp^2-type atomic centers. (b) In analogy to 2D chiral objects that can be transformed into each other through a rotation in higher dimensions (3D), the configuration of 3D-chiral objects can be inverted by simple rotations in 4D (see text for details). (c) Projection mode of higher dimensional objects into lower dimensional space (here visualized as 3D→2D) along the eigenvector associated with the largest eigenvalue λ_3 of the inertia tensor (with $\lambda_1 < \lambda_2 \ldots < \lambda_n$). Similar projections 4D→3D optimally preserve interatomic distances. (d) Temperature dependent scaling factors of projection forces applied to 4D simulated annealing smoothly transforms higher dimensional objects into 3D structures ($\tau_T = 150$ K, see text for details).

The initial input structure is used by DG only for setting up the holonomic bounds and distance matrices (±1% bond lengths), and subsequent configurational and conformational sampling is carried out by our ConArch$^+$/DG approach in an automated sequence of steps. First, molecular structures are generated in four-dimensional (4D) space ("metrization" step, i.e., embedding based on holonomic distance bounds), followed by a 4D "floating-chirality" restrained DG (fc-rDG) and distance bounds driven dynamics (DDD) simulation (simulated annealing). After reduction of dimensionality, the simulated annealing is repeated in 3D space, and each simulation in 4D and 3D is concluded by a gradient-descent type optimization of structures against all restraints, minimizing the total pseudo energy E_{total}. In all dynamics and optimization calculations, the partial derivatives $\partial E_{total}/\partial r_\alpha$ of all energy terms with respect 4D and 3D Cartesian atomic coordinates ($\alpha \in x, y, z(, w)$ for all atoms) are interpreted and used as forces governing the evolution of the system. All derivatives are calculated analytically by ConArch$^+$/DG. During each step of the rDG/DDD runs using RDCs, full updates of the Saupe or alignment tensors are computed based on a singular value decomposition (SVD) algorithm.

Sampling molecular structures first in 4D very efficiently generates diastereomeric geometries as inversion barriers can be overcome easily [70,71]. Configurational inversion in 3D is reduced to a simple rotation in 4D (see Figure 12b), and consequently during simulated annealing in 4D space with chiral restraints removed on all but selected chiral centers (fc-DDD), the transition barriers between diastereomers are significantly lowered or removed altogether.

For an increased sampling efficiency, it is crucial to transport as much 4D information as possible into 3D, in order to produce chemically relevant structure models. Projection from higher to lower dimensionality optimally preserves atom-atom distances when carried out along the eigenvector associated with the largest eigenvalue of the inertia tensor I defined by Equation (4):

$$I = \sum_k ((\vec{r}_k \cdot \vec{r}_k)E - \vec{r}_k \otimes \vec{r}_k), \quad (4)$$

where the sum runs over all atomic positional vectors ($\vec{r}_k$ for k particles) centered about the origin ($\sum \vec{r}_k = 0$) and weighted with unity mass (see Figure 12c) [72]. During 4D simulated annealing, we apply a temperature dependent scaling factor $f = \exp\left(-(T/\tau_T)^2\right)$ with an empirical temperature coupling factor $\tau_T = 150$ K to forces acting along this eigenvector, which gradually restrain the 4D molecular models into a 3D subspace thereof (see Figure 12d). At high temperatures ($T > 300$ K), all structures evolve freely, but are restrained increasingly and smoothly to 3D sub-space during the cooling phase ($T < 300$ K) of the simulated annealing. Finally, all models are projected into pure 3D space and are subjected to an additional simulated annealing therein.

In this study, for each compound **1–5** a total of 1000 structures (configurations and conformations) were generated initially in 4D space. All consecutive simulated annealing simulations in 4D and 3D used 5000 steps of equilibration ($T = 300$ K) and 5000 steps of cooling ($T \rightarrow 0$ K) each (2 fs time steps). The final structures were collected, sorted by their pseudo energy, and a final selection of the ranked structures of lowest energy were used for the plots presented here. For the global energy minimum best-fit structures, errors in calculated RDCs are estimated from Monte-Carlo bootstrapping analysis including tensor updates [22,23]. Total single processor CPU (Intel(R) Core(TM) i7-4790 CPU @ 3.60GHz) wall time used was about 7–8 min. for each compound **1–3**, and up to approx. 50 min for **4** and **5** when three alignment media RDC data sets are used. However, the entire process can be parallelized very efficiently on an arbitrary number of shared memory CPU cores, reducing the total wall time accordingly to a few minutes only.

Supplementary Materials: The following are available online at http://www.mdpi.com/1660-3397/18/6/330/s1, Table S1: NOE data used for Axinellamine A (**1**), Table S2: NOE data used for Tetrabromostyloguanidine (**2**), Table S3: NOE data used for 3,7-*epi*-Massadine chloride (**3**), Table S4: RDC data used for Tubocurarine (**4**), Table S5: NOE data used for **4**, Table S6: RDC data used for Vincristine (**5**), Table S7: NOE data used for **5**, Table S8: Atomic coordinates for rDG structures of compounds **1-5**. Figure S1: rDG structure of compound **1**, Figure S2: Extended rDG simulations of **1**, Figure S3: Structures of **1** obtained from extended rDG simulations, Figure S4: rDG structure of compound **2**, Figure S5: Variations of chiral volume restraints used for **2**, Figure S6: Structures of **2** obtained from unrestrained rDG simulations, Figure S7: Structures of **2** obtained from variations of chiral volume restraints, Figure S8: rDG detailed analysis of **2**, Figure S9: Structures of **2** from rDG detailed analysis, Figure S10: rDG structure of compound **3**, Figure S11: rDG detailed analysis of **3**, Figure S12: Structures of **3** from rDG detailed analysis, Figure S13: rDG structure and back-calculated RDCs for **4**, Figure S14: rDG structure of **4**, Figure S15: rDG structure and back-calculated RDCs for **5**, Figure S16: rDG structure of **5**.

Author Contributions: Conceptualization, M.K. and S.I.; methodology, M.K. and S.I.; software, S.I.; writing—original draft preparation, M.K. and S.I.; writing—review and editing, M.K., M.R., and S.I.; visualization, M.K. and S.I. All authors have read and agreed to the published version of the manuscript.

Funding: This research was funded by the Deutsche Forschungsgemeinschaft (DFG), grant number Re1007/9-1.

Acknowledgments: We would like to thank M.R. Scheek (University of Groningen) for providing his modified version of the DG-II program package. We also thank the Center for Scientific Computing (CSC) of the Goethe University, Frankfurt, for granting access to the high-performance computing cluster and providing the CPU time required for the DFT calculations (Figure 11).

Conflicts of Interest: The authors declare no conflict of interest.

References

1. Köck, M.; Junker, J. Marine natural products—New ways in the constitutional assignment. In *New Aspects in Bioorganic Chemistry*; Diederichsen, U., Lindhorst, T.K., Wessjohann, L., Westermann, B., Eds.; Wiley-VCH: Weinheim, Germany, 1999; pp. 365–378.
2. Lindel, T.; Junker, J.; Köck, M. COCON: From NMR correlation data to molecular constitutions. *J. Mol. Model.* **1997**, *3*, 364–368. [CrossRef]
3. Köck, M.; Junker, J. Determination of the relative configuration of organic compounds using NMR and DG: A systematic approach for a model system. *J. Mol. Model.* **1997**, *3*, 403–407. [CrossRef]
4. Reggelin, M.; Hoffmann, H.; Köck, M.; Mierke, D.F. Determination of conformation and relative configuration of a small, rapidly tumbling molecule in solution by combined application of NOESY and restrained MD calculations. *J. Am. Chem. Soc.* **1992**, *114*, 3272–3277. [CrossRef]
5. Reggelin, M.; Köck, M.; Conde-Frieboes, K.; Mierke, D.F. Determination of the relative configuration by distance geometry calculations with proton-proton distances from NOESY spectra. *Angew. Chem. Int. Ed.* **1994**, *33*, 753–755. [CrossRef]
6. Menna, M.; Imperatore, C.; Mangoni, A.; Della Sala, G.; Taglialatela-Scafati, O. Challenges in the configuration assignment of natural products. A case-selective perspective. *Nat. Prod. Rep.* **2019**, *36*, 476–489. [CrossRef]

7. Schleucher, J.; Schwörer, B.; Zirngibl, C.; Koch, U.; Weber, W.; Egert, E.; Thauer, R.K.; Griesinger, C. Determination of the relative configuration of 5,6,7,8-tetrahydromethanopterin by two-dimensional NMR spectroscopy. *FEBS Lett.* **1992**, *314*, 440–444. [CrossRef]
8. Kaptein, R.; Zuiderweg, E.R.P.; Scheek, R.M.; Boelens, R.; van Gunsteren, W.F. A Protein-Structure From Nuclear Magnetic-Resonance Data - Lac Repressor Headpiece. *J. Mol. Biol.* **1985**, *182*, 179–182. [CrossRef]
9. Clore, G.M.; Gronenborn, A.M.; Brünger, A.T.; Karplus, M. Solution conformation of a heptadecapeptide comprising the DNA binding helix F of the cyclic AMP receptor protein of Escherichia coli: Combined use of 1H nuclear magnetic resonance and restrained molecular dynamics. *J. Mol. Biol.* **1985**, *186*, 435–455. [CrossRef]
10. Navarro-Vázquez, A. When not to rely on Boltzmann populations. Automated CASE-3D structure elucidation of hyacinthacines through chemical shift differences. *Magn. Reson. Chem.* **2020**, *58*, 139–144. [CrossRef]
11. Navarro-Vázquez, A.; Gil, R.R.; Blinov, K. Computer-Assisted 3D Structure Elucidation (CASE-3D) of Natural Products Combining Isotropic and Anisotropic NMR Parameters. *J. Nat. Prod.* **2018**, *81*, 203–210. [CrossRef]
12. Grimme, S. Dispersion Interaction and Chemical Bonding. In *The Chemical Bond*; Frenking, G., Shaik, S., Eds.; Wiley-VCH: Weinheim, Germany, 2014; pp. 477–500.
13. Crippen, G.M.; Havel, T.F. *Distance Geometry and Molecular Conformation*; Research Studies Press LTD: Taunton, UK, 1988.
14. de Vlieg, J.; Scheek, R.M.; van Gunsteren, W.F.; Berendsen, H.J.C.; Kaptein, R.; Thomason, J. Combined procedure of distance geometry and restrained molecular dynamics techniques for protein structure determination from nuclear magnetic resonance data: Application to the DNA binding domain of lac repressor from Escherichia coli. *Proteins Struct. Funct. Genet.* **1988**, *3*, 209–218. [CrossRef]
15. Havel, T.F.; Kuntz, I.D.; Crippen, G.M. The theory and practice of distance geometry. *Bull. Math. Biol.* **1983**, *45*, 665–720. [CrossRef]
16. Kaptein, R.; Boelens, R.; Scheek, R.M.; van Gunsteren, W.F. Protein structures from NMR. *Biochemistry* **1988**, *27*, 5389–5395. [CrossRef]
17. Scheek, R.M.; van Gunsteren, W.F.; Kaptein, R. Molecular dynamics simulation techniques for determination of molecular structures from nuclear magnetic resonance data. *Methods Enzymol.* **1989**, *177*, 204–218.
18. Mierke, D.F.; Reggelin, M. Simultaneous determination of conformation and configuration using distance geometry. *J. Org. Chem.* **1992**, *57*, 6365–6367. [CrossRef]
19. Köck, M.; Junker, J. How many NOE derived restraints are necessary for a reliable determination of the relative configuration of an organic compound? Application to a model system. *J. Org. Chem.* **1998**, *62*, 8614–8615, Erratum in **1998**, *63*, 2409. [CrossRef]
20. Weber, P.L.; Morrison, R.; Hare, D. Determining stereo specific H-1 nuclear magnetic-resonance assignments from distance geometry calculations. *J. Mol. Biol.* **1988**, *204*, 483–487. [CrossRef]
21. Holak, T.A.; Gondol, D.; Otlewski, J.; Wilusz, T. Determination of the complete 3-dimensional structure of the trypsin-inhibitor from squash seeds in aqueous-solution by nuclear magnetic-resonance and a combination of distance geometry and dynamical simulated annealing. *J. Mol. Biol.* **1989**, *210*, 635–648. [CrossRef]
22. Immel, S.; Köck, M.; Reggelin, M. Configurational Analysis by Residual Dipolar Coupling Driven Floating Chirality Distance Geometry Calculations. *Chem. Eur. J.* **2018**, *24*, 13918–13930. [CrossRef]
23. Immel, S.; Köck, M.; Reggelin, M. Configurational analysis by residual dipolar couplings: A critical assessment of diastereomeric differentiabilities. *Chirality* **2019**, *31*, 384–400. [CrossRef]
24. Tolman, J.R.; Flanagan, J.M.; Kennedy, M.A.; Prestegard, J.H. Nuclear magnetic dipole interactions in field-oriented proteins: Information for structure determination in solution. *Proc. Natl. Acad. Sci. USA* **1995**, *92*, 9279–9283. [CrossRef] [PubMed]
25. Tjandra, N.; Grzesiek, S.; Bax, A. Magnetic Field Dependence of Nitrogen-Proton J Splittings in 15N-Enriched Human Ubiquitin Resulting from Relaxation Interference and Residual Dipolar Coupling. *J. Am. Chem. Soc.* **1996**, *118*, 6264–6272. [CrossRef]
26. Li, G.W.; Liu, H.; Qiu, F.; Wang, X.J.; Lei, X.X. Residual Dipolar Couplings in Structure Determination of Natural Products. *Nat. Product. Bioprospect.* **2018**, *8*, 279–295. [CrossRef]
27. Gil, R.R. Residual Dipolar Couplings in Small-Molecule NMR. In *Encyclopedia of Spectroscopy and Spectrometry*; Lindon, J.C., Tranter, G.E., Koppenaal, D.W., Eds.; Academic Press Ltd-Elsevier Science Ltd.: London, UK, 2017; pp. 946–955.

28. Gil, R.R.; Griesinger, C.; Navarro-Vázquez, A.; Sun, H. Structural Elucidation of Small Organic Molecules Assisted by NMR in Aligned Media. In *Structure Elucidation in Organic Chemistry: The Search for the Right Tools*; Cid, M.M., Bravo, J., Eds.; Wiley-VCH: Weinheim, Germany, 2015; pp. 279–323.
29. Luy, B. Distinction of enantiomers by NMR spectroscopy using chiral orienting media. *J. Indian Inst. Sci.* **2010**, *90*, 119–132.
30. Kummerlöwe, G.; Luy, B. Residual Dipolar Couplings for the Configurational and Conformational Analysis of Organic Molecules. In *Annual Reports on NMR Spectroscopy*; Webb, G.A., Ed.; Academic Press: Cambridge, MA, USA, 2009; Volume 68, pp. 193–230.
31. Kummerlöwe, G.; Luy, B. Residual dipolar couplings as a tool in determining the structure of organic molecules. *TrAC Trends Anal. Chem.* **2009**, *28*, 483–493. [CrossRef]
32. Carvalho, D.S.; da Silva, D.G.B.; Hallwass, F.; Navarro-Vázquez, A. Chemically cross-linked polyacrylonitrile. A DMSO compatible NMR alignment medium for measurement of residual dipolar couplings and residual chemical shift anisotropies. *J. Magn. Reson.* **2019**, *302*, 21–27. [CrossRef]
33. Gayathri, C.; Tsarevsky, N.V.; Gil, R.R. Residual Dipolar Couplings (RDCs) Analysis of Small Molecules Made Easy: Fast and Tuneable Alignment by Reversible Compression/Relaxation of Reusable PMMA Gels. *Chem. Eur. J.* **2010**, *16*, 3622–3626. [CrossRef]
34. Gil-Silva, L.F.; Santamaria-Fernandez, R.; Navarro-Vázquez, A.; Gil, R.R. Collection of NMR Scalar and Residual Dipolar Couplings Using a Single Experiment. *Chem. Eur. J.* **2016**, *22*, 472–476. [CrossRef]
35. Garcia, M.E.; Woodruff, S.R.; Hellemann, E.; Tsarevsky, N.V.; Gil, R.R. Di(ethylene glycol) methyl ether methacrylate (DEGMEMA)-derived gels align small organic molecules in methanol. *Magn. Reson. Chem.* **2017**, *55*, 206–209. [CrossRef]
36. Hallwass, F.; Teles, R.R.; Hellemann, E.; Griesinger, C.; Gil, R.R.; Navarro-Vázquez, A. Measurement of residual chemical shift anisotropies in compressed polymethylmethacrylate gels. Automatic compensation of gel isotropic shift contribution. *Magn. Reson. Chem.* **2018**, *56*, 321–328. [CrossRef]
37. Kobzar, K.; Kessler, H.; Luy, B. Stretched gelatin gels as chiral alignment media for the discrimination of enantiomers by NMR spectroscopy. *Angew. Chem. Int. Ed.* **2005**, *44*, 3145–3147. [CrossRef] [PubMed]
38. Kummerlöwe, G.; Knör, S.; Frank, A.O.; Paululat, T.; Kessler, H.; Luy, B. Deuterated polymer gels for measuring anisotropic NMR parameters with strongly reduced artefacts. *Chem. Commun.* **2008**, *44*, 5722–5724. [CrossRef] [PubMed]
39. Kummerlöwe, G.; Behl, M.; Lendlein, A.; Luy, B. Artifact-free measurement of residual dipolar couplings in DMSO by the use of cross-linked perdeuterated poly(acrylonitrile) as alignment medium. *Chem. Commun.* **2010**, *46*, 8273–8275. [CrossRef]
40. Merle, C.; Kummerlöwe, G.; Freudenberger, J.C.; Halbach, F.; Stower, W.; von Gostomski, C.L.; Hopfner, J.; Beskers, T.; Wilhelm, M.; Luy, B. Crosslinked Poly(ethylene oxide) as a Versatile Alignment Medium for the Measurement of Residual Anisotropic NMR Parameters. *Angew. Chem. Int. Ed.* **2013**, *52*, 10309–10312. [CrossRef]
41. Lesot, P.; Aroulanda, C.; Berdague, P.; Meddour, A.; Merlet, D.; Farjon, J.; Giraud, N.; Lafon, O. Multinuclear NMR in polypeptide liquid crystals: Three fertile decades of methodological developments and analytical challenges. *Prog. Nucl. Magn. Reson. Spectrosc.* **2020**, *116*, 85–154. [CrossRef]
42. Ndukwe, I.E.; Wang, X.; Pelczer, I.; Reibarkh, M.; Williamson, R.T.; Liu, Y.; Martin, G.E. PBLG as a versatile liquid crystalline medium for anisotropic NMR data acquisition. *Chem. Commun.* **2019**, *55*, 4327–4330. [CrossRef]
43. Schwab, M.; Schmidts, V.; Thiele, C.M. Thermoresponsive Alignment Media in NMR Spectroscopy: Helix Reversal of a Copolyaspartate at Ambient Temperatures. *Chem. Eur. J.* **2018**, *24*, 14373–14377. [CrossRef]
44. Meyer, N.-C.; Krupp, A.; Schmidts, V.; Thiele, C.M.; Reggelin, M. Polyacetylenes as Enantiodifferentiating Alignment Media. *Angew. Chem. Int. Ed.* **2012**, *51*, 8334–8338. [CrossRef] [PubMed]
45. Lesot, P.; Berdagué, P.; Meddour, A.; Kreiter, A.; Noll, M.; Reggelin, M. 2H and 13C NMR-Based Enantiodetection Using Polyacetylene versus Polypeptide Aligning Media: Versatile and Complementary Tools for Chemists. *ChemPlusChem* **2019**, *84*, 144–153. [CrossRef]
46. Reller, M.; Wesp, S.; Koos, M.R.M.; Reggelin, M.; Luy, B. Biphasic Liquid Crystal and the Simultaneous Measurement of Isotropic and Anisotropic Parameters by Spatially Resolved NMR Spectroscopy. *Chem. Eur. J.* **2017**, *23*, 13351–13359. [CrossRef]

47. Lei, X.X.; Xu, Z.; Sun, H.; Wang, S.; Griesinger, C.; Peng, L.; Gao, C.; Tan, R.X. Graphene Oxide Liquid Crystals as a Versatile and Tunable Alignment Medium for the Measurement of Residual Dipolar Couplings in Organic Solvents. *J. Am. Chem. Soc.* **2014**, *136*, 11280–11283. [CrossRef] [PubMed]
48. Zong, W.; Li, G.W.; Cao, J.M.; Lei, X.X.; Hu, M.L.; Sun, H.; Griesinger, C.; Tan, R.X. An Alignment Medium for Measuring Residual Dipolar Couplings in Pure DMSO: Liquid Crystals from Graphene Oxide Grafted with Polymer Brushes. *Angew. Chem. Int. Ed.* **2016**, *55*, 3690–3693. [CrossRef] [PubMed]
49. Krupp, A.; Reggelin, M. Phenylalanine-based polyarylacetylenes as enantiomer-differentiating alignment media. *Magn. Reson. Chem.* **2012**, *50*, S45–S52. [CrossRef] [PubMed]
50. Parella, T. Current developments in homonuclear and heteronuclear J-resolved NMR experiments. *Magn. Reson. Chem.* **2018**, *56*, 230–250. [CrossRef]
51. Marcó, N.; Souza, A.A.; Nolis, P.; Gil, R.R.; Parella, T. Perfect (1)J(CH)-resolved HSQC: Efficient measurement of one-bond proton-carbon coupling constants along the indirect dimension. *J. Magn. Reson.* **2017**, *276*, 37–42. [CrossRef]
52. Enthart, A.; Freudenberger, J.C.; Furrer, J.; Kessler, H.; Luy, B. The CLIP/CLAP-HSQC: Pure absorptive spectra for the measurement of one-bond couplings. *J. Magn. Reson.* **2008**, *192*, 314–322. [CrossRef]
53. Kramer, F.; Deshmukh, M.V.; Kessler, H.; Glaser, S.J. Residual dipolar coupling constants: An elementary derivation of key equations. *Concepts Magn. Reson. Part A* **2004**, *21A*, 10–21. [CrossRef]
54. Ruan, K.; Briggman, K.B.; Tolman, J.R. De novo determination of internuclear vector orientations from residual dipolar couplings measured in three independent alignment media. *J. Biomol. NMR* **2008**, *41*, 61–76. [CrossRef]
55. Hus, J.C.; Brüschweiler, R. Reconstruction of interatomic vectors by principle component analysis of nuclear magnetic resonance data in multiple alignments. *J. Chem. Phys.* **2002**, *117*, 1166–1172. [CrossRef]
56. Yan, J.L.; Delaglio, F.; Kaerner, A.; Kline, A.D.; Mo, H.P.; Shapiro, M.J.; Smitka, T.A.; Stephenson, G.A.; Zartler, E.R. Complete relative stereochemistry of multiple stereocenters using only residual dipolar couplings. *J. Am. Chem. Soc.* **2004**, *126*, 5008–5017. [CrossRef]
57. Ruan, K.; Tolman, J.R. Composite Alignment Media for the Measurement of Independent Sets of NMR Residual Dipolar Couplings. *J. Am. Chem. Soc.* **2005**, *127*, 15032–15033. [CrossRef] [PubMed]
58. Schwab, M.; Herold, D.; Thiele, C.M. Polyaspartates as Thermoresponsive Enantiodifferentiating Helically Chiral Alignment Media for Anisotropic NMR Spectroscopy. *Chem. Eur. J.* **2017**, *23*, 14576–14584. [CrossRef] [PubMed]
59. Urban, S.; de Almeida Leone, P.; Carroll, A.R.; Fechner, G.A.; Smith, J.; Hooper, J.N.A.; Quinn, R.J. Axinellamines A-D, Novel Imidazo-Azolo-Imidazole Alkaloids from the Australian Marine Sponge *Axinella* sp. *J. Org. Chem.* **1999**, *64*, 731–735. [CrossRef] [PubMed]
60. Grube, A.; Köck, M. Structural assignment of tetrabromostyloguanidine: Does the relative configuration of the palau'amines need revision? *Angew. Chem. Int. Ed.* **2007**, *46*, 2320–2324. [CrossRef] [PubMed]
61. Su, S.; Seiple, I.B.; Young, I.S.; Baran, P.S. Total Syntheses of (±)-Massadine and Massadine Chloride. *J. Am. Chem. Soc.* **2008**, *130*, 16490–16491. [CrossRef] [PubMed]
62. Reynolds, C.D.; Palmer, R.A. Crystal-Structure, Absolute-Configuration and Stereochemistry of (+)-Tubocurarine Dibromide Methanol Solvate—Potent Neuromuscular Blocking-Agent. *Acta Crystallogr. Sect. B* **1976**, *32*, 1431–1439. [CrossRef]
63. Moncrief, J.W.; Lipscomb, W.N. Structure of Leurocristine Methiodide Dihydrate by Anomalous Scattering Methods - Relation to Leurocristine (Vincristine) and Vincaleukoblastine (Vinblastine). *Acta Crystallogr. Sect. A* **1966**, *21*, 322–331. [CrossRef]
64. Kinnel, R.B.; Gehrken, H.P.; Scheuer, P.J. Palau'amine: A cytotoxic and immunosuppressive hexacyclic bisguanidine antibiotic from the sponge Stylotella agminata. *J. Am. Chem. Soc.* **1993**, *115*, 3376–3377. [CrossRef]
65. Kato, T.; Shizuri, Y.; Izumida, H.; Yokoyama, A.; Endo, M. Styloguanidines, new chitinase inhibitors from the marine sponge Stylotella aurantium. *Tetrahedron Lett.* **1995**, *36*, 2133–2136. [CrossRef]
66. Kobayashi, J.; Suzuki, M.; Tsuda, M. Konbu'acidin A, a new bromopyrrole alkaloid with cdk4 inhibitory activity from Hymeniacidon sponge. *Tetrahedron* **1997**, *53*, 15681–15684. [CrossRef]
67. Kinnel, R.B.; Gehrken, H.-P.; Swali, R.; Skoropowski, G.; Scheuer, P.J. Palau'amine and its congeners: A family of bioactive bisguanidines from the marine sponge Stylotella aurantium. *J. Org. Chem.* **1998**, *63*, 3281–3286. [CrossRef]

68. Köck, M.; Grube, A.; Seiple, I.B.; Baran, P.S. The pursuit of Palau'amine. *Angew. Chem. Int. Ed.* **2007**, *46*, 6586–6594. [CrossRef] [PubMed]
69. Köck, M.; Schmidt, G.; Seiple, I.B.; Baran, P.S. Configurational analysis of tetracyclic dimeric pyrrole-imidazole alkaloids using a floating chirality approach. *J. Nat. Prod.* **2012**, *75*, 127–130. [CrossRef] [PubMed]
70. Havel, T.F. An evaluation of computational strategies for use in the determination of protein-structure from distance contraints obtained by nuclear magnetic resonance. *Prog. Biophys. Mol. Biol.* **1991**, *56*, 43–78. [CrossRef]
71. Spellmeyer, D.C.; Wong, A.K.; Bower, M.J.; Blaney, J.M. Conformational analysis using distance geometry methods. *J. Mol. Graphics Modell.* **1997**, *15*, 18–36. [CrossRef]
72. van Schaik, R.C.; Berendsen, H.J.C.; Torda, A.E.; van Gunsteren, W.F. A Structure Refinement Method Based on Molecular Dynamics in Four Spatial Dimensions. *J. Mol. Biol.* **1993**, *234*, 751–762. [CrossRef]

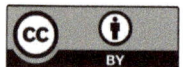

© 2020 by the authors. Licensee MDPI, Basel, Switzerland. This article is an open access article distributed under the terms and conditions of the Creative Commons Attribution (CC BY) license (http://creativecommons.org/licenses/by/4.0/).

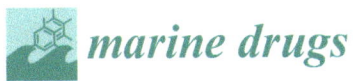

Article

A Phenotarget Approach for Identifying an Alkaloid Interacting with the Tuberculosis Protein Rv1466

Yan Xie [1,2], Yunjiang Feng [1], Angela Di Capua [1], Tin Mak [1], Garry W. Buchko [3,4], Peter J. Myler [5,6], Miaomiao Liu [1] and Ronald J. Quinn [1,*]

1. Griffith Institute for Drug Discovery, Griffith University, Brisbane, Queensland 4111, Australia; yan.xie4@griffithuni.edu.au (Y.X.); Y.Feng@griffith.edu.au (Y.F.); a.dicapua@griffith.edu.au (A.D.C.); t.mak@griffith.edu.au (T.M.); miaomiao.liu@griffith.edu.au (M.L.)
2. Guangxi Key Laboratory of Efficacy Study on Chinese Materia Medica, Guangxi University of Chinese Medicine, Nanning, 530200, China
3. Earth and Biological Sciences Directorate, Pacific Northwest National Laboratory, Richland, WA 99354, USA; garry.buchko@pnnl.gov
4. School of Molecular Biosciences, Washington State University, Pullman, WA 99164, USA
5. Center for Global Infectious Disease Research, Seattle Children's Research Institute, Seattle, WA 98109-5219, USA; peter.myler@seattlechildrens.org
6. Departments of Pediatrics, Global Health, and Biomedical Informatics & Medical Education, University of Washington, Seattle, WA 98195, USA
* Correspondence: r.quinn@griffith.edu.au; Tel.: +61-41-871-3254

Received: 29 December 2019; Accepted: 20 February 2020; Published: 5 March 2020

Abstract: In recent years, there has been a revival of interest in phenotypic-based drug discovery (PDD) due to target-based drug discovery (TDD) falling below expectations. Both PDD and TDD have their unique advantages and should be used as complementary methods in drug discovery. The PhenoTarget approach combines the strengths of the PDD and TDD approaches. Phenotypic screening is conducted initially to detect cellular active components and the hits are then screened against a panel of putative targets. This PhenoTarget protocol can be equally applied to pure compound libraries as well as natural product fractions. Here we described the use of the PhenoTarget approach to identify an anti-tuberculosis lead compound. Fractions from *Polycarpa aurata* were identified with activity against *Mycobacterium tuberculosis* H37Rv. Native magnetic resonance mass spectrometry (MRMS) against a panel of 37 proteins from *Mycobacterium* proteomes showed that a fraction from a 95% ethanol re-extraction specifically formed a protein-ligand complex with Rv1466, a putative uncharacterized *Mycobacterium tuberculosis* protein. The natural product responsible was isolated and characterized to be polycarpine. The molecular weight of the ligand bound to Rv1466, 233 Da, was half the molecular weight of polycarpine less one proton, indicating that polycarpine formed a covalent bond with Rv1466.

Keywords: PhenoTarget approach; MRMS; protein-ligand complex; polycarpine

1. Introduction

Drug discovery research and development has experienced two periods with different centric strategies, namely phenotypic-based drug discovery (PDD) and target-based drug discovery (TDD) (Figure 1). Commonly PDD refers to an approach without prior knowledge of the target. In phenotypic-based screening, compounds that modify a phenotype to generate a positive outcome in cell culture or in a whole organism are identified. TDD examines a specific drug target which is hypothesized to play an important role in disease.

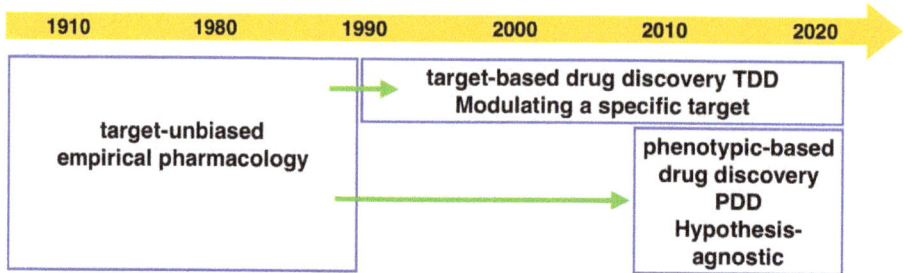

Figure 1. The evolution of technologies and screening strategies in drug discovery from 1910 to 2020. Adapted from [1,2].

Before the 1980s, the era without recombinant DNA technology, PDD was the primary approach in drug discovery. Most drugs at that time were discovered serendipitously by phenotypic assays in live animals or isolated tissues [3]. Examples are penicillin isolated from a *Penicillium* species in 1928 [2,4] and ivermectin isolated from *Streptomyces avermitilis* in 1975 [5]. From the 1990s, the development of genomics allowed the identification of drug target proteins. The advent of high-throughput screening and combinatorial libraries enabled the screening of target proteins in high throughput. Due to the development of technologies including X-ray crystallography, computational modeling and screening (virtual docking), visualization of the interaction of target protein and compound greatly facilitated the later stage of structure-based development. The development of these technologies appealed to the pharmaceutical industry and academic researchers who then switched to focus on TDD during the last three decades.

In the era that mainly focused on TDD, the total number of new molecular entities (NMEs) and new biologics approved by the Food and Drug Administration was far below expectations [6]. The timeline of cumulative NME approvals from 1950 to 2008 was contributed to by the three most productive companies in the industry and showed almost straight lines, indicating that productivity continued at a constant rate for almost 60 years [1]. The introduction of new molecular biology tools such as recombinant DNA technology, deep sequencing, mining of Expressed Sequence Tagged (cDNA) libraries and the draft human genome did not facilitate drug innovation as expected. This was also indicated in a later NMEs analysis with a timeline spanning over five years to 2013 [7]. More dishearteningly, while the number of NMEs per year has remained relatively constant for the past four decades, the investment in pharmaceutical research and development (R&D) has increased dramatically to over 50 billion USD per year. Today the number of NMEs launched per billion dollars of investment is well below the return for an equivalent billion-dollar investment 50 years ago [1]. The asymmetrical output raises questions about the limitation of the popular target centric strategy of R&D in recent decades.

Consequently, there is a revival of interest in PDD. A significant analysis by Swinney demonstrated that the majority of NMEs approved by the FDA during the 10-year period between 1999 and 2008 were discovered using phenotypic assays, where 28 came from phenotypic screening approaches and 17 came from target-based approaches [8]. It was suggested that the lack of successful NMEs in the post-genomic era was mainly due to the limited use of phenotypic screening. Because an organism is a complex biological system, a simplified single protein assay may not efficiently represent the disease pathogenesis [8] The effects on a single protein may not be translated to meaningful therapeutic efficacy. Conversely, phenotypic screening is an approach for unbiased targets. Phenotypic-based screening is, therefore, being reconsidered for screening compounds due to the realization that results for a single target protein may not fully correlate in the context of a complex biological process [9]. Phenotypic screening also holds the unique promise to uncover new mechanisms of action for currently untreated diseases such as rare diseases and/or neglected diseases [2].

The current phenotypic based approach should not be regarded as a step back to the classical phenotypic screening but as a new discipline [7]. Currently, in vivo and in vitro approaches are involved in phenotypic screening, of which in vitro cell-based phenotypic assays can be easily adapted to a high-throughput format for automated phenotypic analysis. New technologies such as gene expression, genetic modifier screening, resistance mutation and computational inference are increasingly being applied in phenotypic screening. These sophisticated phenotypic screening methodologies enhance the identification of novel compounds as well as their mechanism of action [10].

Target identification is a crucial part of drug discovery. Most large pharmaceutical companies strongly recommend target identification because failing to assign the mechanism of action is frequently regarded as a major risk factor for clinical development and regulatory approval [8]. Even with the most advanced phenotypic screens, in most cases, it is still difficult to determine the mechanism of action. Target identification is the key value of TDD [6]. With the target protein in hand, detailed drug-protein characterization is possible and this provides a better understanding of structure-activity relationships, which is a challenge in phenotypic screening without a known target [11].

Considering the strengths and weaknesses of PDD and TDD, these two approaches should not be treated monolithically but as complementary approaches that can work together to increase the productivity of drug discovery and development. This article describes an approach that combines PDD and TDD: PhenoTarget screening to identify active compounds from natural resources. As a proof of principle, we apply this combination approach to probe fractions of natural product libraries for compounds active against *Mycobacterium tuberculosis* H37Rv, the etiological agent responsible for tuberculosis (TB). The active fraction was then screened against a panel of 37 unique mycobacterial proteins to identify the potential compound and protein responsible for the activity against *M. tuberculosis*.

2. Results

A combined approach of phenotypic screening and target screening, which we refer to as a PhenoTarget approach, was used to identify lead compounds against *Mycobacterium tuberculosis* from natural resources. The PhenoTarget approach started from the phenotypic screening of a natural product fraction library to identify fractions that were active in an HTS screen against *M. tuberculosis* H37Rv. Following phenotypic screening, native mass spectrometry was used to simultaneously identify the target protein and the molecular weight of the compound bound to the protein in pooled fractions using a panel of 37 purified mycobacterial proteins. The proteins in the panel were selected because they were all essential enzymes or virulence factors, their three-dimensional structures had been solved by the Seattle Structural Genomics Center for Infectious Diseases (SSGCID); [12,13] and SSGCID was able to supply purified proteins for the PhenoTarget screens. Screening of the pooled fractions against this protein panel of 37 putative anti-TB targets was conducted by a magnetic resonance mass spectrometry (MRMS) system equipped with an automated chip-based Nanomate system. A summary of the PhenoTarget approach is described in Figure 2.

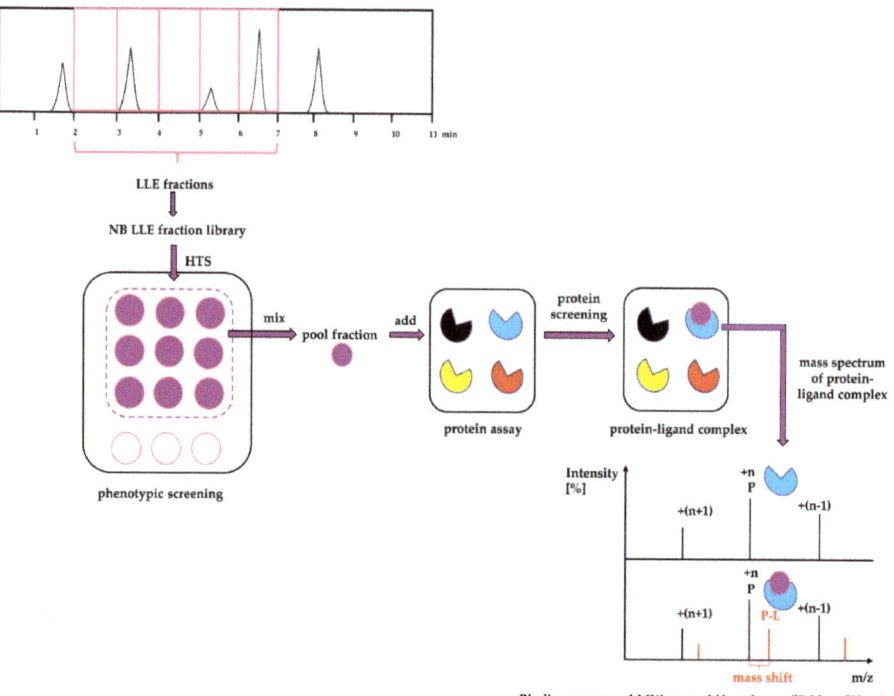

Figure 2. The cascade of PhenoTarget screening for identifying lead compounds and target proteins is shown. The Nature Bank (NB) lead-like enhanced (LLE) fraction library was established following the procedure described by Camp et al. [14]. A high throughput phenotypic screening of 202,983 NB LLE fractions against *M. tuberculosis* H37Rv was initially performed. Active fractions with an MIC value of less than 6.1 µge/µL were identified and chosen for protein screening against a panel of 37 putative anti-TB targets from *Mycobacteria* species. To lower sample consumption, especially protein, nine active fractions were pooled (Pool Fractions 1 to 40) and incubated with each of the target proteins. Native mass spectrometry was then used to identify free target protein (P, blue) and protein-ligand (P-L) complexes. The mass shift between the P (black) and the P-L (red) peaks provided the molecular weight of the bound ligand (L, purple) and this facilitated the isolation and identification of the active compound.

2.1. Native Mass Spectrometry

Figure 3 compares the native MRMS spectra for free Rv1466, a protein associated with [Fe–S] complex assembly and repair (a) and NB LLE Pool Fraction 4 (b) and 5 (c). All three spectra contain clusters of ions with three different charged states (+8, +7, and +6). However, the spectra with Pool Fractions 4 and 5 both contain a cluster of ions shifted to high m/z values by identical amounts relative to the free Rv1466 ions. These new ions are also of higher intensity than the free Rv1466 ions and correspond to Rv1466-ligand (P–L) complexes. From the charge and m/z differences between the cluster of P and P–L ions it is possible to obtain the molecular weight of the ligand-bound to Rv1466, 233 Da. Because the ligand that was bound to Rv1466 from Pool Fraction 4 and 5 had the same molecular weight, and likely the same compound, and appeared to have a high affinity for Rv1466 as deduced by the P:P-L intensity ratio, we chose to pursue the identity of this compound.

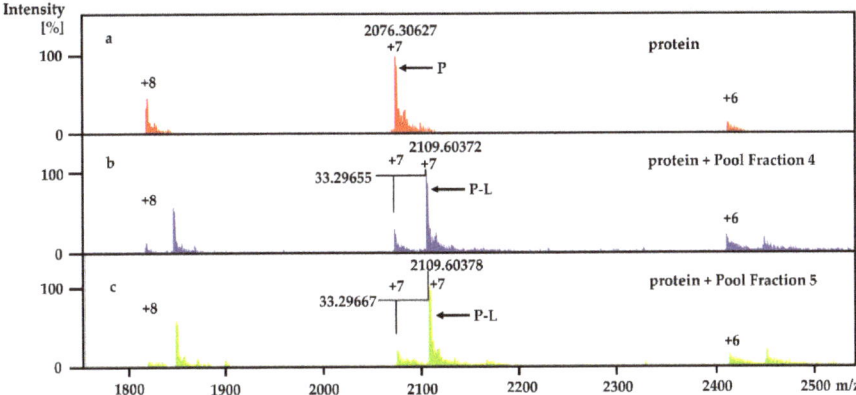

Figure 3. Overlay of the native magnetic resonance mass spectrometry (MRMS) spectra for free Rv1466 (a) and Rv1466 incubated with Pool Fraction 4 (b) and 5 (c). In the spectrum of free Rv1466 (P), clusters of ions corresponding to three different charged states for Rv1466 were observed. The same cluster of ions was observed in the spectra with Pool Fraction 4 and 5 but at lower intensities. Accompanying the ions for free Rv1466 in the spectra with Pool Fractions are clusters of larger intensity ions shifted to high m/z values that correspond to Rv1466-ligand (P-L) complexes. The mass shift for the differently charged cluster pairs (P and P-L) was identical in both Pool Fractions, identifying the molecular weight of the bound ligand: Pool Fraction 4: MW = (2109.60372 − 2076.30627) × 7 = 233 Da; Pool fraction 5: MW = (2109.60378 − 2076.30627) × 7 = 233 Da.

2.2. Target Fraction Confirmation

A feature common to Pool Fractions 4 and 5 was that they contained LLE fractions (LLE-2 and LLE-3, respectively) from the same marine biota, *Polycarpa aurata*, suggesting that a compound from *P. aurata* had interacted with Rv1466. A detailed high-resolution mass spectrometry (HRMS) investigation of all nine fractions from Pool Fraction 5 indicated that no fractions showed an ion at 233 m/z. In this case, MS investigation of the fractions did not confirm the presence of a ligand, so native MS was used to identify the correct fraction for isolation. Thus, five fractions were generated from a re-extraction of *P. aurata* by 95% ethanol and named Fractions A, B, C, D and E (Figure 4a). HRMS analysis of the constituents of Fraction C by a quadrupole-time-of-flight (Q-TOF) mass spectrometer identified an ion at m/z 236 as well as a higher mass ion at m/z 469 corresponding to a 468 + H$^+$ ion (Figure 4b). Another round of native MRMS screening confirmed that a compound in Fraction C interacted with Rv1466 and the molecular weight of the bound species was 233 Da (Figure 4c). Because the molecular weight of the ligand bound to Rv1466 was approximately half the molecular weight of the major species in Fraction C, our attention was drawn towards a potentially symmetrical parent compound with a molecular weight of 468 Da as the agent reacting with Rv1466.

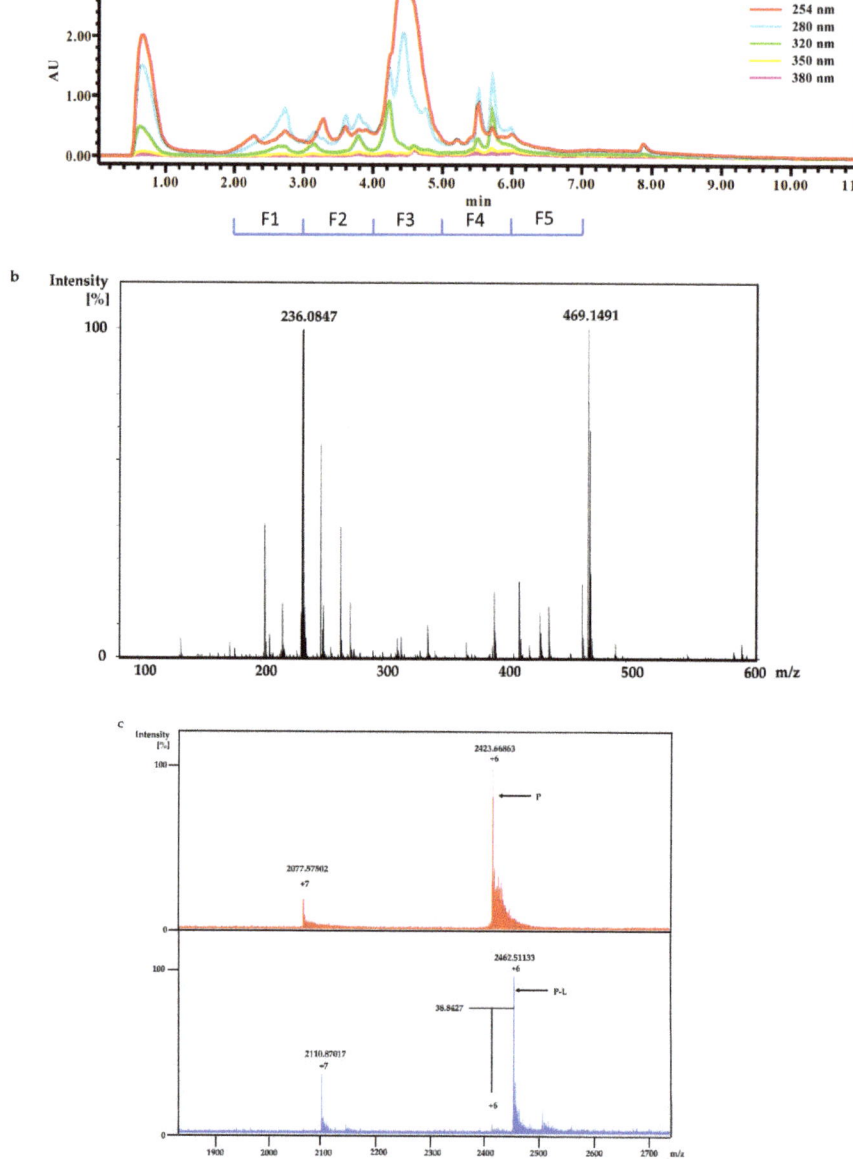

Figure 4. (**a**) Five fractions (Fractions A, B, C, D and E) were collected from a fresh 95% ethanol extraction of *P. aurata*; (**b**) the HRMS analysis of Fraction C identified ions at m/z 236 and 469; (**c**) comparison of the native MRMS spectrum for free Rv1466 (top, red) with the incubation of Rv1466 with Fraction C (bottom, blue). A similar ionization pattern was observed as described in Figure 3 with Pool Fractions 4 and 5. Ions corresponding to free Rv1466 (P) and the Rv1466-ligand complex (P-L) are labeled. Molecular weight of ligand in Fraction C: MW = (2462.51133 − 2423.66863) × 6 = 233 Da.

2.3. Binding Compound Isolation and Structure Elucidation

Separation of *P. aurata* extracts by reverse phase semi-preparative HPLC (Figure 5) gave a compound identified as polycarpine, $C_{22}H_{24}N_6O_2S_2$, a dimeric disulfide alkaloid previously identified from *P. autara* [15] and in a related species, *Polycarpa clavata* [16] (Figure 6). As illustrated in Figure 5a, the resonances observed in the one-dimensional ^1H spectrum of pure polycarpine (bottom, red) are present in the one-dimensional ^1H NMR spectrum for Fraction C (top, black). Moreover, pure polycarpine elutes with a retention time identical to a band in the LC profile for Fraction C (Figure 5b). The mass spectra of both bands are identical (Figure 5c) and consistent with a species with a molecular weight of 468 Da.

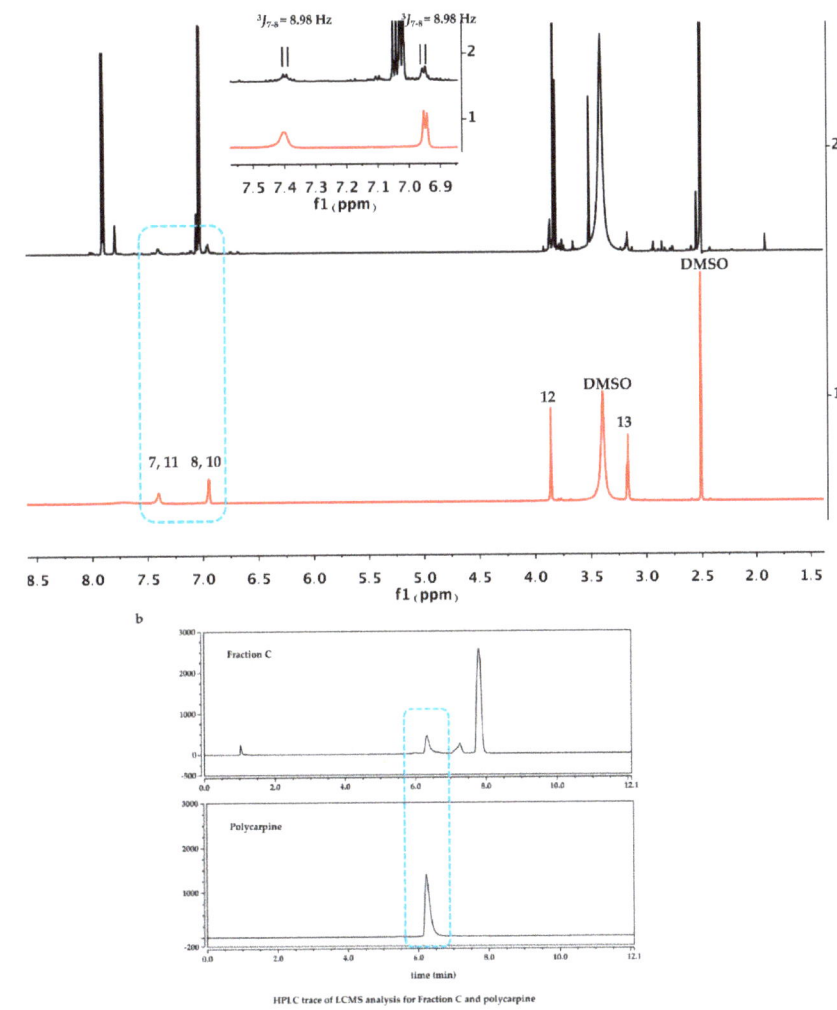

Figure 5. *Cont.*

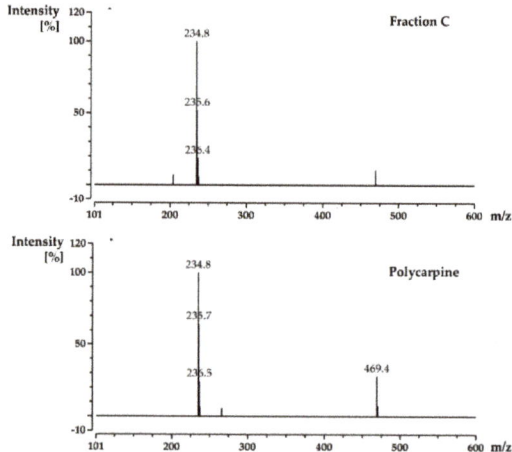

Figure 5. (a) ^{1}H NMR (recorded in DMSO-d_6) of Fraction C (black, top) and polycarpine (red, bottom). The inset, an expansion of the downfield regions of the spectra circled in blue. (b) HPLC analysis of Fraction C (top) and polycarpine (bottom), (c) Mass spectral analysis of both HPLC bands circled in a blue rectangle from Fraction C and polycarpine showed an identical ion at 234 Da.

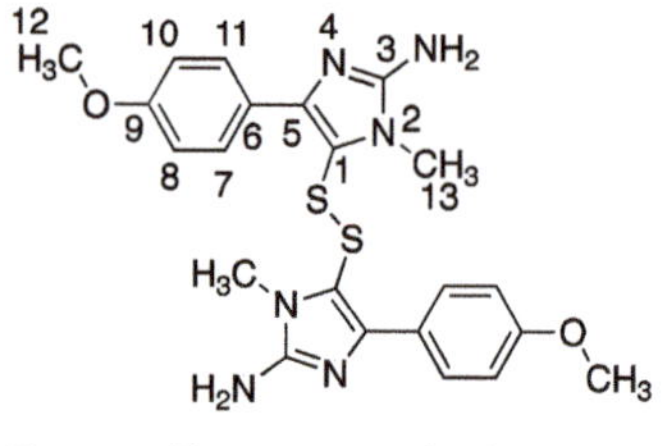

Figure 6. The structure of polycarpine.

2.4. Pseudo-K_D Value Determination of Polycarpine with Rv1466

An advantage of native mass spectrometry is that in addition to the qualitative identification of protein-ligand formation, the technique also provides quantitative information on the strength of the interaction [17,18]. This is because it is possible to estimate the dissociation constant, K_D, from the ratio of free and bound protein observed in the MS chromatograms. It is accomplished by collecting MRMS data at a fixed protein concentration with increasing concentrations of the ligand (Figure 7a). Figure 7b displays twelve mass spectra of samples containing 9 µM Rv1466 and increasing amounts of polycarpine (0.1–300 µM). A ligand concentration was reached where the intensity of the protein-ligand complex reached a plateau. The ratios of the intensity of protein-ligand peak and sum of protein peak and protein-ligand peak were plotted against the concentration of polycarpine (Figure 7c). Using these ratios and Equations 1 and 2, a pseudo-K_D of 5.3 ± 0.4 µM was calculated for polycarpine binding to Rv1466. A real K_D cannot be calculated because after binding a covalent bond forms between the ligand and Rv1466 in a time-dependent manner, pushing the equilibrium to the product.

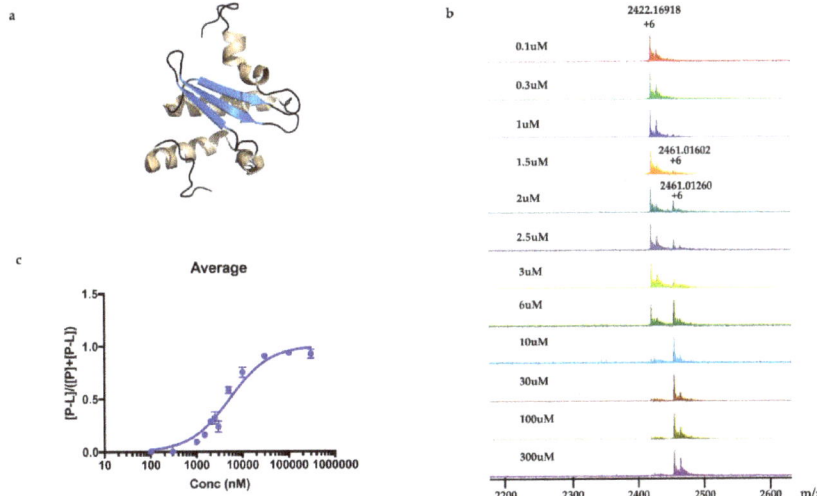

Figure 7. Direct determination of pseudo-K_D for polycarpine using a dose-response curve. (**a**) Cartoon representation of the Rv1466 structure (5IRD) closest to the average structure in the calculated ensemble. The α-helices and β-strands are colored gold and blue, respectively; (**b**) Overlay of twelve mass spectra of samples containing Rv1466 (9 μM) incubated with varying concentrations of polycarpine (0.1–300 μM); (**c**) The relative mass responses of protein-ligand complex with protein, [P-L]/([P-L]+[P]), plotted against the concentration of polycarpine. The pseudo-K_D was determined to be 5.29 ± 0.39 μM.

3. Discussion

Using the PhenoTarget approach, a ligand from a natural product fraction library was identified that bound to the *M. tuberculosis* protein Rv1466. The ligand molecular weight from the native MRMS spectrum was 233 Da. The compound was shown to be polycarpine with a molecular mass of 468 Da. The ligand MW of 233 Da was half the molecular weight of polycarpine less one proton, indicating that polycarpine formed a covalent bond with Rv1466. Under mild silica chromatography, the polycarpine disulfide bond has been shown to be cleaved [15,16]. Rv1466 has a single cysteine and the structure of Rv1466 (5IRD) indicates this residue is exposed on the surface of the protein so that it could attack the disulfide bond of polycarpine to form a covalent disulfide linked complex. The polycarpine-Rv1466 pseudo-K_D was determined to be 5.3 ± 0.4 μM. *P. aurata*, a species of tunicate in the family Styelidae, is rich in alkaloids containing sulfur such as polycarpine, polycarpaurine A, polycarpaurine B and polycarpaurine C [15,16,19,20].

In the PhenoTarget approach, phenotypic screening is conducted initially to detect cellular active components. In our case a natural product fraction library was used, however, this could be equally applied to pure compound libraries. Mass spectrometry using a protein panel of putative targets provided sufficient throughput to analyze the phenotypic hits. Native mass spectrometry offers the further advantage that it can be used for cloned, expressed and purified proteins that lack structural information. This opens the option to explore the proteome of many species, in our case, the *Mycobacterium* proteome. As well as its high sensitivity, high-throughput capability and in time observation of protein-ligand interaction, it can also provide exact mass information of the binding compound [21]. The mass information is useful for isolating the compound from the fraction mixture using mass-guided isolation. In addition, mass spectrometry has been reported as an alternative technique for the quantitative characterization of protein–ligand interactions in solution, that is, the determination of equilibrium constants for protein–ligand association (Ka) or dissociation (Kd = 1/Ka) [22,23]. Among all the mass spectrometers, MRMS provides the highest accuracy and resolution. Nanoelectrospray was used for sample delivery. Compared to conventional electrospray, its benefits include an increased sensitivity signal, lower consumption of ligand and protein, and no sample-to-sample cross-contamination, a faster speed and a higher degree of nozzle-to-nozzle reproducibility [24]. A high degree of nozzle-to-nozzle reproducibility is important for quantitative studies such as K_D determination. It has been proven that K_D results from chip-based electrospray are consistent with conventional techniques [17].

While there are advantages in the phenotypic drug discovery approach it should be noted that there are also some disadvantages. Foremost is the procurement of pure protein panels for target identification. For example, the genome of *M. tuberculosis* contains over 4000 genes [25] and our exploratory panel contained only 37 different proteins. This bottleneck can be partly circumvented by using orthologous proteins from related species [26]. Indeed, in addition to *M. tuberculosis* (12 proteins), our mycobacterial panel contained proteins from *Mycobacterium smegmatis* (5), *Mycobacterium abscessus* (4), *Mycobacterium laprae* (3), *Mycobacterium marinum* (3), *Mycobacterium ulcerans* (3), *Mycobacterium fotuitum* (3), *Mycobacterium avium* (2), and *Mycobacterium paratuberculosis* (2). Advantages, on the other hand, lie in the sensitivity and specificity of MRMS for ligand identification.

In summary, while the PhenoTarget approach has some limitations, this article is an example of the powerful potential of the PhenoTarget approach in identifying new lead compounds, from a natural product fraction library, as well as the target protein of the lead compound. In the PhenoTarget approach, phenotypic screening is conducted initially to detect cellular active components. The hits are then screened against a panel of putative targets. This PhenoTarget protocol can be equally applied to pure compound libraries as well as natural product fractions and may prove to be a valuable alternative strategy for developing new intervention therapies.

4. Materials and Methods

4.1. General Experimental Procedures

NMR spectra were recorded in DMSO-d_6 (δ_H 2.50 and δ_C 39.5), CD$_3$OD (δ_H 3.31, 4.78) at 25 °C on the Bruker AVANCE III HDX 800 MHz NMR spectrometer (Fällanden, Zürich, Switzerland) equipped with a triple resonance cryoprobe. The low-resolution LC-MS was acquired using Ultimate 3000 RS UHPLC coupled to a Thermo Fisher MSQ Plus single quadruple ESI mass spectrometer (Waltham, MA, USA) with a Thermo Accucore C$_{18}$ column (2.6 μm, 2.1 × 150 mm). High-resolution mass spectra (HRESIMS) were recorded on a Bruker maXis II ETD ESI- qTOF (Bremen, Germany). The HPLC system for LLE fractions for phenotypic screening included a Waters 600 pump (Milford, MA, USA) fitted with a 996-photodiode array detector and Gilson FC204 fraction collector (Middleton, WI, USA). The HPLC system for Fractions A~E from re-extraction by ethanol was the Thermo Ultimate 3000 system (Waltham, MA, USA). Semi-preparative HPLC was also programmed on Thermo Ultimate 3000 with a PDA detector. A Phenomenex C$_{18}$ Monolithic column (5 μm, 4.6 × 100 mm) was used for analytical HPLC; a Thermo Electron Betasil C$_{18}$ column (5 μm, 21.2 × 150 mm) was used for semi-preparative HPLC.

The fraction library (202,983 fractions) was from Nature Bank (Griffith Institute for Drug Discovery, Brisbane, Australia). All the solvents used for extraction, chromatography and MS were Lab-Scan HPLC grade, and the H$_2$O was Millipore Milli-Q PF filtered.

Ammonium acetate was purchased from. Sigma-Aldrich (St Louis, O.M., USA). Rv1466 and the other 36 unique proteins in the target panel were supplied by the Seattle Structural Genomics Center for Infectious Diseases (SSGCID, Seattle, WA, USA). These were "well behaved" proteins whose structures have been solved by SSGCID and are publicly available in the PDB. All proteins contained a non-natural, N-terminal tag for purification (MAHHHHHHMGTLEAQTQGPGS-). For protein buffer exchange, Nalgene NAP-5 size G25, from GE Healthcare (Parramatta, NSW, Australia) was used (purchased through Thermo Fisher Scientific Australia Pty Ltd., Scoresby, VIC, Australia). The screening of protein-ligand complexes was conducted using Bruker Daltonics SolariX 12 T Magnetic

Resonance Mass Spectrometry (Bruker Daltonics Inc., Billerica, MA, USA) equipped with automatic Nanoelectrospray system (TriVersa NanoMate, Advion Biosciences, Ithaca, NY, USA).

4.2. Lead-Like Enhanced Fraction Library

The lead-like enhanced fraction library was prepared as previously described [14].

4.3. Phenotypic Screening-Activity against Replicating M. tuberculosis H37Rv

Growth inhibition of *M. tuberculosis* was monitored using a 1 μL of fraction (250 μge/μL) dispensed into each well of a 384-well plate. To this, 40 μL of *M. tuberculosis* ATCC 27294 H37Rv ($3–5 \times 10^5$/mL in Middlebrook 7H9 broth with 0.05% Tween 80, 10 *v/v* ADC and Casamino acids) was added with a Multidrop dispenser. The plates were then incubated at 37 °C for 7 days. A 10 μL solution of Resazurin (20 mg/100 mL diluted 1:1 with 10% Tween 80) was added and incubated further for an additional 24 h at 37 °C for color development. Absorbance was monitored at two wavelengths (575 and 610 nm) using Spectramax and the ratios were determined to calculate the % inhibition. Growth controls in the absence of compound as well as media controls served as inhibition ~0% and −100% respectively.

Single point screen: samples (1 μL) which gave ≥80% inhibition were considered positive. MIC: the least concentration which gave ≥80% inhibition was considered as MIC (start conc. = 1 μL of fraction (250 μge/μL).

4.4. Re-extraction and Fractionation

The dry powder of *P. aurata* (1.8 g) was extracted with 95% ethanol (3×150 mL) to afford a crude extract (1.48 g). A portion of the crude extract (40 mg) was dissolved *in DMSO-d_6* (600 μL). Twice injection (2×100 μL) was performed for each sample. HPLC separations were performed on a Phenomenex C_{18} Monolithic HPLC column (4.6×100 mm) using conditions that consisted of a linear gradient (curve 6) from 90% H_2O (0.1% TFA)/10% MeOH (0.1% TFA) to 50% H_2O (0.1% TFA)/50% MeOH (0.1% TFA) in 3 min at a flow rate of 4 mL/min; A convex gradient (curve 6) to 50% H_2O (0.1% TFA)/50% MeOH (0.1% TFA) at a flow rate of 3 mL/min in 0.01 min, then a linear gradient (curve 5) to 100% MeOH (0.1% TFA) in 3.50 min; A held at 100% MeOH (0.1% TFA) (curve 6) for 1.50 min at a flow rate of 3 mL/min, then held at 100% MeOH (0.1% TFA) (curve 6) with a flow rate increasing to 4 mL/min in 0.01 min; A held at 100% MeOH (0.1% TFA) (curve 6) at a flow rate of 4 mL/min for a further 1 min; A linear gradient (curve 6) back to 90% H_2O (0.1% TFA)/10% MeOH (0.1% TFA) in 1 min at a flow rate of 4 mL/min, then held at 90% H_2O (0.1% TFA)/10% MeOH (0.1% TFA) (curve 6) for 2 min at a flow rate of 4 mL/min. The total run time for each injection was 11 min, and 5 fractions were collected between 2.0 and 7.0 min, i.e., Fraction A (time = 2.01-3.00 min), Fraction B (time = 3.01-4.00 min), Fraction C (time = 4.01-5.00 min), Fraction D (time = 5.01-6.00 min) and Fraction E (time = 6.01-7.00 min). Each fraction was dissolved in 200 μL of DMSO-d_6 and was run for ^{1}H NMR fingerprint in a 3 mm NMR tube on a Bruker AVANCE III HDX 800 MHz NMR instrument.

4.5. Automatic Chip-Based MRMS High Throughtput Screening

Proteins were buffer-exchanged into a suitable volatile buffer (ammonium acetate) under near physiological conditions using size exclusion chromatography prior to MRMS analysis. Depending on the protein, the buffer and its concentration were chosen to obtain the highest sensitivity in the mass spectrometer. Final concentration was 10 μM protein in 10 mM ammonium acetate after buffer change.

All screening samples were prepared fresh on the day for analyzing data to avoid the precipitation or decomposition in the sample.

Each 9 LLE fractions (9×1 μL) were combined as a Pool Fraction. Every Pool Fraction was dried, re-suspended in 9 μL MeOH. For the screening of Pool Fractions, 1 μL MeOH solution of pool fraction was mixed with 9 μL of 10 μM protein and then incubated for 1 h at room temperature before being analyzed by MRMS.

For screening the incubation of Fraction C of *P. aurata* with Rv1466-Putative uncharacterized protein, Fraction C was dried and re-suspended in 400 μL MeOH. An aliquot solution (1 μL) was added to protein (9 μL at 10 μM) for 15 min at room temperature and then analyzed by MRMS.

For the screening of pure compound-polycarpine, the stock solution of polycarpine, 3000 μM dissolved in DMSO-d_6, was further diluted to additional varied concentrations between 1–1000 μM for dose-response measurement. Polycarpine solution in DMSO-d_6 was dried and then dissolved in MeOH. A 40 μL sample of these polycarpine solutions was lyophilized and resuspended in 40 μL of MeOH. An aliquot (1 μL) of varied concentration of polycarpine in MeOH was incubated with 9μL of protein (10 μM) for 15 min at room temperature and then analyzed by MRMS.

Experiments were performed on a Bruker SolariX XR 12T MRMS (Bruker Daltonics Inc., Billerica, MA) equipped with an external automated chip-based nanoelectrospray. The ESI mass spectra were recorded in positive mode with a mass range from 294 to 10,000 m/z. Each spectrum was composed of 2 M data points. All the aspects of instrument parameter and data acquisition were controlled by Solarix control software under Windows operating system. Instrument parameters were tuned as follows for Pool Fraction screening: sample flow rate 120 μL/min, nebulizer gas (N_2) pressure 3, end plate offset voltage 0 V, capillary voltage 1000 V, drying gas (N_2) flow rate 1.5 L/min, drying gas temperature 100 °C, capillary exit voltage 220 V, skimmer 1 voltage 60 V, collision voltage −5, time of flight 2.1 s, scan 8 and accumulation time 0.5 s. For the screening of Rv1466-Putative uncharacterized protein with Fraction C and polycarpine, six parameters change including skimmer 1 voltage (30 V), collision voltage (−10 V), time of flight (1.8 s), scan (32) and accumulation time (2 s).

All sample solutions were injected by fully automated chip-based nanoelectrospray, which was mounted to the mass spectrometer. A Triversa NanoMate incorporating ESI chip technology (Advion Biosciences, Ithaca, NY) was used as an automatic chip system. The automated chip system consists of a 384-well plate, a rack of 96 disposable, conductive pipette tips, and the chip, which was positioned a few millimeters from the sampling cone. The system was programmed by ChipSoft software (Version 8.3.1, Advion BioSciences), which sequentially picks up a new pipette tip, aspirates 3 μL of sample from the 384-well plate followed by 1.5 μL of air and then delivers to the inlet side of ESI chip. Nanoelectrospray was carried out by applying a 1.60 kV spray voltage and a 1.0 psi gas pressure to the sample in the pipette tip. Sample solutions for screening were transferred into the 384-well plate. For every sample, a fresh tip and nozzle were used, thus preventing cross-contamination of samples. Following sample infusion and MS analysis, the pipet tip was disposed.

When the protein-ligand complex was found, the molecular weight of the binding ligand was estimated from the spectrum using the following equation: MW ligand = Δ m/z × z.

4.6. Isolation

Crude ethanolic extract of *P. aurata* (200 mg) was dissolved in MeOH. HPLC separation was conducted on a Thermo Electron Betasil C_{18} column (5 μm, 21.2 × 150 mm) at a flow rate of 9 mL/min: using gradient solvent system (10–100% MeOH in 50 min, 100% MeOH from 50–60min) and 60 fractions were collected by minutes. Fraction 33 and 34 were further purified on the same column using gradient solvent from 30–80% MeOH to afford polycarpine.

Polycarpine was obtained as yellow powder. HRMS (positive mode): m/z 469 [M + H]$^+$ (calculated for $C_{22}H_{25}N_6O_2S_2$, 469.1475). ^{1}H NMR (CD$_3$OD, 800MHz) δ 7.49 (2H, d, *J* = 8.98Hz, H-7/11), 7.03 (2H, d, *J* = 8.98Hz, H-8/10), 3.91 (3H, s, 12-CH$_3$), 3.25 (3H, s, 13-CH$_3$). Carbon chemical shift was confirmed from 2D NMR, δ 109.8 (C-1), 148.1 (C-3), 137.6 (C-5), 117.6 (C-6), 127.7 (C-7/11), 113.7 (C-8/10), 161.4 (C-9), 54.4 (C-12) and 27.8 (C-13).

4.7. Dose-Response Data Analysis

The relative abundances of protein-ligand complex to total protein in the mass spectra correlated to the relative equilibrium concentrations of ligand to total protein in solution. The pseudo K_D of polycarpine with Rv1466 was determined using the following equations [18]:

$$\frac{\Sigma\,I(P-L)^{n+}/n}{\Sigma\,I\,(P)^{n+}/n + \Sigma\,I\,(P-L)^{n+}/n} = \frac{[P-L]}{[P]_t} \quad (1)$$

$$\frac{\Sigma\,I(P-L)^{n+}/n}{\Sigma\,I\,(P)^{n+}/n + \Sigma\,I\,(P-L)^{n+}/n} = \frac{[P]_t + [L]_t + K_D - \sqrt{([P]_t + [L]_t + K_D)^2 - 4[P]_t[L]_t}}{2[P]_t} \quad (2)$$

Experimental relative ratios of protein-ligand complex and total protein ion abundances were plotted against the total concentration of ligand. The pseudo K_D could be obtained as a parameter of a nonlinear least-squares curve fitting.

Author Contributions: Conceptualization, R.J.Q. and M.L.; methodology, Y.X., A.D.C., T.M., Y.F., G.W.B. and P.J.M.; resources, R.J.Q. and Y.F.; data curation, M.L.; writing—original draft preparation, Y.X.; writing—review and editing, R.J.Q. All authors have read and agreed to the published version of the manuscript.

Funding: This research was funded by the Bill and Melinda Gates Foundation (OPP1035218, OPP1174957). This research was supported by an Australian Research Council Discovery and Linkage Projects funding (DP160101429, LP120100485) and equipment support (LE120100170, LE140100119). This research was funded by the National Institute of Allergy and Infectious Diseases, National Institutes of Health, Department of Health and Human Services under Federal Contract number HHSH27220120025C, HHSN272200700057C, and HHSN272201700059C.

Acknowledgments: We acknowledge the NatureBank biota repository that is housed at the Griffith Institute for Drug Discovery, Griffith University (www.griffith.edu.au/gridd). We thank Vasanthi Ramachandran, Sreevalli Sharma, Supreeth Guptha, Sunita DeSousa from the former AstraZeneca Bangalore for the *M. tuberculosis* H37Rv assay. Part of the research was conducted at the W.R. Wiley Environmental Molecular Sciences Laboratory, a national scientific user facility sponsored by U.S. Department of Energy's Office of Biological and Environmental Research (BER) program located at Pacific Northwest National Laboratory (PNNL). Battelle operates PNNL for the U.S. Department of Energy.

Conflicts of Interest: The authors declare no conflict of interest.

References

1. Munos, B. Lessons from 60 years of pharmaceutical innovation. *Nat. Rev. Drug Discov.* **2009**, *8*, 959–968. [CrossRef] [PubMed]
2. Zheng, W.; Thorne, N.; McKew, J.C. Phenotypic screens as a renewed approach for drug discovery. *Drug Discov. Today* **2013**, *18*, 1067–1073. [CrossRef]
3. Swinney, D.C. Phenotypic vs. target-based drug discovery for first-in-class medicine. *Clin. Pharmacol. Ther.* **2013**, *93*, 299–301. [CrossRef] [PubMed]
4. Wainwright, M. The mystery of the plate: Fleming's discovery and contribution to the early development of penicillin. *J. Med. Biogr.* **1993**, *1*, 59–65. [CrossRef] [PubMed]
5. Campbell, W.C.; Burg, R.W.; Fisher, M.H.; Dybas, R.A. The discovery of ivermectin and other avermectins. *ACS Symp. Ser.* **1984**, *255*, 5–20.
6. Eder, J.; Sedrani, R.; Wiesmann, C. The discovery of first-in-class drugs: Origins and evolution. *Nat. Rev. Drug Discov.* **2014**, *13*, 577–587. [CrossRef] [PubMed]
7. Lee, J.A.; Berg, E.L. Neoclassic drug discovery: The case for lead generation using phenotypic and functional approaches. *J. Biomol. Screen.* **2013**, *18*, 1143–1155. [CrossRef]
8. Swinney, D.C.; Anthony, J. How were new medicines discovered? *Nat. Rev. Drug Discov.* **2011**, *10*, 507–519. [CrossRef]
9. Moffat, J.G.; Vincent, F.; Lee, J.A.; Eder, J.; Prunotto, M. Opportunities and challenges in phenotypic drug discovery: An industry perspective. *Nat. Rev. Drug Discov.* **2017**, *16*, 531–543. [CrossRef]
10. Wagner, B.K.; Schreiber, S.L. The power of sophisticated phenotypic screening and modern mechanism-of-action methods. *Cell Chem. Biol.* **2016**, *23*, 3–9. [CrossRef]
11. Croston, G.E. The utility of target-based discovery. *Expert Opin. on Drug Discov.* **2017**, *12*, 427–429. [CrossRef]

12. Myler, P.J.; Stacy, R.; Stewart, L.J.; Staker, B.L.; Voorhis, W.C.V.; Varani, G.; Buchko, G.W. The seattle structural genomics center for infectious disease (SSGCID). *Infect. Disord. Drug Targets* **2009**, *9*, 493–506. [CrossRef]
13. Stacy, R.; Begley, D.; Phan, I.; Staker, B.; Voorhis, W.C.V.; Varani, G.; Buchko, G.W.; Stewart, L.C.; Myler, P.J. Structural genomics of infectious disease drug targets: The SSGCID. *Acta Crystallogr.* **2011**, *F67*, 979–984. [CrossRef]
14. Camp, D.; Davis, R.A.; Campitelli, M.; Ebdon, J.; Quinn, R.J. Drug-like properties: Guiding principles for the design of natural product libraries. *J. Nat. Prod.* **2012**, *75*, 72–81. [CrossRef]
15. Abbas, S.A.; Hossain, M.B.; van der Helm, D.; Schmitz, F.J.; Laney, M.; Cabuslay, R.; Schatzman, R.C. Alkaloids from the tunicate *Polycarpa aurata* from Chuuk Atoll. *J. Org. Chem.* **1996**, *61*, 2709–2712. [CrossRef]
16. Kang, H.; Fenical, W. Polycarpine dihydrochloride: A cytotoxic dimeric disulfide alkaloid from the indian ocean ascidian *Polycarpa clavata*. *Tetrahedron Lett.* **1996**, *37*, 2369–2372. [CrossRef]
17. Zhang, S.; Van Pelt, C.K.; Wilson, D.B. Quantitative determination of noncovalent binding interactions using automated nanoelectrospray mass spectrometry. *Anal. Chem.* **2003**, *75*, 3010–3018. [CrossRef]
18. Pedro, L.; Van Voorhis, W.C.; Quinn, R.J. Optimization of electrospray ionization by statistical design of experiments and response surface methodology: Protein-ligand equilibrium dissociation constant determinations. *J. Am. Soc. Mass Spectrom.* **2016**, *27*, 1520–1530. [CrossRef]
19. Pham, C.D.; Weber, H.; Hartmann, R.; Wray, V.; Lin, W.; Lai, D.; Proksch, P. New cytotoxic 1,2,4-thiadiazole alkaloids from the ascidian *Polycarpa aurata*. *Org. Lett.* **2013**, *15*, 2230–2233. [CrossRef]
20. Wang, W.; Oda, T.; Fujita, A.; Mangindaan, R.E.P.; Nakazawa, T.; Ukai, K.; Kobayashi, H.; Namikoshi, M. Three new sulfur-containing alkaloids, polycarpaurines A, B, and C, from an Indonesian ascidian *Polycarpa aurata*. *Tetrahedron* **2007**, *63*, 409–412. [CrossRef]
21. Pacholarz, K.J.; Garlish, R.A.; Taylor, R.J.; Barran, P.E. Mass spectrometry based tools to investigate protein-ligand interactions for drug discovery. *Chem. Soc. Rev.* **2012**, *41*, 4335–4355. [CrossRef] [PubMed]
22. El-Hawiet, A.; Kitova, E.N.; Arutyunov, D.; Simpson, D.J.; Szymanski, C.M.; Klassen, J.S. Quantifying ligand binding to large protein complexes using electrospray ionization mass spectrometry. *Anal. Chem.* **2012**, *84*, 3867–3870. [CrossRef] [PubMed]
23. Breuker, K. New Mass Spectrometric Methods for the Quantification of Protein-Ligand Binding in Solution. *Angew. Chem. Int. Ed. Engl.* **2004**, *43*, 22–25. [CrossRef] [PubMed]
24. Zhang, S.; Van Pelt, C.K. Chip-based nanoelectrospray mass spectrometry for protein characterization. *Expert Rev Proteom.* **2004**, *1*, 449–468. [CrossRef] [PubMed]
25. Clark-Curtiss, J.E.; Haydel, S.E. Molecular genetics of *Mycobacterium tuberculosis* pathogenesis. *Annu. Rev. Microbiol.* **2003**, *57*, 517–549. [CrossRef]
26. Baugh, L.; Phan, I.; Begley, D.W.; Clifton, M.C.; Gardberg, A.S.; Armour, B.; Dieterich, S.H.; Dranow, D.M.; Taylo, J.B.M.; Muruthi, M.M.; et al. Increasing the structural coverage of tuberculosis drug targets. *Tuberculosis* **2015**, *95*, 142–148. [CrossRef]

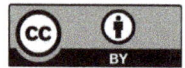

© 2020 by the authors. Licensee MDPI, Basel, Switzerland. This article is an open access article distributed under the terms and conditions of the Creative Commons Attribution (CC BY) license (http://creativecommons.org/licenses/by/4.0/).

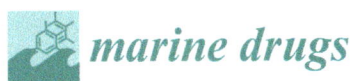

Article

Anti-Inflammatory Cembranoids from a Formosa Soft Coral *Sarcophyton cherbonnieri*

Chia-Chi Peng [1,†], Chiung-Yao Huang [1,†], Atallah F. Ahmed [2,3], Tsong-Long Hwang [4,5,6] and Jyh-Horng Sheu [1,7,8,*]

1. Department of Marine Biotechnology and Resources, National Sun Yat-sen University, Kaohsiung 804, Taiwan; Chia-Chi.Peng@hki-jena.de (C.-C.P.); huangcy@mail.nsysu.edu.tw (C.-Y.H.)
2. Department of Pharmacognosy, College of Pharmacy, King Saud University, Riyadh 11451, Saudi Arabia; afahmed@ksu.edu.sa
3. Department of Pharmacognosy, Faculty of Pharmacy, Mansoura University, Mansoura 35516, Egypt
4. Graduate Institute of Natural Products, College of Medicine, Chang Gung University, Taoyuan 333, Taiwan; htl@mail.cgu.edu.tw
5. Research Center for Industry of Human Ecology and Graduate Institute of Health Industry Technology, Chang Gung University of Science and Technology, Taoyuan 333, Taiwan
6. Department of Anesthesiology, Chang Gung Memorial Hospital, Taoyuan 333, Taiwan
7. Graduate Institute of Natural Products, Kaohsiung Medical University, Kaohsiung 807, Taiwan
8. Department of Medical Research, China Medical University Hospital, China Medical University, Taichung 404, Taiwan
* Correspondence: sheu@mail.nsysu.edu.tw; Tel.: +886-7-525-2000 (ext. 5030); Fax: +886-7-525-5020
† These authors contributed equally to this work.

Received: 25 September 2020; Accepted: 13 November 2020; Published: 19 November 2020

Abstract: The present investigation on chemical constituents of the soft coral *Sarcophyton cherbonnieri* resulted in the isolation of seven new cembranoids, cherbonolides F–L (**1–7**). The chemical structures of **1–7** were determined by spectroscopic methods, including infrared, one- and two-dimensional (1D and 2D) NMR (COSY, HSQC, HMBC, and NOESY), MS experiments, and a chemical reduction of hydroperoxide by triphenylphosphine. The anti-inflammatory activities of **1–7** against neutrophil proinflammatory responses were evaluated by measuring their inhibitory ability toward *N*-formyl-methionyl-leucyl-phenylalanine/cytochalasin B (fMLF/CB)-induced superoxide anion generation and elastase release in primary human neutrophils. The results showed that all isolates exhibited moderate activities, while cherbonolide G (**2**) and cherbonolide H (**3**) displayed a more active effect than others on the inhibition of elastase release (48.2% ± 6.2%) and superoxide anion generation (44.5% ± 4.6%) at 30 µM, respectively.

Keywords: *Sarcophyton cherbonnieri*; cembranoid; anti-inflammatory activity; elastase release; superoxide anion generation

1. Introduction

Series of cembranoidal secondary metabolites from soft corals have been shown to exhibit attractive biological activities including cytotoxicity [1–14] and anti-inflammatory ability [6,7,9,11,13–18]. From previous investigations of exploring bioactive natural products from soft corals, many cembranoids were discovered from organisms of the genera *Sarcophyton*, [1–8,16], *Sinularia* [9–12,17,18], and *Lobophyton* [13–15]. In some cases, two cembranoid units could be linked to produce biscembranoids via various reactions [18–24], marking the high diversity and complexity in chemical structures of cembrane-related soft coral natural products.

Many studies have revealed that soft corals of the genus *Sarcophyton* are important sources of various types of natural products, some of them with notable bioactives [25–28]. Our previous chemical study on *Sarcophyton cherbonnieri* led to the isolation of six new cembranoids cherbonolides A–E and one biscembranoid bischerbolide peroxide, along with a known compound, isosarcophine [24]. In continuation of our effort on discovery of new and bioactive compounds from marine animals, we further explored the chemical constituents of *S. cherbonnieri*. This investigation again led to the discovery of new cembranoids, cherbonolides F–L (**1–7**). The structures of **1–7** (Figure 1) were determined by spectroscopic analysis, including two-dimensional (2D) NMR experiments and a chemical reaction. Compounds **2** and **4** were elucidated as cembranoids possessing an allylic peroxy group. Cembranoids of isosarcophine-type have been reported frequently [24,27–30].

The screening of the in vitro anti-inflammatory activities through the inhibition of superoxide anion generation and elastase release in N-formyl-methionyl-leucyl-phenylalanine/cytochalasin B (fMLF/CB)-induced primary human neutrophils was also performed in order to unveil the anti-inflammatory ability of these compounds. We report herein the isolation, structure determination, and bioactivity of the new metabolites **1–7**.

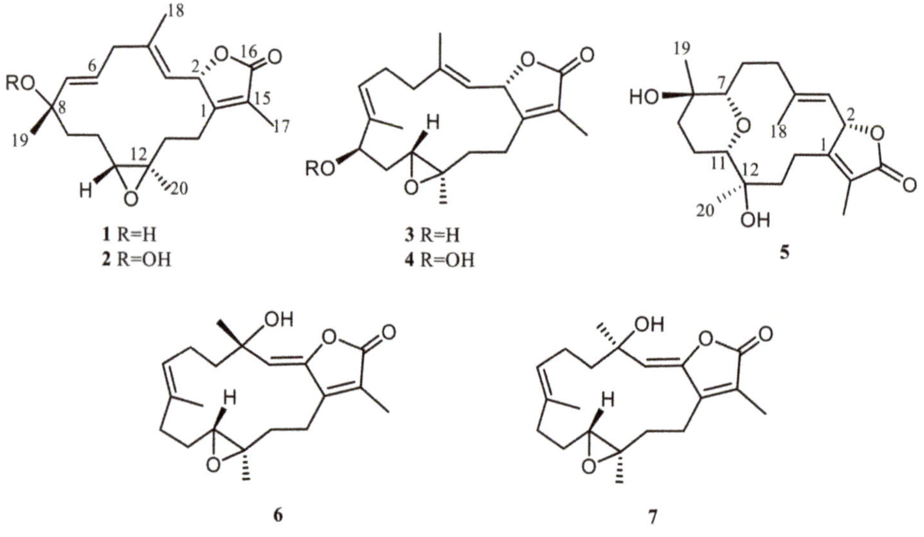

Figure 1. New cembranoids isolated from *Sarcophyton cherbonnieri*.

2. Results and Discussion

Solvent-free residue of the ethyl acetate extract of the soft coral *S. cherbonnieri* was separated and further purified by chromatographic methods to yield metabolites **1–7**. The structures were established by extensive analyses of MS and NMR spectra (Figures S1–S49, Supplementary Materials). ^{13}C- and ^{1}H-NMR data which were essential for structure determination of **1–7** are listed in Tables 1–3.

Cherbonolide F (**1**) was obtained as a colorless oil. The molecular formula of **1**, $C_{20}H_{28}O_4$, was established by high-resolution electrospray ionization mass spectrometry (HR-ESI-MS) (m/z calculated 355.1880; found 355.1879, [M + Na]$^+$), implying seven degrees of unsaturation. The IR spectrum of **1** revealed the absorptions of a hydroxy (ν_{max} 3460 cm^{-1}) and a lactonic carbonyl group (ν_{max} 1748 cm^{-1}). The ^{13}C-NMR spectrum of **1** showed 20 signals which were assigned to four methyls, five sp^3 methylenes, two sp^3 oxygenated methines, three sp^2 methines, and two sp^3 and four sp^2 nonprotonated carbon atoms (Table 1) with the assistance of distortionless enhancement by polarization transfer (DEPT) spectra. Carbon signals resonating at δ_C 173.9 (C), 160.5 (C), 123.6 (C), 78.6 (CH), and 9.0 (CH$_3$) and proton signals resonating at δ_H 4.95 (1H, dd, J = 10.0, 1.6 Hz) and δ_H 1.66 (3H, s) were attributed to signals of an α-methyl-α,β-unsaturated-γ-lactone ring by comparing the NMR data of the γ-lactone ring of the known compound isosarcophine (**7**). Signals at δ_C 61.2

(CH), 60.2 (C), and δ_H 2.54 (1H, dd, J = 6.0, 6.0 Hz) showed the appearance of a trisubstituted epoxide. One trisubstituted and one disubstituted double bond were identified by NMR signals resonating at δ_C 120.9 (CH), 142.4 (C) and δ_H 4.54 (1H, dd, J = 10.0, 0.8 Hz), and at δ_C 140.3 (CH), 124.5 (CH) and δ_H 5.32 (1H, d, J = 16.0 Hz) and 5.38 (1H, ddd, J = 16.0, 6.8, 6.8 Hz), respectively. ^{1}H–^{1}H correlation spectroscopy (COSY) correlations established four separate proton sequences, which were connected by heteronuclear multiple bond correlation (HMBC) correlations (Figure 2). Essential HMBC correlations from H-2 to C-1 and C-4, H$_2$-14 to C-1 and C-2, H$_3$-17 to C-1, C-15, and C-16, H$_3$-18 to C-3, C-4, and C-5, H$_3$-19 to C-7, C-8, and C-9, and H$_3$-20 to C-11, C-12, and C-13 established the 14-membered ring carbon skeleton of **1**, which also indicated the presence of a hydroxyl at C-8.

Furthermore, analysis of nuclear Overhauser effect (NOE) correlations was applied to establish the relative configuration of **1**, as shown in Figure 3. It was revealed that H-2 showed NOE correlation with H$_3$-18, but not with H-3; therefore, assuming the β-orientation of H-2, H$_3$-18 should be located on the β face. Moreover, H$_3$-18 exhibited NOE correlation with H-7, but not with H-6, revealing the β-orientation of H-7 and the α-orientation of H-6. Both H-6 and H-7 exhibited NOE interactions with H$_3$-19, thus established the β-orientation of H$_3$-19 as shown in Figure 3. One methylene proton at C-13 exhibited NOE correlation with H-2 and was characterized as H-13β (δ_H 0.99, m), while the other proton was assigned as H-13α (δ_H 1.49, m). NOE correlations of H-13β with H-11 and H-13α with H$_3$-20 reflected the β-orientation of H-11 and the α-orientation of H$_3$-20. The E geometries of the trisubstituted C-3/C-4 and C-6/C-7 double bonds were also assigned from the NOE correlations of H$_3$-18 (δ_H 1.35, s) with H-2, but not with H-3, as well as the large coupling constant J = 16.0 Hz between H-6 and H-7, and the observed more shielded signal of C-18 (δ_C 16.7). According to the above observations, the relative configuration of this compound was established. As **1** was isolated together with the previous reported compounds isosarcophine and cherbonolides A–E [24] from the same organism, it should possess the same (2S,8S,11R,12R)-configuration from the shared biosynthetic pathway.

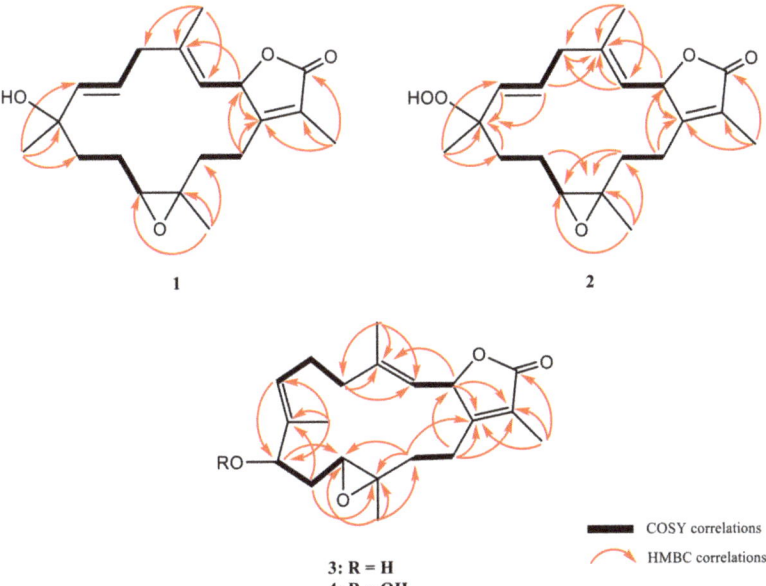

Figure 2. The selected COSY and HMBC correlations of **1**–**4**.

Table 1. ^{13}C-NMR spectroscopic data of compounds 1–7.

Position	1 [a]	2 [a]	3 [a]	4 [c]	5 [a]	6 [d]	7 [d]
1	160.5 (C)	160.4 (C)	159.9 (C)	160.2 (C)	162.4 (C)	151.2 (C)	151.2 (C)
2	78.6 (CH) [b]	78.5 (CH)	77.7 (CH)	78.0 (CH)	79.5 (CH)	147.2 (C)	147.2 (C)
3	120.9 (CH)	121.2 (CH)	121.8 (CH)	122.3 (CH)	120.7 (CH)	116.2 (CH)	116.1 (CH)
4	142.4 (C)	142.1 (C)	143.2 (C)	143.4 (C)	143.2 (C)	72.7 (C)	72.6 (C)
5	41.5 (CH$_2$)	41.9 (CH$_2$)	38.4 (CH$_2$)	38.7 (CH$_2$)	36.4 (CH$_2$)	42.5 (CH$_2$)	42.2 (CH$_2$)
6	124.5 (CH)	128.6 (CH)	23.9 (CH$_2$)	24.4 (CH$_2$)	24.7 (CH$_2$)	23.1 (CH$_2$)	23.2 (CH$_2$)
7	140.3 (CH)	135.9 (CH)	127.3 (CH)	130.9 (CH)	84.1 (CH)	127.2 (CH)	126.5 (CH)
8	71.7 (C)	83.7 (C)	137.1 (C)	133.8 (C)	69.4 (C)	133.9 (C)	133.8 (C)
9	39.7 (CH$_2$)	35.7 (CH$_2$)	76.2 (CH)	88.9 (CH)	40.7 (CH$_2$)	36.3 (CH$_2$)	36.2 (CH$_2$)
10	24.3 (CH$_2$)	24.2 (CH$_2$)	32.4 (CH$_2$)	28.4 (CH$_2$)	23.5 (CH$_2$)	24.4 (CH$_2$)	24.3 (CH$_2$)
11	61.3 (CH)	61.1 (CH)	59.2 (CH)	59.4 (CH)	80.1 (CH)	60.5 (CH)	60.5 (CH)
12	60.2 (C)	60.2 (C)	60.1 (C)	60.6 (C)	72.6 (C)	60.2 (C)	60.3 (C)
13	35.7 (CH$_2$)	35.6 (CH$_2$)	36.9 (CH$_2$)	37.3 (CH$_2$)	37.2 (CH$_2$)	35.1 (CH$_2$)	35.1 (CH$_2$)
14	23.2 (CH$_2$)	22.9 (CH$_2$)	23.6 (CH$_2$)	24.0 (CH$_2$)	20.2 (CH$_2$)	19.6 (CH$_2$)	19.8 (CH$_2$)
15	123.6 (C)	123.6 (C)	123.7 (C)	124.1 (C)	123.4 (C)	123.6 (C)	123.7 (C)
16	173.9 (C)	173.9 (C)	173.8 (C)	174.2 (C)	174.4 (C)	169.5 (C)	169.8 (C)
17	9.0 (CH$_3$)	8.9 (CH$_3$)	8.7 (CH$_3$)	9.1 (CH$_3$)	8.9 (CH$_3$)	9.1 (CH$_3$)	9.0 (CH$_3$)
18	16.7 (CH$_3$)	16.2 (CH$_3$)	14.4 (CH$_3$)	14.7 (CH$_3$)	16.2 (CH$_3$)	29.9 (CH$_3$)	29.4 (CH$_3$)
19	28.0 (CH$_3$)	21.6 (CH$_3$)	9.6 (CH$_3$)	10.3 (CH$_3$)	20.4 (CH$_3$)	15.3 (CH$_3$)	15.5 (CH$_3$)
20	16.7 (CH$_3$)	16.9 (CH$_3$)	16.0 (CH$_3$)	16.2 (CH$_3$)	23.7 (CH$_3$)	17.5 (CH$_3$)	17.4 (CH$_3$)

[a] Spectra recorded in C$_6$D$_6$ at 100 MHz at 25 °C. [b] Attached protons were deduced by distortionless enhancement by polarization transfer (DEPT) experiments. [c] Spectra recorded in C$_6$D$_6$ at 125 MHz. [d] Spectra recorded in CDCl$_3$ at 100 MHz.

Table 2. ^{1}H-NMR spectral data for compounds 1–4.

Position	1 [a]	2 [a]	3 [a]	4 [b]
2	4.95, dd (10.0, 1.6) [c]	4.92, dd (10.0, 1.6)	4.99, dd (10.4, 1.6)	4.96, d (10.5)
3	4.54, dd (10.0, 0.8)	4.47, d (10.0)	4.49, d (10.4)	4.47, d (10.5)
5	2.40, dd (13.2, 6.8)	2.41, dd (13.6, 7.2)	1.84, dd (13.2, 4.4)	1.80, dd (13.5, 4.5)
	2.26, dd (13.2, 6.8)	2.27, dd (13.6, 7.2)	1.92, m	1.91, m
6	5.38, ddd (16.0, 6.8, 6.8)	5.47, ddd (16.8, 7.2, 7.2)	1.73, m	1.75, m
			2.03, m	2.02, m
7	5.32, d (16.0)	5.35, d (16.8)	4.74, dd (10.0, 1.2)	4.91, d (9.5)
9	1.52, m	1.57, m	3.68, dd (11.6, 4.0)	4.06, dd (12.0, 4.0)
	1.59, m	1.59, m		
10	1.43, m	1.56, m	1.47, m	1.53, m
	1.71, m	1.56, m	2.16, ddd	2.03, m
11	2.54, dd (6.0, 6.0)	2.44, dd (6.4, 6.4)	2.03, m	2.09, dd (10.5, 3.0)
13	1.49, m	1.69, m	1.59, dd (13.2, 5.6)	1.56, m
	0.99, m	0.99, m	0.72, ddd (13.2, 13.2, 2.8)	0.69, dd (13.5, 13.5, 2.5)
14	1.81, m	1.78, m	1.93, m	1.89, m
	1.67, m	1.68, m	1.49, m	1.43, m
17	1.66, s	1.66, s	1.65, s	1.65, s
18	1.35, s	1.29, s	1.13, s	1.11, s
19	1.05, s	1.19, s	1.37, s	1.37, s
20	1.03, s	1.02, s	1.03, s	1.01, s

[a] Spectra recorded in C$_6$D$_6$ at 400 MHz at 25 °C. [b] Spectra recorded in C$_6$D$_6$ at 500 MHz at 25 °C. [c] Coupling constants (J values) in Hz are shown in parentheses.

Table 3. ^{1}H-NMR spectral data for compounds 5–7.

Position	5[a]	6[b]	7[b]
2	4.92, d (11.2)[c]		
3	4.85, d (11.2)	5.50, s	5.52, s
5	2.07, m	1.83, m	1.94, m
	1.93, m	1.98, m	1.94, m
6	1.31, m	2.41, m	2.46, m
	1.70, m	2.21, m	2.14, m
7	2.79, dd (10.0, 2.4)	5.26, dd (6.0, 6.0)	5.25, dd (7.2, 7.2)
9	1.59, m	2.28, m	2.26, m
	1.31, m	2.08, m	2.06, m
10	1.22, m	1.53, m	1.54, m
	1.50, m	1.85, m	1.86, m
11	2.96, d (11.2)	2.71, dd (6.8, 5.6)	2.73, dd (7.6, 4.6)
13	1.59, m	2.16, m	2.19, m
	1.21, m	1.63, m	1.62, m
14	2.16, ddd (12.4, 12.4, 6.4)	2.26, m	2.24, m
	1.59, m	2.42, m	2.45, m
17	1.72, s	1.95, s	1.92, s
18	1.47, s	1.41, s	1.51, s
19	0.94, s	1.66, s	1.65, s
20	0.89, s	1.30, s	1.28, s

[a] Spectra recorded in C$_6$D$_6$ at 400 MHz at 25 °C. [b] Spectra recorded in CDCl$_3$ at 400 MHz at 25 °C. [c] Coupling constants (J values) in Hz are shown in parentheses.

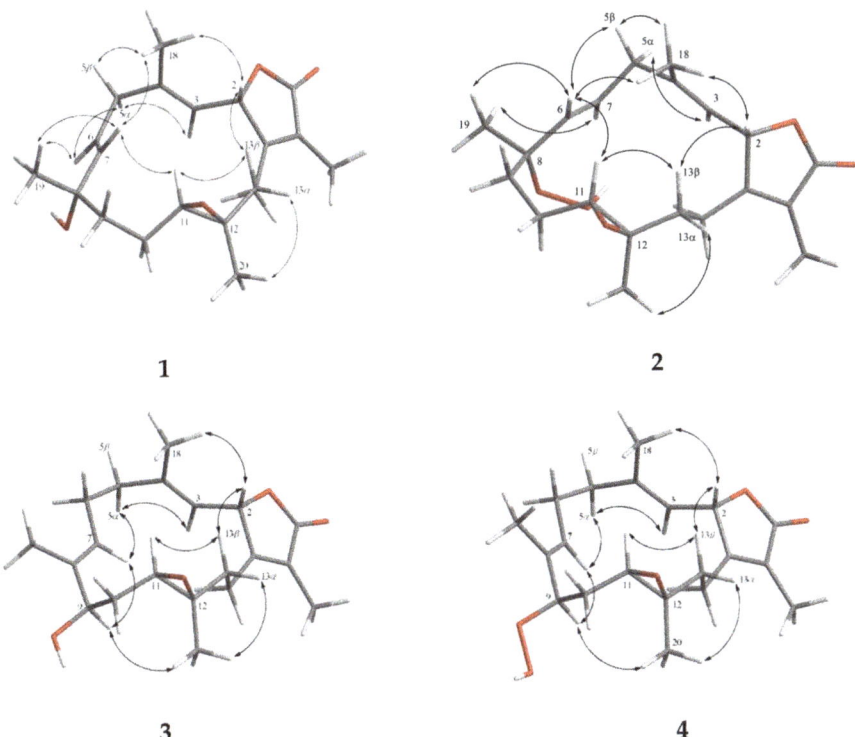

Figure 3. Key NOE correlations for 1–4.

The molecular formula of cherbonolide G (**2**) was found to be $C_{20}H_{28}O_5$ by analysis of HR-ESI-MS (*m/z* calculated 371.1829; found 371.1830, [M + Na]$^+$), revealing that **2** possesses an additional oxygen atom to that of **1**. Moreover, both **1** and **2** showed the very similar ^{1}H- and ^{13}C-NMR data (Table 1), except that the chemical shift of C-8 was shifted from δ_C 71.7 of **1** to δ_C 83.7 of **2**. The very similar COSY, HMBC (Figure 2), and NOE (Figure 3) correlations of **1** and **2** also revealed the very close structures for both compounds. However, the hydroxy group of **1** at C-8 was replaced by a hydroperoxy group in **2**, with a broad singlet appearing at δ_H 6.72 and the downfield shift of C-8. Accordingly, the molecular skeleton and the (2*S*,8*S*,11*R*,12*R*)-configuration of **2** were determined.

Cherbonolide H (**3**) has the same molecular formula as that of **1**, as determined by HR-ESI-MS experiment. Moreover, most of the ^{1}H–^{1}H COSY and HMBC correlations (Figure 2) of **3** were similar to those of isoscarcophine except for the presence of a hydroxyl at C-9 leading to the shift of CH-9 to lower field (δ_C 76.2; δ_H 3.68), and the shift of C-6/C-7 double bond of **1** to C-7/C-8 double bond of **3**. Analysis of NOE correlations (Figure 3) showed that the β-oriented H-2 exhibited NOE interactions with both H$_3$-18 and H-13β, but not with H-3, assigning the *E*-geometry of the trisubstituted C-3/C-4 double bond. These results, along with the found NOE correlations (Figure 3) of H-13α/ H$_3$-20, H$_3$-20/H-9, led to the assignment of the α-orientation of H-9.

Cherbonolide I (**4**) was found to contain one additional oxygen atom than **3**, according to HR-ESI-MS experiment. These two compounds also showed very similar ^{1}H–^{1}H COSY and HMBC correlations, revealing the identical molecular framework of both compounds. NMR data of **3** and **4** were similar (Table 1), except for those of CH-9, suggesting that **4** is possibly the C-9 hydroperoxy derivative of **3**. By analysis of NOE correlations (Figure 3), the *E* geometries of both C-3/C-4 and C-7/C-8 double bonds of **4** and the (2*S*,9*R*,11*R*,12*R*)-configuration were also established. Reduction of **4** by triphenylphosphine yielded **3**, further confirming the structure of **4**.

Cherbonolide J (**5**) was given as a colorless oil with a molecular formula $C_{20}H_{30}O_5$ on the basis of HR-ESI-MS data (*m/z* calculated for $C_{20}H_{30}O_5Na$ 373.1986; found 373.1984), revealing six degrees of unsaturation. The IR absorptions at 3443 and 1748 cm^{-1} were due to hydroxy and ester carbonyl groups, respectively. The ^{13}C- and ^{1}H-NMR spectroscopic data (Tables 1 and 3) of **5** measured at C_6D_6 were very close to a known compound sarcophyolide E [29], and the 2D NMR (COSY, HSQC, and HMBC) correlation analysis revealed that both compounds had the same molecular framework (Figure 4). Detailed analysis of the NOE correlations (Figure 5) showed that both compounds possessed the same relative configuration. However, the $[\alpha]_{25}^D$ values in CHCl$_3$ (−6 for **5** and +4.4 for sarcophyolide E) were close but with different signs, suggesting that **5** is the enantiomer of this known compound. The absolute configurations of **5** and sarcophyolide E were deduced by comparison of the circular dichroism (CD) spectroscopic data. As shown in Figure 6, the negative Cotton effect at 247 nm and positive effect at 228 nm for **5** in comparison with the positive and negative Cotton effects at 252 and 226 nm for sarcophyolide E [29], respectively, confirmed that **5** is the newly found enantiomer of sarcophyolide E.

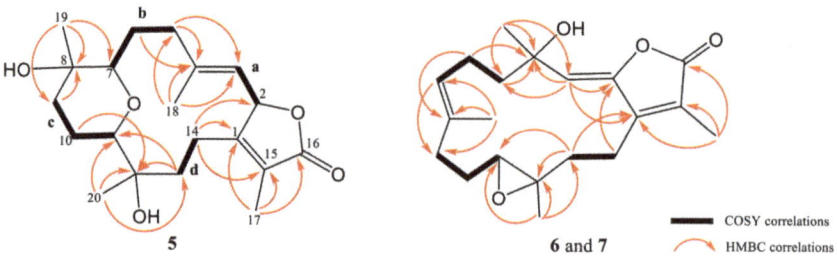

Figure 4. Selected COSY and HMBC correlations of **5**–**7**.

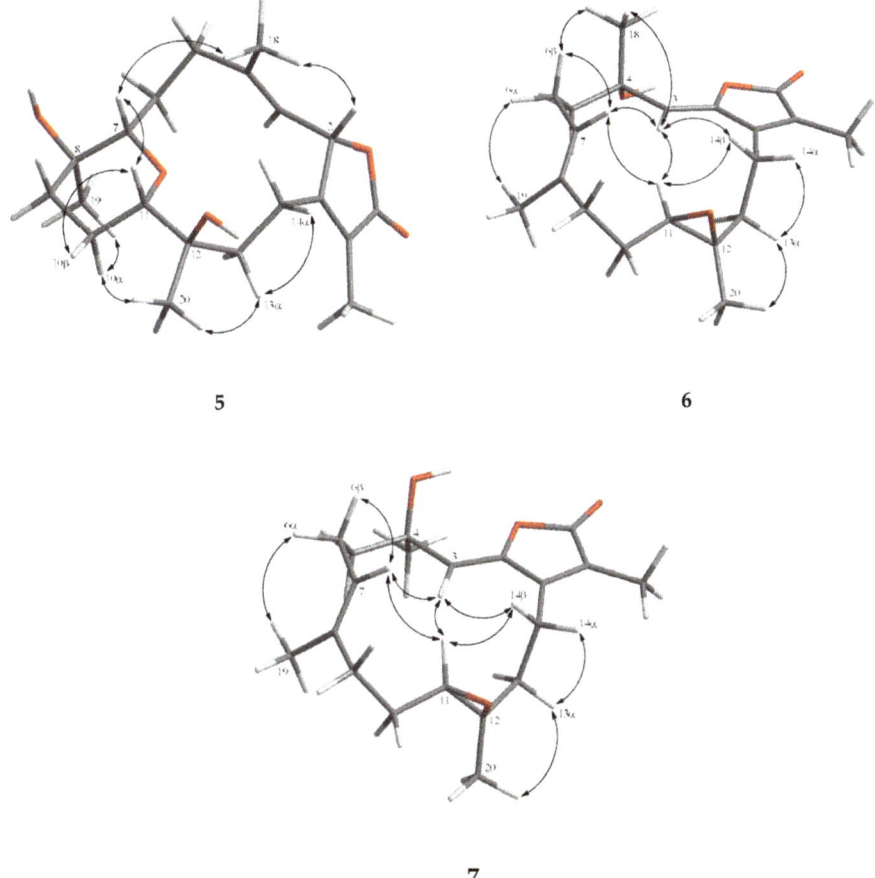

Figure 5. Selected NOE correlations for **5**–**7**.

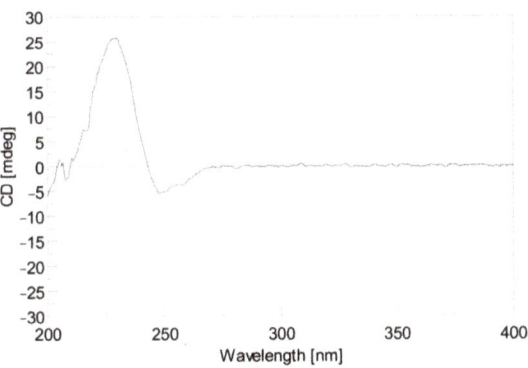

Figure 6. the CD spectrum of **5** (1.2 × 10^{-4} M, MeOH).

Cherbonolide K (**6**) is a colorless oil which was shown to have the molecular formula $C_{20}H_{28}O_4$ by HR-ESI-MS experiment, appropriate for seven degrees of unsaturation. The infrared (IR) spectrum of **6** showed peaks of hydroxy and estercarbonyl groups at 3444 and 1763 cm^{-1}, respectively. ^{13}C-NMR data (Table 1) with signals at δ_C 151.2 (C), 147.2 (C), 116.2 (CH), 72.7 (C), 123.6 (C), 169.5 (C), 9.1 (CH$_3$), and 29.9 (CH$_3$) and ^{1}H NMR data (Table 3) with signals at δ_H 5.50 (s, 1H), 1.95 (s, 3H), and 1.41 (s, 3H) were attributed to the cembranoidal α-methyl-α,β-unsaturated-γ lactone ring with a conjugated 2,3-double bond that further connected with the methyl and hydroxyl substituted C-4. The above results were supported by HMBC correlations of **6** (Figure 4) from H-3 (δ_H 5.50) to C-1 (δ_C 151.2), C-2 (δ_C 147.2), and C-4 (δ_C 72.7), H$_3$-17 (δ_H 1.95) to C-1, C-15 (δ_C 123.6), and C-16 (δ_C 169.5), and H$_3$-18 (δ_H 1.41) to C-3 (δ_C 116.2) and C-4 (δ_C 72.6). The remainder of the structure from C-5 to C-14 was found to be identical to isosarcophine [24]. Thus, the planar structure of **6** was established. Furthermore, the NOE correlation analysis shown in Figure 5 revealed the α-orientations of 4-OH and 12-CH$_3$, β-orientation of H-11, (Z)-2,3-double bond, and (E)-7,8-double bond. An isomer of **6**, cherbonolide L (**7**), was also subsequently isolated. The metabolite **7** had nearly the same NMR data as **6** except for CH$_2$-5 and CH$_2$-6. Thus, it can be assumed that **7** is the C-4 epimer of **6**. Analysis of the 2D NMR correlations of **7** (Figures 4 and 6) further supported this assumption.

For the screening of bioactivities, the anti-inflammation activities of **1–7** toward inhibition of N-formyl-methionyl-leucyl-phenylalanine/cytochalasin B (fMLF/CB)-induced generation of superoxide anion (O$_2^{\bullet-}$) and release of elastase in primary human neutrophils were measured. The results (Table 4) showed that, although none of the isolates exhibited strong inhibitory activities in the assay, **2** and **3** were found to display notable ability to inhibit the elastase release (48.2% ± 6.2%) and superoxide anion generation (44.5% ± 4.6%) at 30 µM, respectively. In comparison with (+)-isosarcophine, cherbonolides A–E, and bischerbonolide peroide discovered previously from *S. cherbonnieri* [24], it was found that, although **2** and **3** exhibited weaker activities than bischerbonolide peroxide, they displayed comparable activities to those of cherbonolides A and C. In general, allylic oxidation at the 7,8-double bond of (+)-isosarcophine might be able to produce derivatives with stronger bioactivities.

Table 4. Inhibitory effects of metabolites **1–7** against elastase release and superoxide anion generation in N-formyl-methionyl-leucyl-phenylalanine/cytochalasin B (fMLF/CB)-induced primary human neutrophils. IC$_{50}$, half maximal inhibitory concentration.

Compound	Superoxide Anion		Elastase Release	
	IC$_{50}$ (µM) [a]	Inh [b] %	IC$_{50}$ (µM) [a]	Inh [b] %
1	>30	11.0 ± 8.7	>30	35.1 ± 10.6 ***
2	>30	29.8 ± 9.8 **	>30	48.2 ± 12.5 ***
3	>30	44.5 ± 7.9 ***	>30	35.6 ± 10.7 ***
4	>30	6.4 ± 7.3	>30	27.6 ± 12.8 **
5	>30	6.2 ± 5.5	>30	29.7 ± 11.1 **
6	>30	12.9 ± 11.4	>30	16.7 ± 10.2 *
7	>30	17.1 ± 11.6 *	>30	27.6 ± 12.0 **
Idelalisib	0.07 ± 0.03	102.8 ± 5.4 ***	0.07 ± 0.02	99.6 ± 10.3 ***

[a] Concentration necessary for 50% inhibition (IC$_{50}$). [b] Percentage of inhibition (Inh %) at 30 µM. Results presented as mean ± S.D. The anti-inflammatory assays were performed with eight biological replicates. * $p < 0.05$, ** $p < 0.01$, and *** $p < 0.001$ compared with the control.

3. Materials and Methods

3.1. General Experimental Procedures

Values of the specific optical rotation of the isolates were measured with a JASCO P-1020 polarimeter (JASCO Corporation, Tokyo, Japan). Infrared spectra were recorded using a JASCO FT/IR-4100 infrared spectrophotometer (JASCO Corporation, Tokyo, Japan). The CD spectrum was recorded on a Jasco J-815 circular dichroism (CD) spectropolarimeter (JASCO, Tokyo, Japan) in MeOH. ^{1}H- and ^{13}C-NMR spectra were acquired on a Varian 400MR FT-NMR (or Varian Unity INOVA500 FT-NMR) instrument (Varian Inc., Palo Alto, CA, USA) at 400 MHz (or 500 MHz) and 100 MHz (or 125 MHz), respectively, in CDCl$_3$ or C$_6$D$_6$. LR-ESI-MS and HR-ESI-MS experiments were carried out using a Bruker APEX II (Bruker, Bremen, Germany) mass spectrometer. Silica gel (230–400 mesh) was used as the adsorbent for normal-phase column chromatography. Thin-layer chromatography (TLC) analyses were performed with precoated silica gel plates (Kieselgel 60 F-254, 0.2 mm, Merck, Darmstadt, Germany). Further purification of impure fractions or compounds was further achieved by high-performance liquid chromatography on a Hitachi L-7100 HPLC instrument (Hitachi Ltd., Tokyo, Japan) with a Merck Hibar Si-60 column (250 mm × 21 mm, 7 μm; Merck, Darmstadt, Germany) and on a Hitachi L-2455 HPLC apparatus (Hitachi, Tokyo, Japan) with a Supelco C18 column (250 mm × 21.2 mm, 5 μm; Supelco, Bellefonte, PA, USA).

3.2. Animal Materials

The marine organism *S. cherbonnieri* was collected and preserved as described previously [24].

3.3. Extraction and Isolation

By using the procedure reported previously, 1.2 kg (wet weight) of organism *S. cherbonnieri* was dehydrated, minced, extracted, and concentrated to afford 10.2 g of residue. The residue was fractionated by chromatography to yield 19 fractions [24]. Fraction 10, eluting with *n*-hexane–acetone (4:1), was further purified over silica gel using *n*-hexane–acetone (6:1) to afford seven subfractions (A1–A7). Subfraction A3 was further separated by reverse-phase HPLC using acetonitrile–H$_2$O (1:1.1) to afford **2** (1.4 mg). Subfraction A4 was purified by reverse-phase HPLC using acetonitrile–H$_2$O (1:1.2) to afford **4** (8.8 mg), and subfraction A6 was purified by reverse-phase HPLC acetonitrile–H$_2$O (2:1) to afford **5** (3.1 mg). Fractions 11 and 12, obtained by eluting with *n*-hexane–acetone 3:1 and 2:1, respectively, were combined and further eluted with acetone by a Sephadex LH-20 column to afford six subfractions (B1–B6). The purification of subfractions B4 and B5 using reverse-phase HPLC by elution of acetonitrile–H$_2$O (1:1.3) and MeOH–H$_2$O (3:2) afforded **6** (12.4 mg) and **7** (33.1 mg), respectively. Fraction 13, eluting with *n*-hexane–acetone (1:1), was purified by eluting with acetone on Sephadex LH-20 to yield five subfractions (C1–C5). Subfraction C2 was further separated by reverse-phase HPLC using acetonitrile–H$_2$O (1:1.4) to afford **1** (3.3 mg) and **3** (10.8 mg).

Cherbonolide F (**1**): colorless oil; $[\alpha]_{25}^{D}$ +177 (*c* 0.50, CHCl$_3$); IR (neat) ν_{max} 3460, 2967, 2928, 2864, 1748, 1677, 1452, 1385, 1096, 984, and 755 cm^{-1}; for ^{13}C- and ^{1}H-NMR data (400 MHz; C$_6$D$_6$), see Tables 1 and 2; ESI-MS *m/z* 355 [M + Na]$^+$; HR-ESI-MS *m/z* 355.1879 [M + Na]$^+$ (calculated for C$_{20}$H$_{28}$O$_4$Na, 355.1880).

Cherbonolide G (**2**): colorless oil; $[\alpha]_{25}^{D}$ +25 (*c* 0.33, CHCl$_3$); IR (neat) ν_{max} 3419, 2925, 2855, 1748, 1678, 1454, 1387, 1096, 987, and 755 cm^{-1}; for ^{13}C- and ^{1}H-NMR data (400 MHz; C$_6$D$_6$), see Tables 1 and 2; ESI-MS *m/z* 371 [M + Na]$^+$; HR-ESI-MS *m/z* 371.1830 [M + Na]$^+$ (calculated for C$_{20}$H$_{28}$O$_5$Na, 371.1829).

Cherbonolide H (**3**): colorless oil; $[\alpha]_{25}^{D}$ +41 (*c* 1.00, CHCl$_3$); IR (neat) ν_{max} 3445, 2928, 2864, 1747, 1679, 1455, 1387, 1094, 996, and 755 cm^{-1}; for ^{13}C- and ^{1}H-NMR data (400 MHz; C$_6$D$_6$), see Tables 1 and 2; ESI-MS *m/z* 355 [M + Na]$^+$; HR-ESI-MS *m/z* 355.1878 [M + Na]$^+$ (calculated for C$_{20}$H$_{28}$O$_4$Na, 355.1880).

Cherbonolide I (**4**): colorless oil; $[\alpha]_{25}^{D}$ +13 (*c* 1.00, CHCl$_3$); IR (neat) ν_{max} 3420, 2925, 2855, 1747, 1541, 1390, 992, and 756 cm^{-1}; for ^{13}C- and ^{1}H-NMR data (500 MHz; C$_6$D$_6$), see Tables 1 and 2; ESI-MS *m/z* 371 [M + Na]$^+$; HR-ESI-MS *m/z* 371.1828 [M + Na]$^+$ (calculated for C$_{20}$H$_{28}$O$_5$Na, 371.1829).

Cherbonolide J (**5**): white powder; $[\alpha]_{25}^{D}$ −6 (*c* 0.50, CHCl$_3$); IR (neat) ν_{max} 3443, 2937, 2860, 1755, 1675, 1381, 1076, 990, and 755 cm^{-1}; CD (1.2 × 10^{-4} M, MeOH) λ_{max} ($\Delta\varepsilon$) 247 (−5.2), and 228 (+26.5) nm; for ^{13}C- and ^{1}H-NMR data (400 MHz; C$_6$D$_6$), see Tables 1 and 3; ESI-MS *m/z* 373 [M + Na]$^+$; HR-ESI-MS *m/z* 373.1984 [M + Na]$^+$ (calculated for C$_{20}$H$_{30}$O$_5$Na, 373.1986).

Cherbonolide K (**6**): yellow oil; $[\alpha]_{25}^{D}$ +12 (*c* 1.00, CHCl$_3$); IR (neat) ν_{max} 3444, 2927, 1763, 1435, 1386, 1241, 1083, 931, and 756 cm^{-1}; for ^{13}C- and ^{1}H-NMR data (400 MHz; CDCl$_3$), see Tables 1 and 3; ESI-MS *m/z* 355 [M + Na]$^+$; HR-ESI-MS *m/z* 355.1880 [M + Na]$^+$ (calculated for C$_{20}$H$_{28}$O$_4$Na, 355.1880).

Cherbonolide L (**7**): yellow oil; $[\alpha]_{25}^{D}$ +33 (c 1.00, CHCl$_3$) ; IR (neat) ν_{max} 3445, 2929, 2872, 1752, 1665, 1455, 1384, 1050, 927, and 756 cm^{-1}; for ^{13}C- and ^{1}H-NMR data (400 MHz; CDCl$_3$), see Tables 1 and 3; ESI-MS m/z 355 [M + Na]$^+$; HR-ESI-MS m/z 355.1877 [M + Na]$^+$ (calculated for C$_{20}$H$_{28}$O$_4$Na, 355.1880).

3.4. Reduction of Cherbonolide I (**4**)

The solution of compound **4** (1.4 mg) in diethyl ether (5.0 mL) was added to an excess amount of triphenylphosphine (1.3 mg), and the mixture was stirred at room temperature for 4 h. The solvent of the solution was evaporated under reduced pressure to afford a residue, which was purified by silica gel column chromatography using n-hexane–acetone (3:1) as an eluent to yield **3** (1.0 mg, 75%).

3.5. In Vitro Anti-Inflammatory Assay

3.5.1. Primary Human Neutrophils

Blood was obtained from the elbow vein of healthy adult volunteers (with ages 20–30). Neutrophils were enriched by means of dextran sedimentation, Ficoll–Hypaque centrifugation, and hypotonic lysis. Neutrophils were incubated in an ice-cold Ca^{2+}-free Hank's Balanced Salt Solution (HBSS buffer, pH 7.4) [31]. The research protocol was granted approval by the institutional review board of Chang Gung Memorial Hospital (IRB No: 201601307A3, 20161124-20191123; 201902217A3, 20200501-20240630). All subjects gave their informed consent for inclusion before they participated in the study. The study was conducted in accordance with the Declaration of Helsinki.

3.5.2. Superoxide Anion Generation

Neutrophils (6 × 10^5 cells·mL^{-1}) incubated in HBSS with ferricytochrome c (0.5 mg·mL^{-1}) and Ca^{2+} (1 mM) at 37 °C were treated with dimethyl sulfoxide (DMSO), as control, or with the tested compound for 5 min. Neutrophils were primed by cytochalasin B (CB, 1 µg·mL^{-1}) for 3 min before activating fMLF (100 nM) for 10 min (fMLF/CB). The change in superoxide anion generation was spectrophotometrically measured at 550 nm (U-3010, Hitachi, Tokyo, Japan) [32,33].

3.5.3. Elastase Release

Neutrophils (6 × 10^5 cells·mL^{-1}) incubated in HBSS with MeO-Suc-Ala-Ala-Pro-Val-p- nitroanilide (100 µM) and Ca^{2+} (1 mM) at 37 °C were treated with DMSO or the tested compound for 5 min. Neutrophils were challenged by fMLF (100 nM)/CB (0.5 µg·mL^{-1}) for 10 min. The change in elastase release was spectrophotometrically measured at 405 nm (U-3010, Hitachi, Tokyo, Japan) [32].

3.5.4. Statistical Analysis

Data were displayed as the mean ± SD, and comparisons were performed by one-way ANOVA with Dunnett analysis. All results were obtained from eight biological replicates. A probability value of 0.05 or less was considered to be significant. The Prism software (Version 5.0, GraphPad Software, San Diego, CA, USA) was used for the statistical analysis.

4. Conclusions

Our present examination of the chemical constituents of the soft coral *S. cherbonnieri* led to the discovery of new cembranoid compounds **1–7**. All compounds were found to possess anti-inflammatory activity by exhibiting inhibitory effects on the generation of superoxide anion and elastase release in fMLF/CB-induced primary human neutrophils, and cherbonolides G and H (**2** and **3**) were found to be the most active in the inhibition of elastase release and superoxide anion generation, respectively. As the marine environment is an important source of bioactive substances, and due to the high chemical diversity and specimen diversity of the *Sarcophyton* genus [27,28,34,35], it can be expected that new natural products and activities from soft corals of this genus can be continuously discovered in the future.

Supplementary Materials: The following are available online at http://www.mdpi.com/1660-3397/18/11/573/s1. HR-ESI-MS, ^{1}H-NMR, ^{13}C-NMR, DEPT, HMQC, COSY, HMBC, and NOESY spectra of new compounds **1–7** are available online at http://www.mdpi.com/1660-3397/16/8/276/s1. Figure S1: HR-ESI-MS spectrum of **1**; Figure S2. ^{1}H-NMR spectrum of **1** in C$_6$D$_6$; Figure S3. ^{13}C-NMR spectrum of **1** in C$_6$D$_6$; Figure S4. HSQC spectrum of **1** in C$_6$D$_6$; Figure S5. ^{1}H–^{1}H COSY spectrum of **1** in C$_6$D$_6$; Figure S6. HMBC spectrum of **1** in C$_6$D$_6$; Figure S7. NOESY spectrum of **1** in C$_6$D$_6$; Figure S8. HR-ESI-MS spectrum of **2**; Figure S9. ^{1}H-NMR spectrum of **2** in C$_6$D$_6$; Figure S10. ^{13}C-NMR spectrum of **2** in C$_6$D$_6$; Figure S11. HSQC spectrum of **2** in C$_6$D$_6$; Figure S12. ^{1}H–^{1}H COSY spectrum of **2** in C$_6$D$_6$; Figure S13. HMBC spectrum of **2** in C$_6$D$_6$; Figure S14. NOESY spectrum of **2** in C$_6$D$_6$; Figure S15. HR-ESI-MS spectrum of **3**; Figure S16. ^{1}H-NMR spectrum of **3** in C$_6$D$_6$; Figure S17. ^{13}C-NMR spectrum of **3** in C$_6$D$_6$; Figure S18. HSQC spectrum of **3** in C$_6$D$_6$; Figure S19. ^{1}H–^{1}H COSY spectrum of **3** in C$_6$D$_6$; Figure S20. HMBC spectrum of **3** in C$_6$D$_6$; Figure S21. NOESY spectrum of **3** in C$_6$D$_6$; Figure S22. HR-ESI-MS spectrum of **4**; Figure S23. ^{1}H-NMR spectrum of **4** in C$_6$D$_6$; Figure S24. ^{13}C-NMR spectrum of **4** in C$_6$D$_6$; Figure S25. HSQC spectrum of **4** in C$_6$D$_6$; Figure S26. ^{1}H-^{1}HCOSY spectrum of **4** in C$_6$D$_6$; Figure S27. HMBC spectrum of **4** in C$_6$D$_6$; Figure S28. NOESY spectrum of **4** in C$_6$D$_6$; Figure S29. HR-ESI-MS spectrum of **5**; Figure S30. ^{1}H-NMR spectrum of **5** in C$_6$D$_6$; Figure S31. ^{13}C-NMR spectrum of **5** in C$_6$D$_6$; Figure S32. HSQC spectrum of **5** in C$_6$D$_6$; Figure S33. ^{1}H–^{1}H COSY spectrum of **5** in C$_6$D$_6$; Figure S34. HMBC spectrum of **5** in C$_6$D$_6$; Figure S35. NOESY spectrum of **5** in C$_6$D$_6$; Figure S36. HR-ESI-MS spectrum of **6**; Figure S37. ^{1}H-NMR spectrum of **6** in CDCl$_3$; Figure S38. ^{13}C-NMR spectrum of **6** in CDCl$_3$; Figure S39. HSQC spectrum of **6** in CDCl$_3$; Figure S40. ^{1}H–^{1}H COSY spectrum of **6** in CDCl$_3$; Figure S41. HMBC spectrum of **6** in CDCl$_3$; Figure S42. NOESY spectrum of **6** in CDCl$_3$; Figure S43. HR-ESI-MS spectrum of **7**; Figure S44. ^{1}H-NMR spectrum of **7** in CDCl$_3$; Figure S45. ^{13}C-NMR spectrum of **7** in CDCl$_3$; Figure S46. HSQC spectrum of **7** in CDCl$_3$; Figure S47. ^{1}H–^{1}H COSY spectrum of **7** in CDCl$_3$; Figure S48. HMBC spectrum of **7** in CDCl$_3$; Figure S49. NOESY spectrum of **7** in CDCl$_3$.

Author Contributions: Conceptualization, J.-H.S.; investigation, C.-C.P.; analysis, C.-C.P. and C.-Y.H.; writing—original draft, C.-Y.H., J.-H.S., and A.F.A.; writing—review and editing, J.-H.S.; anti-inflammatory assay, T.-L.H. All authors read and agreed to the published version of the manuscript.

Funding: Financial support of this work from the Ministry of Science and Technology of Taiwan (MOST 104-2113-M-110-006, 104-2320-B-110-001-MY2, and 107-2320-B-110-001-MY3) to J.-H.S. and further funding from the Deanship of Scientific Research at King Saud University through research group RG-1440-127.

Conflicts of Interest: The authors declare no conflict of interest.

References

1. Farag, M.A.; Fekry, M.I.; Al-Hammady, M.A.; Khalil, M.N.; El-Seedi, H.R.; Meyer, A.; Porzel, A.; Westphal, H.; Wessjohann, L.A. Cytotoxic effects of *Sarcophyton* sp. soft corals-is there a correlation to their NMR fingerprints? *Mar. Drugs* **2017**, *15*, 211. [CrossRef]
2. Chao, C.H.; Li, W.L.; Huang, C.Y.; Ahmed, A.F.; Dai, C.F.; Wu, Y.C.; Lu, M.C.; Liaw, C.C.; Sheu, J.H. Isoprenoids from the soft coral *Sarcophyton glaucum*. *Mar. Drugs* **2017**, *15*, 202. [CrossRef]
3. Hegazy, M.E.F.; Elshamy, A.I.; Mohamed, T.A.; Hamed, A.R.; Ibrahim, M.A.A.; Ohta, S.; Paré, P.W. Cembrene diterpenoids with ether linkages from *Sarcophyton ehrenbergi*: An anti-proliferation and molecular-docking assessment. *Mar. Drugs* **2017**, *15*, 192. [CrossRef]
4. Elkhateeb, A.; El-Beih, A.A.; Gamal-Eldeen, A.M.; Alhammady, M.A.; Ohta, S.; Paré, P.W.; Hegazy, M.E.F. New terpenes from the Egyptian soft coral *Sarcophyton ehrenbergi*. *Mar. Drugs* **2014**, *12*, 1977–1986. [CrossRef]
5. Eltahawy, N.A.; Ibrahim, A.K.; Radwan, M.M.; ElSohly, M.A.; Hassanean, H.A.; Hassanean, H.A.; Ahmed, S.A. Cytotoxic cembranoids from the Red Sea soft coral, *Sarcophyton auritum*. *Tetrahedron Lett.* **2014**, *55*, 3984–3988. [CrossRef]
6. Lin, W.Y.; Lu, Y.; Su, J.H.; Wen, Z.H.; Dai, C.F.; Kuo, Y.H.; Sheu, J.H. Bioactive cembranoids from the dongsha atoll soft coral *Sarcophyton crassocaule*. *Mar. Drugs* **2011**, *9*, 994–1006. [CrossRef]
7. Lin, W.Y.; Su, J.H.; Lu, Y.; Wen, Z.H.; Dai, C.F.; Kuo, Y.H.; Sheu, J.H. Cytotoxic and anti-inflammatory cembranoids from the Dongsha Atoll soft coral *Sarcophyton crassocaule*. *Bioorg. Med. Chem.* **2010**, *18*, 1936–1941. [CrossRef]
8. Hassan, H.M.; Rateb, M.E.; Hassan, M.H.; Sayed, A.M.; Shabana, S.; Raslan, M.; Amin, E.; Behery, F.A.; Ahmed, O.M.; Bin Muhsinah, A.; et al. New antiproliferative cembrane diterpenes from the Red Sea *Sarcophyton* species. *Mar. Drugs* **2019**, *17*, 411. [CrossRef]
9. Huang, C.Y.; Tseng, Y.J.; Chokkalingam, U.; Hwang, T.L.; Hsu, C.H.; Dai, C.F.; Sung, P.J.; Sheu, J.H. Bioactive isoprenoid-derived natural products from a Dongsha Atoll soft coral *Sinularia erecta*. *J. Nat. Prod.* **2016**, *79*, 1339–1346. [CrossRef]

10. Tseng, Y.J.; Yang, Y.C.; Wang, S.K.; Duh, C.Y. Numerosol A–D, new cembranoid diterpenes from the soft coral *Sinularia numerosa*. *Mar. Drugs* **2014**, *12*, 3371–3380. [CrossRef]
11. Lillsunde, K.-E.; Festa, C.; Adel, H.; De Marino, S.; Lombardi, V.; Tilvi, S.; Nawrot, D.A.; Zampella, A.; D'Souza, L.; D'Auria, M.V.; et al. Bioactive cembrane derivatives from the Indian Ocean soft coral, *Sinularia kavarattiensis*. *Mar. Drugs* **2014**, *12*, 4045–4068. [CrossRef]
12. Li, G.; Zhang, Y.; Deng, Z.; van Ofwegen, L.; Proksch, P.; Lin, W. Cytotoxic cembranoid diterpenes from a soft coral *Sinularia gibberosa*. *J. Nat. Prod.* **2005**, *68*, 649–652. [CrossRef]
13. Cheng, S.Y.; Wen, Z.H.; Wang, S.K.; Chiou, S.F.; Hsu, C.H.; Dai, C.F.; Chiang, M.Y.; Duh, C.Y. Unprecedented hemiketal cembranolides with anti-inflammatory activity from the soft coral *Lobophytum durum*. *J. Nat. Prod.* **2009**, *72*, 152–155. [CrossRef]
14. Chao, C.H.; Wen, Z.H.; Wu, Y.C.; Yeh, H.C.; Sheu, J.H. Cytotoxic and anti-inflammatory cembranoids from the soft coral *Lobophytum crassum*. *J. Nat. Prod.* **2008**, *71*, 1819–1824. [CrossRef]
15. Lai, K.H.; You, W.J.; Lin, C.C.; El-Shazly, M.; Liao, Z.J.; Su, J.H. Anti-inflammatory cembranoids from the soft coral *Lobophytum crassum*. *Mar. Drugs* **2017**, *15*, 327. [CrossRef] [PubMed]
16. Lin, K.H.; Tseng, Y.J.; Chen, B.W.; Hwang, T.L.; Chen, H.Y.; Dai, C.F.; Sheu, J.H. Tortuosenes A and B, new diterpenoid metabolites from the Formosan soft coral *Sarcophyton tortuosum*. *Org. Lett.* **2014**, *16*, 1314–1317. [CrossRef]
17. Chao, C.H.; Wu, C.Y.; Huang, C.Y.; Wang, H.C.; Dai, C.F.; Wu, Y.C.; Sheu, J.H. Cubitanoids and cembranoids from the soft coral *Sinularia nanolobata*. *Mar. Drugs* **2016**, *14*, 150. [CrossRef]
18. Chen, B.W.; Chao, C.H.; Su, J.H.; Huang, C.Y.; Dai, C.F.; Wen, Z.H.; Sheu, J.H. A novel symmetric sulfur-containing biscembranoid from the Formosan soft coral *Sinularia flexibilis*. *Tetrahedron Lett.* **2010**, *51*, 764–766. [CrossRef]
19. Huang, C.Y.; Sung, P.J.; Uvarani, C.; Su, J.H.; Lu, M.C.; Hwang, T.L.; Dai, C.F.; Wu, S.L.; Sheu, J.H. Glaucumolides A and B, biscembranoids with new structural type from a cultured soft coral *Sarcophyton glaucum*. *Sci. Rep.* **2015**, *5*, 15624. [CrossRef]
20. Jia, R.; Kurtan, T.; Mandi, A.; Yan, X.H.; Zhang, W.; Guo, Y.W. Biscembranoids formed from an alpha, β-unsaturated gamma-lactone ring as a dienophile: Structure revision and establishment of their absolute configurations using theoretical calculations of electronic circular dichroism spectra. *J. Org. Chem.* **2013**, *78*, 3113–3119. [CrossRef]
21. Kusumi, T.; Igari, M.; Ishitsuka, M.O.; Ichikawa, A.; Itezono, Y.; Nakayama, N.; Kakisawa, H. A novel chlorinated biscembranoid from the marine soft coral *Sarcophyton glaucum*. *J. Org. Chem.* **1990**, *55*, 6286–6289. [CrossRef]
22. Tseng, Y.J.; Ahmed, A.F.; Dai, C.F.; Chiang, M.Y.; Sheu, J.H. Sinulochmodins A–C, three novel terpenoids from the soft coral *Sinularia lochmodes*. *Org. Lett.* **2005**, *7*, 3813–3816. [CrossRef] [PubMed]
23. Li, Y.; Pattenden, G. Biomimetic syntheses of ineleganolide and sinulochmodin C from 5-episinuleptolide via sequences of transannular Michael reactions. *Tetrahedron* **2011**, *67*, 10045–10052. [CrossRef]
24. Peng, C.C.; Huang, C.Y.; Ahmed, A.F.; Hwang, T.L.; Dai, C.F.; Sheu, J.H. New cembranoids and a iscembranoid peroxide from the soft coral *Sarcophyton cherbonnieri*. *Mar. Drugs* **2018**, *16*, 276. [CrossRef] [PubMed]
25. Sang, V.T.; Dat, T.; Vinh, L.B.; Cuong, L.; Oanh, P.; Ha, H.; Kim, Y.H.; Anh, H.; Yang, S.Y. Coral and coral-associated microorganisms: A prolific source of potential bioactive natural products. *Mar. Drugs* **2019**, *17*, 468. [CrossRef] [PubMed]
26. Rodrigues, I.G.; Miguel, M.G.; Mnif, W. A brief review on new naturally occurring cembranoid diterpene derivatives from the soft corals of the genera *Sarcophyton*, *Sinularia*, and *Lobophytum* since 2016. *Molecules* **2019**, *24*, 781. [CrossRef] [PubMed]
27. Elkhawas, Y.A.; Elissawy, A.M.; Elnaggar, M.S.; Mostafa, N.M.; Al-Sayed, E.; Bishr, M.M.; Singab, A.N.B.; Salama, O.M. Chemical diversity in species belonging to soft coral genus *Sacrophyton* and its impact on biological activity: A review. *Mar. Drugs* **2020**, *18*, 41. [CrossRef]
28. Maloney, K.N.; Botts, R.T.; Davis, T.S.; Okada, B.K.; Maloney, E.M.; Leber, C.A.; Alvarado, O.; Brayton, C.; Caraballo-Rodríguez, A.M.; Chari, J.V.; et al. Cryptic species account for the seemingly idiosyncratic secondary metabolism of *Sarcophyton glaucum* specimens collected in Palau. *J. Nat. Prod.* **2020**, *83*, 693–705. [CrossRef]
29. Xi, Z.; Bie, W.; Chen, W.; Liu, D.; van Ofwegen, L.; Proksch, P.; Lin, W. Sarcophyolides B–E, new cembranoids from the soft coral *Sarcophyton elegans*. *Mar. Drugs* **2013**, *11*, 3186–3196. [CrossRef]

30. Kusumi, T.; Yamada, K.; Ishitsuka, M.O.; Fujita, Y.; Kakisawa, H. New cembranoids from the Okinawan soft coral *Sinularia mayi*. *Chem. Lett.* **1990**, *19*, 1315–1318. [CrossRef]
31. Hwang, T.L.; Su, Y.C.; Chang, H.L.; Leu, Y.L.; Chung, P.J.; Kuo, L.M.; Chang, Y.J. Suppression of superoxide anion and elastase release by C18 unsaturated fatty acids in human neutrophils. *J. Lipid Res.* **2009**, *50*, 1395–1408. [CrossRef] [PubMed]
32. Yang, S.C.; Chung, P.J.; Ho, C.M.; Kuo, C.Y.; Hung, M.F.; Huang, Y.T.; Chang, W.Y.; Chang, Y.W.; Chan, K.H.; Hwang, T.L. Propofol inhibits superoxide production, elastase release, and chemotaxis in formyl peptide-activated human neutrophils by blocking formyl peptide receptor 1. *J. Immunol.* **2013**, *190*, 6511–6519. [CrossRef] [PubMed]
33. Yu, H.P.; Hsieh, P.W.; Chang, Y.J.; Chung, P.J.; Kuo, L.M.; Hwang, T.L. 2-(2-Fluorobenzamido) benzoate ethyl ester (EFB-1) inhibits superoxide production by human neutrophils and attenuates hemorrhagic shock-induced organ dysfunction in rats. *Free Radic. Biol. Med.* **2011**, *50*, 1737–1748. [CrossRef] [PubMed]
34. Wei, W.-C.; Sung, P.-J.; Duh, C.-Y.; Chen, B.-W.; Sheu, J.-H.; Yang, N.-S. Anti-inflammatory activities of natural products isolated from soft corals of Taiwan between 2008 and 2012. *Mar. Drugs* **2013**, *11*, 4083–4126. [CrossRef] [PubMed]
35. Ahmad, B.; Shah, M.; Choi, S. Oceans as a source of immunotherapy. *Mar. Drugs* **2019**, *17*, 282. [CrossRef] [PubMed]

Publisher's Note: MDPI stays neutral with regard to jurisdictional claims in published maps and institutional affiliations.

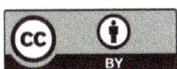

© 2020 by the authors. Licensee MDPI, Basel, Switzerland. This article is an open access article distributed under the terms and conditions of the Creative Commons Attribution (CC BY) license (http://creativecommons.org/licenses/by/4.0/).

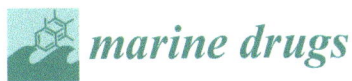

Article

Biologically Active Metabolites from the Marine Sediment-Derived Fungus *Aspergillus flocculosus*

Anton N. Yurchenko [1,*], Phan Thi Hoai Trinh [2], Elena V. Girich (Ivanets) [1], Olga F. Smetanina [1], Anton B. Rasin [1], Roman S. Popov [1], Sergey A. Dyshlovoy [1,3,4,5], Gunhild von Amsberg [4,5], Ekaterina S. Menchinskaya [1], Tran Thi Thanh Van [2] and Shamil Sh. Afiyatullov [1]

1. G.B. Elyakov Pacific Institute of Bioorganic Chemistry, Far Eastern Branch of the Russian Academy of Sciences, Prospect 100-letiya Vladivostoka, 159, Vladivostok 690022, Russia; ev.ivanets@yandex.ru (E.V.G.); smetof@rambler.ru (O.F.S.); abrus__54@mail.ru (A.B.R.); prs_90@mail.ru (R.S.P.); dyshlovoy@gmail.com (S.A.D.); ekaterinamenchinskaya@gmail.com (E.S.M.); afiyat@piboc.dvo.ru (S.S.A.)
2. Department of Marine Biotechnology, Nhatrang Institute of Technology Research and Application, Vietnam Academy of Science and Technology, 650000 Nha Trang, Vietnam; phanhoaitrinh84@gmail.com (P.T.H.T.); tranthanhvan@nitra.vast.vn (T.T.T.V.)
3. School of Natural Science, Far Eastern Federal University, Sukhanova St., 8, Vladivostok 690000, Russia
4. Laboratory of Experimental Oncology, Department of Oncology, Hematology and Bone Marrow Transplantation with Section Pneumology, Hubertus Wald-Tumorzentrum, University Medical Center Hamburg-Eppendorf, 20246 Hamburg, Germany; g.von-amsberg@uke.de
5. Martini-Klinik Prostate Cancer Center, University Hospital Hamburg-Eppendorf, 20246 Hamburg, Germany
* Correspondence: yurchant@ya.ru; Tel.: +7-423-231-1168

Received: 10 September 2019; Accepted: 9 October 2019; Published: 11 October 2019

Abstract: Four new compounds were isolated from the Vietnamese marine sediment-derived fungus *Aspergillus flocculosus*, one aspyrone-related polyketide aspilactonol G (**2**), one meroterpenoid 12-epi-aspertetranone D (**4**), two drimane derivatives (**7,9**), together with five known metabolites (**1,3,5,6,8,10**). The structures of compounds **1–10** were established by NMR and MS techniques. The absolute stereoconfigurations of compounds **1** and **2** were determined by a modified Mosher's method. The absolute configurations of compounds **4** and **7** were established by a combination of analysis of ROESY data and coupling constants as well as biogenetic considerations. Compounds **7** and **8** exhibited cytotoxic activity toward human prostate cancer 22Rv1, human breast cancer MCF-7, and murine neuroblastoma Neuro-2a cells.

Keywords: marine-derived fungi; secondary metabolites; polyketides; drimanes; meroterpenoids; cytotoxicity

1. Introduction

Marine fungi are rich sources of new biologically active compounds [1]. Fungi of the genus *Aspergillus*, section *Circumdati* (*Aspergillus insulicola*, *Aspergillus flocculosus*, *Aspergillus ochraceus*, *Aspergillus ochraceopetaliformis*, and others) [2], are known to produce metabolites belonging to various chemical classes: aspyrone-related pentaketides [3,4], meroterpenoids [5,6], diketopiperazine alkaloids [7], drimane sesquiterpenoids and their nitrobenzoyl derivatives [8,9], steroids, and cerebrosides [10]. Many of them possess antimicrobial [4,10], antiviral [11], cytotoxic [8,11], and neuroprotective [12] activities.

Aspyrone-related pentaketides are polyketide metabolites commonly found in this fungal group [13]. Usually, they are divided into three structural types: linear (aspinonene) [3], δ-lactones (aspyrone) [3], and γ-lactones (iso-aspinonene, aspilactonols) [3,14]. Meroterpenoid metabolites of *Aspergillus*, section *Circumdati* fungi are represented mainly by triketidesesquiterpenoids with rare α-pyrone-contained linear or angular skeleton. To date, only several representatives of this chemical class belonging to the aspertetranones [5] and ochraceopones [6] series were reported. Nitrobenzoyl derivatives of drimane-sesquiterpenoids were initially found in *A. insulicola* species but can also be produced by other related fungi [15]. These compounds are characterized by a small structural diversity with two isomeric backbones (cinnamolide- and confertifolin-based) and various locations of acyl groups. A residue of *p*-nitrobenzoic acid usually can be found at positions 9-OH or 14-OH. Nitrobenzoyl derivatives are relatively unstable compounds that cannot be hydrolyzed to form the corresponding sesquiterpenoids [8]. Acetylation of these compounds with acetic anhydride results in rearrangement and formation of several products [16].

Recently, we have started a project focusing on the search for producers of novel bioactive compounds among fungi isolated from various substrates found in the Vietnamese waters of the South China Sea [17,18]. Thus, from a sediment sample collected in Nha Trang Bay, we have isolated a strain of fungus *A. flocculosus*. Recently, we described the new neuroprotective alkaloid mactanamide produced by this strain [12]. Herein, we report the isolation, structure elucidation and cytotoxic activity of four new (**2,4,7,9**) and six known (**1,3,5,6,8,10**) metabolites produced by the same fungus (Figure 1).

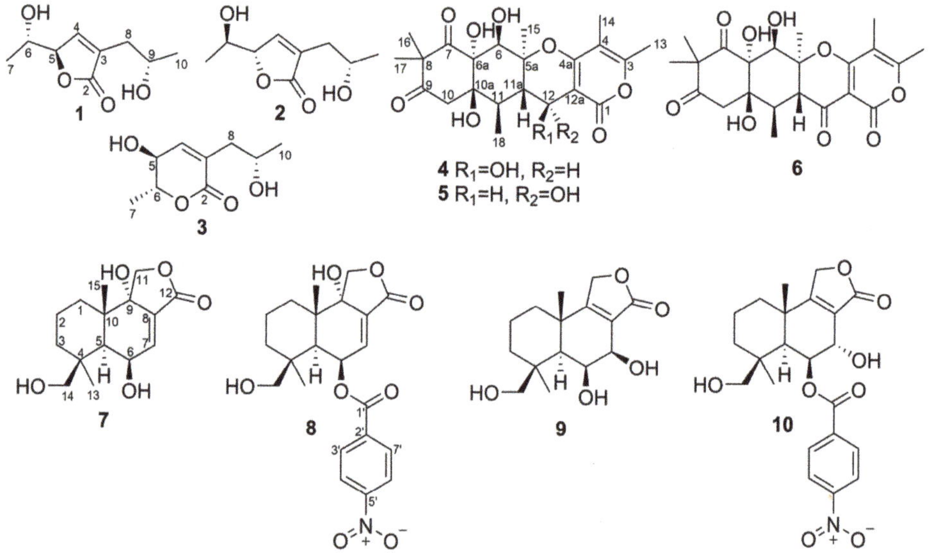

Figure 1. Chemical structures of the isolated compounds **1–10**.

2. Results and Discussion

The molecular formula of compound **1** was determined as $C_9H_{14}O_4$ by an HRESIMS peak at *m/z* 209.0785 [M + Na]$^+$, which was supported by the ^{13}C NMR spectrum.

A close inspection of the ^{1}H and ^{13}C NMR data of **1** (Table 1, Figures S1–S3) revealed the presence of two methyls (δ_C 23.3, 18.8; δ_H 1.31, 1.25), one methylene (δ_C 34.9; δ_H 2.52, 2.45), three oxygen-bearing sp^3-methines (δ_C 84.9, 67.8, 66.2; δ_H 4.85, 4.08, 4.05) and one sp^2-methine (δ_C 147.4; δ_H 7.27). Two remaining signals at δ_C 132.8 and 174.2 ppm corresponded to a quaternary sp^2-carbon and a carboxyl carbon, respectively.

The HMBC correlations (Figure 2 and Figure S6) from H-4 (δ_H 7.27) to C-2 (δ_C 174.2), C-3 (δ_C 132.8), and C-5 (δ_C 84.9) and from H-5 (δ_H 4.85) to C-2, C-3, and C-4 (δ_C 147.4) suggested the presence of a dihydrofuran ring. The structure of the 1-hydroxyethyl side chain and its location at C-5 in **1** was established by COSY correlations of H-6/H-5 and H-7 and HMBC correlations from H-6 (δ_H 4.05) to C-4, C-5, and C-7 (δ_C 18.8). The data of COSY spectrum (Figure S4) and HMBC correlations from H-10

(δ_H 1.25) to C-8 (δ_C 34.9), C-9 (δ_C 66.2), and from both H$_2$-8 (δ_H 2.52, 2.45) to C-3, C-4, C-9, and C-10 (δ_C 23.3) determined the structure of the 2-hydroxypropyl side chain and its location at C-3.

Table 1. ^{1}H and ^{13}C NMR data (δ in ppm, CDCl$_3$) for aspilactonols G (1) and F (2).

Position	1		2	
	δ_C, mult	δ_H (J in Hz)	δ_C, mult	δ_H (J in Hz)
2	174.2, C		174.1, C	
3	132.8, C		132.9, C	
4	147.4, CH	7.27, d (1.4)	147.3, CH	7.25, d (1.2)
5	84.9, CH	4.85, dd (4.4, 1.4)	84.8, CH	4.86, dd (4.2, 1.4)
6	67.8, CH	4.05, qd (6.4, 4.4)	67.6, CH	4.08, qd (6.6, 4.2)
7	18.8, CH$_3$	1.31, d (6.4)	18.8, CH$_3$	1.31, d (6.6)
8	34.9, CH$_2$	2.52, ddt (15.0, 3.8, 1.4) 2.45, ddt (15.0, 7.8, 1.4)	35.2, CH$_2$	2.55, ddt (14.6, 3.6, 1.4) 2.40, dd (14.6, 8.5)
9	66.2, CH	4.08, m	65.8, CH	4.04, m
10	23.3, CH$_3$	1.25, d (6.3)	23.2, CH$_3$	1.25, d (6.2)

^{1}H NMR and ^{13}C NMR spectroscopic data were measured at 500 MHz and 125 MHz, respectively.

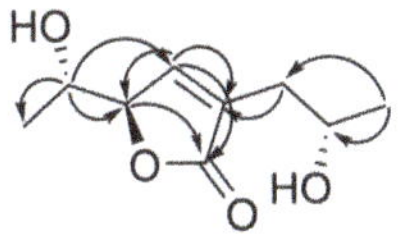

Figure 2. The key HMBC correlations of 1.

The absolute configuration of the chiral centers C-6 and C-9 of **1** was established using a modified Mosher's method. Esterification of the C-6 and C-9 hydroxy moieties of **1** with (R)- and (S)-MTPA chloride afforded the (S)- and (R)-bis-MTPA-esters, respectively. The observed chemical shift differences $\Delta\delta$ ($\delta_S - \delta_R$) (Figure 3A) indicated 6S, 9S configurations. The absolute configuration of C-5 stereocenter in **1** was proven as R on the basis of a characteristic Cotton's effect at λ_{217} + 11.35 in the CD spectrum (Experimental Section and Figure S8) and a coupling constant value $^3J_{H5-H6}$ = 4.4 Hz [14,19]. Compound **1** was recently reported as aspilactonol F, that was a component of unseparated mixture of epimers at C-9. Our study is the first determination of the absolute configurations of all stereocenters of aspilactonol F.

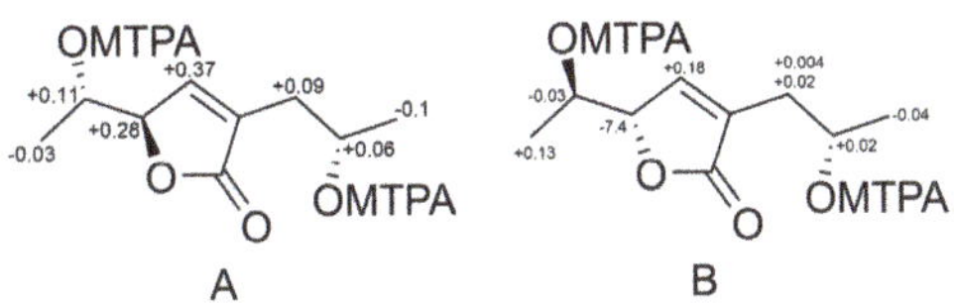

Figure 3. $\Delta\delta$ ($\delta_S - \delta_R$) values (in ppm) for the MTPA ester of 1 (A) and 2 (B).

The molecular formula of compound **2** was determined as C$_9$H$_{14}$O$_4$ (the same as **1**) on the basis of HRESIMS data and confirmed by ^{13}C NMR. The NMR data of **2** were very similar to those of **1** (Table 1, Figures S9–S16). Thus, the planar structure of **2** was suggested to be the same as that of aspilactonol F (**1**).

Esterification of the C-6 and C-9 hydroxy moieties of **2** with (R)- and (S)-MTPA chloride afforded the (S)- and (R)-bis-MTPA-esters, respectively. The observed chemical shift differences $\Delta\delta$ ($\delta_S - \delta_R$) (Figure 3B) indicated 6R, 9S configurations. The absolute configuration of the C-5 stereocenter in **2** was suggested as S on the basis of a strong negative Cotton's effect at λ_{216} −11.51 in the CD spectrum (Experimental Section and Figure S17) [19]. Compound **2** was named aspilactonol G.

The molecular formula of compound 4 was established as $C_{22}H_{28}O_9$ on the basis of HRESIMS, containing a peak at m/z 459.1628 $[M + Na]^+$, and was supported by the ^{13}C NMR spectrum.

An analysis of NMR data of 4 (Table 2, Figures S20–S24) revealed the presence of six methyl groups (δ_C 25.1, 24.0, 18.5, 17.3, 10.8, 9.5; δ_H 2.24, 1.89, 1.43, 1.41, 1.39, 1.31), one sp^3-methylene group (δ_C 45.6; δ_H 2.86, 2.76), two sp^3-methines (δ_C 39.5, 39.3; δ_H 2.32, 2.00), two oxygen-bearing ones (δ_C 75.15, 63.5; δ_H 4.63, 4.36), one quaternary sp^3-carbon (δ_C 55.5), three oxygen-bearing quaternary sp^3-carbons (δ_C 83.0, 76.5, 75.07), two quaternary sp^2-carbons (δ_C 107.3, 102.2), three oxygen-bearing quaternary sp^2-carbons (δ_C 164.4, 162.5, 157.9), and two ketone groups (δ_C 211.4, 209.1).

Table 2. ^1H and ^{13}C NMR data (δ in ppm, CDCl$_3$) for 12-*epi*-aspertetranone D (4).

Position	δ_C, Mult	δ_H (J in Hz)	HMBC
1	164.4, C		
3	157.9, C		
4	107.3, C		
4a	162.5, C		
5a	83.0, C		
6	75.15, CH	4.36, s	5a, 6a, 7, 10a, 11a, 15
6a	76.5, C		
7	211.4, C		
8	55.5, C		
9	209.1, C		
10	45.6, CH$_2$	2.86, d (17.7)	6a, 9, 10a
		2.76, dd (17.7, 2.7)	9, 10a
10a	75.07, C		
11	39.5, CH	2.00, dd (12.0, 6.8)	5a, 10a, 11a, 18
11a	39.3, CH	2.32, dd (12.0, 9.4)	5a, 6, 10a, 11, 12, 18
12	63.5, CH	4.63, d (9.4)	1, 4a, 11, 11a, 12a
12a	102.2, C		
13	17.3, CH$_3$	2.24, s	3, 4, 4a
14	9.5, CH$_3$	1.89, s	3, 4, 4a
15	18.5, CH$_3$	1.43, s	5a, 6, 11a
16	25.1, CH$_3$	1.39, s	7, 8, 9, 17
17	24.0, CH$_3$	1.41, s	7, 8, 9, 16
18	10.8, CH$_3$	1.31, d (6.8)	10a, 11, 11a
6-OH		3.57, brs	
6a-OH		3.12, brs	
10a-OH		4.01, d (2.7)	10, 10a
12-OH		4.43, brs	11a, 12

^1H NMR and ^{13}C NMR spectroscopic data were measured at 500 MHz and 125 MHz, respectively.

The HMBC correlations of 4 (Figure 4 and Figure S25, Table 2) suggested the presence of a linear tetracyclic backbone like in the recently reported merosesquiterpenoids aspetetranones A-D [5]. The general features of the ^{13}C NMR spectrum of 4 (Table 2, Figures S21–S22) were similar to those of aspertetranone D (5) [5], with the exception of the C-6, C-11, C-11a, C-12, C-15, and C-18 carbon signals. The main patterns of the experimental CD spectrum of 4 in methanol (Experimental section, Figure S27) matched well with those of aspertetranone D (5) [5]. The value of the vicinal coupling constant between H-11a and H-12 (9.4 Hz) in 4 instead of $^3J_{H11a-H12}$ = 3.9 Hz in aspertetranone D (5) indicated a β orientation of the OH group at C-12 in 4. Thus, the absolute configurations of chiral centers in 4 were suggested as 5a*S*, 6*R*, 6a*R*, 10a*R*, 11*R*, 11a*S*, 12*S*. Compound 4 was named 12-*epi*-aspertetranone D.

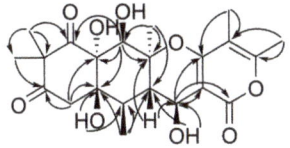

Figure 4. The key HMBC correlations of **4**.

The molecular formula of compound **7** was established as $C_{15}H_{22}O_5$ on the basis of an HRESIMS peak at m/z 305.1361 [M + Na]$^+$, which was supported by the ^{13}C NMR spectrum and corresponded to four double-bond equivalents.

A close inspection of the ^{1}H and ^{13}C NMR data of **7** (Table 3, Figures S30–S32) revealed the presence of two methyl groups (δ_C 26.8, 20.8; δ_H 1.23, 1.15), three sp^3-methylene groups (δ_C 42.0, 32.6, 17.6; δ_H 2.13, 1.63, 1.50 (2H), 1.38, 1.24), two oxygen-bearing sp^3-methylene groups (δ_C 75.0, 68.4; δ_H 4.44, 4.41, 4.24, 3.42), two sp^3-methine groups (δ_C 63.5, 47.1; δ_H 4.62, 2.00), including one oxygen-bearing, one sp^2-methine group (δ_C 139.1; δ_H 6.96), three quaternary sp^3-carbons (δ_C 77.5, 39.0, 38.3), including one oxygen-bearing, and two quaternary sp^2-carbons (δ_C 169.6, 130.1).

Table 3. ^{1}H and ^{13}C NMR data (δ in ppm) for 6β,9α,14-trihydroxycinnamolide (**7**) and 6β,7β,14-trihydroxyconfertifolin (**9**).

Position	7 a			9 b		
	δ_C, mult	δ_H (J in Hz)	HMBC	δ_C, mult	δ_H (J in Hz)	HMBC
1	32.6, CH$_2$	1.24, m; 2.13, td (12.7, 5.7)	2, 3, 5, 9, 10, 15	37.8, CH$_2$	1.59, m; 1.54, m	2, 3, 5, 15
2	17.6, CH$_2$	1.50, m	1, 3, 4	18.0, CH$_2$	1.71, m; 1.45, m	1, 3
3	42.0, CH$_2$	1.38, td (12.9, 5.3); 1.63, m	2, 4, 13, 14; 1, 2, 4, 5, 14	37.8, CH$_2$	1.32, td (13.0, 3.8); 1.10, td (13.6, 4.3)	1, 2, 13, 14
4	38.3, C			38.3, C		
5	47.1, CH	2.00, d (4.0)	4, 6, 9, 13, 14, 15	48.6, CH	1.57, brs	1, 6, 9, 10, 14, 15
6	63.5, CH	4.62, t (4.2)	7, 8, 10	70.0, CH	3.99, brs	5, 7, 8, 9, 10
7	139.1, CH	6.96, d (4.0)	5, 9, 12	64.1, CH	4.00, d (2.1)	5, 6, 12
8	130.1, C			122.1, C		
9	77.5, C			173.1, C		
10	39.0, C			36.3, C		
11	75.0, CH$_2$	4.24, d (9.8); 4.44, d (9.8)	8, 9, 12	68.1, CH$_2$	4.94, dd (17.6, 1.7); 4.79, brd (17.6)	7, 8, 9
12	169.6, C			173.4, C		
13	26.8, CH$_3$	1.15, s	3, 4, 5, 14	27.9, CH$_3$	0.97, s	3, 4, 5, 14
14	68.4, CH$_2$	3.42, d (11.4); 4.41, d (11.4)	3, 4, 5, 13	65.6, CH$_2$	3.94, dd (11.3, 3.8); 3.26, dd (11.3, 6.0)	3, 4, 5, 13
15	20.8, CH$_3$	1.23, s	1, 5, 9, 10	21.6, CH$_3$	1.40, s	1, 5, 9, 10

^{1}H NMR and ^{13}C NMR spectroscopic data were measured ^{a} in CDCl$_3$ at 500 MHz and 125 MHz, respectively, and ^{b} in DMSO-d$_6$ at 700 MHz and 176 MHz, respectively.

The ^{13}C NMR data of **7** were similar to those of the drimane moiety of insulicolide A (**8**) [15], also reported as 9α-14-dihydroxy-6β-p-nitrobenzoylcinnamolide [8], with the exception of the C-3, C-6, C-7, C-8, and C-14 carbon signals. The COSY spectrum data (Figure S33) and HMBC correlations (Figure S35, Table 3) from H-6 (δ_H 4.62) to C-7 (δ_C 139.1), C-8 (δ_C 130.1), and C-10 (δ_C 39.0), from H-7 (δ_H 6.96) to C-5 (δ_C 47.1), C-9, and C-12 (δ_C 169.6), from H$_3$-13 (δ_H 1.15) to C-3 (δ_C 42.0), C-4 (δ_C 38.3), C-5 (δ_C 47.1), and C-14 (δ_C 68.4), and from H$_3$-15 (δ_H 1.23) to C-1 (δ_C 32.6), C-5, C-9, and C-10 proved the drimane framework of **7** the same as in insulicolide A (**8**).

The ROESY correlations (Figure S36) of H$_3$-13 with H-5 (δ_H 2.00) and H-6, long-range COSY correlation H$_3$-15/H-5, together with the vicinal coupling constant $^3J_{H5-H6}$ = 4.4 Hz established the relative configurations of the C-4, C-5, C-6, and C-10 chiral centers. The absolute configurations of the stereocenters in **7** were suggested as depicted in Figure 1 from CD spectra similarity (Figures S37 and

S38) and biogenetic relationship with insulicolide A (8), whose absolute configurations were determined previously by X-ray analysis [15]. Compound 7 was named 6β,9α,14-trihydroxycinnamolide.

The molecular formula of compound 9 was established as $C_{15}H_{22}O_5$ on the basis of an HRESIMS peak at m/z 305.1361 $[M + Na]^+$, which was supported by the ^{13}C NMR spectrum.

A close inspection of the ^1H and ^{13}C NMR data of 9 (Table 3, Figures S39–S41) revealed the presence of two methyl groups (δ_C 27.9, 21.6; δ_H 1.40, 0.97), three sp^3-methylene groups (δ_C 37.8 (2C), 18.0; δ_H 1.71, 1.59, 1.54, 1.45, 1.32, 1.10), two oxygen-bearing sp^3-methylene groups (δ_C 68.1, 65.6; δ_H 4.94, 4.79, 3.94, 3.26), three sp^3-methine groups (δ_C 70.0, 64.1, 48.6; δ_H 4.00, 3.99, 1.57), including two oxygen-bearing, two quaternary sp^3-carbons (δ_C 38.3, 36.3), and three quaternary sp^2-carbons (δ_C 173.4, 173.1, 122.1).

The HMBC correlations (Table 3, Figure S42) from H-6 (δ_H 3.99) to C-5 (δ_C 48.6), C-7 (δ_C 64.1), C-8 (δ_C 122.1), C-9 (δ_C 173.1), and C-10 (δ_C 36.3), from H-7 (δ_H 4.00) to C-12 (δ_C 173.4), from H_2-11 (δ_H 4.94, 4.79) to C-8, C-9, and C-12, from H_3-13 (δ_H 0.97) to C-3 (δ_C 37.8), C-4 (δ_C 38.3), C-5, and C-14 (δ_C 65.6), from H_3-15 (δ_H 1.40) to C-1 (δ_C 37.8), C-5, C-9, and C-10 indicated the drimane moiety in 9 being the same as in 7α,14-dihydroxy-6β-p-nitrobenzoylconfertifolin [8].

The ROESY correlations (Figure 5 and Figure S43) of H_3-13 with H-5 (δ_H 1.57), H-6 (δ_H 3.99), and H-7 (δ_H 4.00), of H_3-15 with H_2-14 (δ_H 3.94, 3.26), together with the coupling constant $^3J_{H6-H7}$ = 2.1 Hz indicated the related configurations of the chiral centers in 9 as depicted (Figure 1). Compound 9 was named 6β,7β,14-trihydroxyconfertifolin.

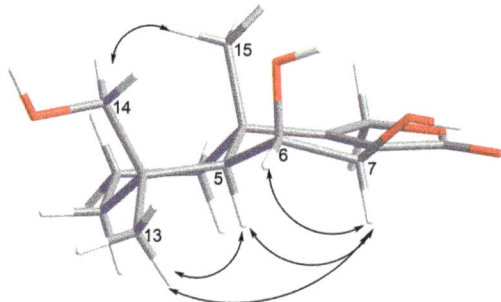

Figure 5. Key ROESY correlations of 9.

Besides the new compounds **1,2,4,7**, and **9**, the known dihydroaspirone (**3**) [14], aspertetranones D (**5**) [5,6] and A (**6**) [5], insulicolide A (**8**) [15], and 7α,14-dihydroxy-6β-p-nitrobenzoylconfertifolin (**10**) [8] were isolated from this fungal strain.

All isolated compounds were tested for cytotoxicity toward murine neuroblastoma Neuro-2a cells (Table 4). Compound 7 demonstrated cytotoxic activity toward Neuro-2a cell, with the IC_{50} of 24.1 µM, while its analogue 9 was non-cytotoxic up to 100 µM. The highest activity was demonstrated for 9α,14-dihydroxy-6β-p-nitrobenzoylcinnamolide (**8**), with IC_{50} of 4.9 µM, while its analogue **10** did not affect the viability of Neuro-2a cells. Compounds **1–6** were non-cytotoxic against Neuro-2a cells at concentrations up to 100 µM.

Then, we investigated the effect of the compounds **1–10** on the viability and colony formation ability of human drug-resistant prostate cancer 22Rv1 cells (Table 4). MTT assay revealed the compounds **7** and **8** to be cytotoxic in 22Rv1 cells, with IC_{50} values of 31.5 µM and 3.0 µM, respectively. Compounds **1–6, 9**, and **10** were non-cytotoxic against these cells at concentrations up to 100 µM. In this model, docetaxel (positive control) showed cytotoxicity, with IC_{50} of 0.02 µM. At the same time, compounds **4** and **9** were able to inhibit the colony formation of 22Rv1 prostate cancer cells (in vitro prototype of in vivo anti-metastatic activity) for 41% and 36%, respectively, at 100 µM. It is known that 22Rv1 cells are resistant to hormone therapy because they express the androgen receptor splice variant AR-V7 [20].

The compounds which demonstrated cytotoxic activity toward AR-V7-positive 22Rv1 cells therefore may be promising for the therapy of human drug-resistant prostate cancer.

Table 4. Cytotoxic effects of the isolated compounds 1–10.

Compounds	Cytotoxicity IC$_{50}$, µM			Colony Formation, %
	Neuro-2a	22Rv1	MCF-7	22Rv1
1	>100	>100	nt	-
2	>100	>100	nt	-
3	>100	>100	nt	-
4	>100	>100	nt	41
5	>100	>100	nt	-
6	>100	>100	nt	-
7	24.1	31.5	>100	-
8	4.9	3.0	59.6	-
9	>100	>100	>100	36
10	>100	>100	>100	-
Docetaxel	nt	0.02	nt	nt

"nt": compound was not tested; "-": compound did not demonstrate any effect at the concentration of 100 µM.

Finally, the new compounds **7** and **9** were tested for cytotoxicity toward human breast cancer cells MCF-7 and did not show any effect up to 100 µM (Table 4). Additionally, the known compounds **8** and **10** were examined in this experiment as reference substances. Compound **8** showed a weak cytotoxic effect, with IC$_{50}$ of 59.6 µM, whereas, previously, a higher cytotoxicity of **8** toward MCF-7 cells was reported (IC$_{50}$ = 6.08 µM) [11]. This could be explained by different treatment times used by us (24 h) in comparison with those used by Fang and colleagues (72 h) [11]. Moreover, different amounts of cells per well were used. Note, compound **10** was non-cytotoxic up to 100 µM.

The analysis of structure–activity relationships of compounds **7–10**, together with literature data, showed that these compounds have three relevant structural sites. First, a double bond at C7=C8 as part of an α,β-unsaturated lactone. Previously, it was shown that the cytotoxicity of such moiety can be explained by a nucleophilic Michael addition reaction with biological nucleophiles [8,21]. In the case of the non-cytotoxic compounds **9** and **10**, the double bond of the α,β-unsuturated lactone may be inaccessible for a nucleophile attack because of steric obstacles. Second, a hydroxyl group at C-9 in the drimane core is also essential for cytotoxicity. In fact, a recent report of a series of similar compounds revealed the most pronounced cytotoxicity for compounds possessing a 9-OH group [9]. Finally, our results strongly suggest that the presence of a *p*-nitrobenzoyl moiety significantly enhances the cytotoxic activity. Previously, Tan et al. [9] demonstrated that the nitrobezoylation of 6-OH increased the cytotoxicity of related compounds towards human renal cell carcinoma cells compared with that of 14-OH-derivatives. At the same time, it should be noted that another study of 6- and 14-nitrobenzoate derivatives cytotoxicity toward other cancer cell lines did not support this observation [11].

3. Materials and Methods

3.1. General Experimental Procedures

Optical rotations were measured on a Perkin-Elmer 343 polarimeter (Perkin Elmer, Waltham, MA, USA). UV spectra were recorded on a Specord UV–vis spectrometer (Carl Zeiss, Jena, Germany) in methanol. NMR spectra were recorded in CDCl$_3$, acetone-d_6 and DMSO-d_6 with Bruker DPX-500 (Bruker BioSpin GmbH, Rheinstetten, Germany) and Bruker DRX-700 (Bruker BioSpin GmbH, Rheinstetten, Germany) spectrometers, using TMS as an internal standard. HRESIMS spectra were measured on a Maxis impact mass spectrometer (Bruker Daltonics GmbH, Rheinstetten, Germany).

Low-pressure liquid column chromatography was performed using silica gel (50/100 µm, Imid, Russia). Plates (4.5 cm × 6.0 cm) precoated with silica gel (5–17 µm, Imid) were used for thin-layer chromatography. Preparative HPLC was carried out with a Shimadzu LC-20 chromatograph (Shimadzu

USA Manufacturing, Canby, OR, USA) using YMC ODS-AM (YMC Co., Ishikawa, Japan) (5 μm, 10 mm × 250 mm) and YMC SIL (YMC Co., Ishikawa, Japan) (5 μm, 10 mm × 250 mm) columns with a Shimadzu RID-20A refractometer (Shimadzu Corporation, Kyoto, Japan).

3.2. Fungal Strain

The strain of *A. flocculosus* was isolated from a sediment sample (Nha Trang Bay, South China Sea, Vietnam) and identified as described earlier [12]. The strain is stored at the collection of microorganisms of Nha Trang Institute of Technology and Research Application VAST (Nha Trang, Vietnam) under the code 01NT.1.12.3.

3.3. Cultivation of the Fungus

The fungus was cultured at 28 °C for three weeks in 50 × 500 mL Erlenmeyer flasks, each containing rice (20.0 g), yeast extract (20.0 mg), KH_2PO_4 (10 mg), and natural sea water from Nha Trang Bay (40 mL).

3.4. Extraction and Isolation

The fungal mycelia of *A. flocculosus* with the medium were extracted for 24 h with 15 L of EtOAc. Evaporation of the solvent, under reduced pressure, gave a dark brown oil (5.0 g), to which 250 mL H_2O–EtOH (4:1) was added, and the mixture was thoroughly stirred to yield a suspension. It was extracted, successively, with hexane (150 mL × 2), EtOAc (150 mL × 2), and n-BuOH (150 mL × 2). After evaporation of the EtOAc layer, the residual materials (3.36 g) were passed over a silica gel column (35.0 cm × 2.5 cm), which was eluted with a hexane–EtOAc gradient (1:0–0:1). The n-hexane–EtOAc (80:20, 1.3 g) fraction was purified by a Sephadex LH-20 column (80 cm × 2 cm, 50 g) with $CHCl_3$ to yield compound **8** (245 mg). The n-hexane–EtOAc (75:25) fraction AF-1-64 (393 mg) was purified by HPLC on a YMC-SIL column eluting with $CHCl_3$–MeOH–NH_4OAc (97:3:1) to yield compounds **3** (220 mg) and **4** (11 mg). The n-hexane–EtOAc (75:25) fraction AF-1-67 (483 mg) was purified by HPLC on a YMC-SIL column eluting with $CHCl_3$–MeOH–NH_4OAc (97:3:1) to yield compounds **5** (5.9 mg), **7** (9.0 mg), and **10** (3.1 mg). The n-hexane–EtOAc (75:25) fraction AF-1-88 (68.3 mg) was purified by HPLC on a YMC-SIL column eluting with $CHCl_3$–MeOH–NH_4OAc (97:3:1) to yield compounds **1** (2.9 mg) and **2** (3.8 mg). The n-hexane–EtOAc (70:30) fraction AF-1-93 (784 mg) was purified by HPLC first on a YMC-SIL column eluting with $CHCl_3$–MeOH–NH_4OAc (97:3:1) and then on a YMC ODS-AM column, eluting with MeOH–H_2O (55:45) to yield compound **9** (5.5 mg). The n-hexane–EtOAc (60:40, 282 mg) fraction was purified by Sephadex LH-20 column (80 cm × 2 cm, 50 g) with $CHCl_3$-EtOH (3:1) to yield compound **6** (68 mg).

Aspilactonol F (**1**): white powder; $[\alpha]_D^{20}$ +98 (c 0.20, MeOH); UV (MeOH) λ_{max} (log ε) 214 (4.03) nm; ECD (0.9 mM, MeOH) λ_{max} (Δε) 217 (+11.35) nm; ^1H and ^{13}C NMR data see Table 1, Figures S1–S7; HR ESIMS m/z 209.0785 [M + Na]$^+$ (calcd. for $C_9H_{14}O_4Na$, 209.0784, Δ −0.1 ppm).

Aspilactonol G (**2**): white powder; $[\alpha]_D^{20}$ −49 (c 0.49, MeOH); UV (MeOH) λ_{max} (log ε) 214 (4.05) nm; ECD (1.1 mM, MeOH) λ_{max} (Δε) 216 (−11.51) nm; ^1H and ^{13}C NMR data see Table 1, Figures S9–S16; HRESIMS m/z 209.0782 [M + Na]$^+$ (calcd. for $C_9H_{14}O_4Na$, 209.0784, Δ +1.1 ppm).

12-*Epi*-aspertetranone D (**4**): white powder; $[\alpha]_D^{20}$ +78 (c 0.07, MeOH); UV (MeOH) λ_{max} (log ε) 290 (3.93), 208 (4.53) nm; ECD (0.5 mM, MeOH) λ_{max} (Δε) 209 (+25.54), 284 (+1.86) nm; ^1H and ^{13}C NMR data see Table 2, Figures S20–S26; HRESIMS m/z 459.1628 [M + Na]$^+$ (calcd. for $C_{22}H_{28}O_9Na$, 459.1626, Δ −0.2 ppm).

6β,9α,14-trihydroxycinnamolide (**7**): white crystals; $[\alpha]_D^{20}$ −7.3 (c 0.15, MeOH); UV (MeOH) λ_{max} (log ε) 206 (3.61) nm; ECD (2.8 mM, MeOH) λ_{max} (Δε) 224 (−2.33) nm; ^1H and ^{13}C NMR data see Table 3, Figures S30–S36; HRESIMS m/z 305.1361 [M + Na]$^+$ (calcd. for $C_{15}H_{22}O_5Na$, 305.1359, Δ −0.5 ppm).

6β,7β,14-trihydroxyconfertifolin (**9**): white crystals; $[\alpha]_D^{20}$ +93.5 (*c* 0.36, MeOH); UV (MeOH) λ_{max} (log ε) 214 (4.00) nm; ECD (1.1 mM, MeOH) λ_{max} (Δε) 217 (+3.68), 243 (+1.51) nm; ^{1}H and ^{13}C NMR data see Table 3, Figures S39–S47; HRESIMS *m/z* 305.1361 [M + Na]$^+$ (calcd. for $C_{15}H_{22}O_5Na$, 305.1359, Δ −0.5 ppm).

3.5. Preparation of (S)-MTPA and (R)-MTPA Esters of Aspilactonol F (1)

The compounds 4-dimethylaminopyridine (a few crystals) and (*R*)-MTPA-Cl (4 μL) were added to a solution of **1** (1.0 mg) in pyridine at room temperature and stirred for 5 h. After evaporation of the solvent, the residue was purified by HPLC on a YMC SIL column (EtOAc–hexane, 20:80) to afford the (*S*)-MTPA ester (0.5 mg). The (*R*)-MTPA ester (0.5 mg) was prepared in a similar manner using (*S*)-MTPA-Cl.

(*S*)-MTPA ester of **1**: ^{1}H NMR (CDCl$_3$, 500.13 MHz) δ: 6.88 (1H, brs, H-4), 5.28-5.34 (2H, m, H-6, H-9), 4.84 (1H, dd, *J* = 3.9; 1.7 Hz, H-5), 3.48 (3H, s, OMe), 3.43 (3H, s, OMe), 2.56-2.60 (2H, m, H$_2$-8), 1.26 (3H, d, *J* = 6.5 Hz, Me-7), 1.24 (3H, d, *J* = 6.3 Hz, Me-10), 7.39–7.48 (10H, m, 2Ph). HRESIMS *m/z* 641.1576 [M + Na]$^+$ (calcd for $C_{29}H_{28}F_6Na$, 641.1581, Δ = 0.8 ppm).

(*R*)-MTPA ester of **1**: ^{1}H NMR (CDCl$_3$, 500.13 MHz) δ: 6.52 (1H, brs, H-4), 5.25 (1H, m, H-9), 5.20 (1H, dd, *J* = 6.6, 4.3 Hz, H-6), 4.56 (1H, dd, *J* = 4.3, 1.6 Hz, Hz, H-5), 3.56 (3H, s, OMe), 3.50 (3H, s, OMe), 2.48-2.51 (2H, m, H$_2$-8), 1.35 (3H, d, *J* = 6.2 Hz, Me-10), 1.29 (3H, d, *J* = 6.6 Hz, Me-7), 7.38–7.52 (10H, m, 2Ph). HRESIMS *m/z* 641.1577 [M + Na]$^+$ (calcd for $C_{29}H_{28}F_6Na$, 641.1581, Δ = 0.6 ppm).

3.6. Preparation of (S)-MTPA and (R)-MTPA Esters of Aspilactonol G (2)

(*R*)-MTPA-Cl (9 μL) was added to a solution of **2** (1.9 mg) in pyridine at room temperature and stirred for 2 h. After evaporation of the solvent, the residue was purified by HPLC on a YMC SIL column (acetone–hexane, 25:75) to afford the (*S*)-MTPA ester (1.4 mg). The (*R*)-MTPA ester (1.5 mg) was prepared in a similar manner using (*S*)-MTPA-Cl.

(*S*)-MTPA ester of **2**: ^{1}H NMR (CDCl$_3$, 700 MHz) δ: 6.86 (1H, brs, H-4), 5.32 (1H, m, H-9), 5.23 (1H, m, H-6), 4.81 (1H, brd, *J* = 5.0 Hz, H-5), 3.52 (3H, s, OMe), 3.47 (3H, s, OMe), 2.65 (1H, dd, *J* = 15.8; 6.9, H-8), 2.48 (1H, ddt, *J* = 15.9; 5.0; 1.5, H-8), 1.39 (3H, d, *J* = 6.5 Hz, Me-7), 1.29 (3H, d, *J* = 6.2 Hz, Me-10), 7.38–7.50 (10H, m, 2Ph). HRESIMS *m/z* 641.1576 [M + Na]$^+$ (calcd for $C_{29}H_{28}F_6Na$, 641.1581, Δ = 0.8 ppm).

(*R*)-MTPA ester of **2**: ^{1}H NMR (CDCl$_3$, 700 MHz) δ: 6.68 (1H, brs, H-4), 5.30 (1H, m, H-9), 5.26 (1H, m, H-6), 4.82 (1H, m, Hz, H-5), 3.53 (3H, s, OMe), 3.48 (3H, s, OMe), 2.61 (1H, dd, *J* = 15.9; 7.2, H-8), 2.46 (1H, dd, *J* = 15.9; 4.7, H-8), 1.33 (3H, d, *J* = 6.3 Hz, Me-10), 1.25 (3H, d, *J* = 6.7 Hz, Me-7), 7.37–7.52 (10H, m, 2Ph). HRESIMS *m/z* 641.1576 [M + Na]$^+$ (calcd for $C_{29}H_{28}F_6Na$, 641.1581, Δ = 0.8 ppm).

3.7. Cell Culture

All cell lines used in this investigation were purchased from ATCC.

The neuroblastoma cell line Neuro-2a and the human breast cancer cell line MCF-7 were cultured in DMEM medium containing 10% fetal bovine serum (Biolot, St. Petersburg, Russia) and 1% penicillin/streptomycin (Invitrogen, Carlsbad, CA, USA).

The human prostate cancer cell line 22Rv1 was cultured according to the manufacturer's instructions in 10% FBS/RPMI medium (Invitrogen). Cells were continuously kept in culture for a maximum of 3 months, were routinely inspected microscopically for stable phenotype, and regularly checked for contamination with mycoplasma. Cell line authentication was performed by DSMZ (Braunschweig, Germany) using highly polymorphic short tandem repeat loci [22].

All cells were incubated at 37 °C in a humidified atmosphere containing 5% (*v/v*) CO_2.

3.8. Cytotoxicity Assay

The in vitro cytotoxicity of individual substances was evaluated using the MTT assay, which was performed as previously described [23]. Docetaxel was used as a control.

3.9. Colony Formation Assay

The colony formation assay was performed as described before with slight modifications [22]. 22Rv1 cells were treated with the testing compounds for 48 h and then were trypsinized. The number of alive cells was counted with the trypan blue exclusion assay as described before [24]. In total, 100 viable cells were plated into each well of six-well plates in complete fresh medium (3 mL/well) and were incubated for 14 days. Then, the medium was aspirated, and the surviving colonies were fixed with 100% MeOH, followed by washing with PBS, and air-drying at RT. Next, the cells were incubated with a Giemsa staining solution was for 25 min at RT, the staining solution was aspirated, and the wells were rinsed with dH$_2$O and air-dried. The number of cell colonies was counted by naked eye.

4. Conclusions

A new aspyrone-related polyketide, aspilactonol G (**2**), a new meroterpenoid, 12-*epi*-aspertetranone D (**4**), two new drimane derivatives (**7,9**), together with six known metabolites were isolated from the Vietnamese marine sediment-derived fungus *A. flocculosus*. The structures of compounds **1–10** were established using spectroscopic methods. The absolute configurations of chiral centers were determined using either a modified Mosher's method (for compounds **1** and **2**) or a combination of ROESY data, coupling constants analysis and biogenetic considerations for compounds **4, 7** and **9**. Drimane sesquiterpenoid derivatives **7** and **8** showed cytotoxicity toward human prostate cancer 22Rv1, human breast cancer MCF-7, and murine neuroblastoma Neuro-2a cells. The analysis of structure–activity relationships of compounds **7–10** together with literature data showed that these compounds have three sites in their structures related to cytotoxicity, i.e., a double bond at C7=C8, a hydroxyl group at C-9, and a *p*-nitrobenzoyl moiety.

Supplementary Materials: The following are available online at http://www.mdpi.com/1660-3397/17/10/579/s1, Figures S1–S57: 1D and 2D NMR spectra and ECD spectra of compounds **1–10**.

Author Contributions: Conceptualization, A.N.Y.; Data curation, P.T.H.T. and S.A.D.; Formal analysis, E.V.G., O.F.S., A.B.R., R.S.P., S.A.D. and E.S.M.; Funding acquisition, G.v.A., T.T.T.V. and S.S.A.; Investigation, P.T.H.T., E.V.G., O.F.S., A.B.R., R.S.P., S.A.D. and E.S.M.; Methodology, A.N.Y.; Project administration, T.T.T.V. and S.S.A.; Resources, A.N.Y., G.v.A. and S.S.A.; Supervision, G.v.A., T.T.T.V. and S.S.A.; Validation, A.N.Y. and S.A.D.; Visualization, A.N.Y.; Writing—original draft, A.N.Y., P.T.H.T. and S.A.D.; Writing—review ' editing, A.N.Y., G.v.A., T.T.T.V. and S.S.A.

Funding: The study was supported by the Russian Science Foundation (grant No 19-74-10014 for the chemical study of compounds **7–10**), by the Russian Foundation of Basic Research (grants No 18-34-00737 for the cytotoxicity study on MCF-7 and Neuro-2A, No 19-53-54002 for the chemical study of compounds **1–6** and cytotoxicity study), and by the Vietnam Academy of Science and Technology (grant No QTRU01.03/19-20) for microbiology.

Acknowledgments: The study was carried out on the equipment of the Collective Facilities Center "The Far Eastern Center for Structural Molecular Research (NMR/MS) PIBOC FEB RAS". The authors thank Ekaterina A. Yurchenko (PIBOC FEB RAS, Vladivostok, Russia) for valuable comments in the work and writing of the article and Natalya Yu. Kim (PIBOC FEB RAS, Vladivostok, Russia) for CD spectra acquisition. The authors are grateful to Andrea Speckmann and Dipl.-Ing. Jessica Hauschild (Universitätsklinikum Hamburg-Eppendorf, Hamburg, Germany) for assistance in the performance of the biological experiments and data analysis

Conflicts of Interest: The authors declare no conflict of interest.

References

1. Carroll, A.R.; Copp, B.R.; Davis, R.A.; Keyzers, R.A.; Prinsep, M.R. Marine natural products. *Nat. Prod. Rep.* **2019**, *36*, 122–173. [CrossRef] [PubMed]
2. Varga, J.; Tóth, B.; Rigó, K.; Téren, J.; Hoekstra, R.F.; Kozakiewicz, Z. Phylogenetic analysis of *aspergillus* section *circumdati* based on sequences of the internal transcribed spacer regions and the 5.8 S rRNA gene. *Fungal Genet. Biol.* **2000**, *30*, 71–80. [CrossRef] [PubMed]
3. Fuchser, J.; Zeeck, A. Secondary metabolites by chemical screening, 34—Aspinolides and Aspinonene/Aspyrone co-metabolites, new pentaketides produced by *aspergillus ochraceus*. *Liebigs Ann.* **1997**, *1997*, 87–95. [CrossRef]

4. Liu, Y.; Li, X.M.; Meng, L.H.; Wang, B.G. Polyketides from the marine mangrove-derived fungus *aspergillus ochraceus* ma-15 and their activity against aquatic pathogenic bacteria. *Phytochem. Lett.* **2015**, *12*, 232–236. [CrossRef]
5. Wang, Y.; Qi, S.; Zhan, Y.; Zhang, N.; Wu, A.A.; Gui, F.; Guo, K.; Yang, Y.; Cao, S.; Hu, Z.; et al. Aspertetranones a-d, putative meroterpenoids from the marine algal-associated fungus *aspergillus* sp. ZL0-1b14. *J. Nat. Prod.* **2015**, *78*, 2405–2410. [CrossRef]
6. Wang, J.; Wei, X.; Qin, X.; Tian, X.; Liao, L.; Li, K.; Zhou, X.; Yang, X.; Wang, F.; Zhang, T.; et al. Antiviral merosesquiterpenoids produced by the antartic fungus *aspergillus ochraceopetaliformis* SCSIO 05702. *J. Nat. Prod.* **2016**, *79*, 59–65. [CrossRef] [PubMed]
7. Shin, H.J.; Choi, B.K.; Trinh, P.T.H.; Lee, H.S.; Kang, J.S.; Van, T.T.T.; Lee, H.S.; Lee, J.S.; Lee, Y.J.; Lee, J. Suppression of rankl-induced osteoclastogenesis by the metabolites from the marine fungus *aspergillus flocculosus* isolated from a sponge *stylissa* sp. *Mar. Drugs* **2018**, *16*, 14. [CrossRef]
8. Belofsky, G.N.; Jensen, P.R.; Renner, M.K.; Fenical, W. New cytotoxic sesquiterpenoid nitrobenzoyl esters from a marine isolate of the fungus *aspergillus versicolor*. *Tetrahedron* **1998**, *54*, 1715–1724. [CrossRef]
9. Tan, Y.; Yang, B.; Lin, X.; Luo, X.; Pang, X.; Tang, L.; Liu, Y.; Li, X.; Zhou, X. Nitrobenzoyl sesquiterpenoids with cytotoxic activities from a marine-derived *aspergillus ochraceus* fungus. *J. Nat. Prod.* **2018**, *81*, 92–97. [CrossRef]
10. Zheng, J.; Wang, Y.; Wang, J.; Liu, P.; Li, J.; Zhu, W. Antimicrobial ergosteroids and pyrrole derivatives from halotolerant *aspergillus flocculosus* PT05-1 cultured in a hypersaline medium. *Extrem. Life Under Extrem. Cond.* **2013**, *17*, 963–971. [CrossRef]
11. Fang, W.; Lin, X.; Zhou, X.; Wan, J.; Lu, X.; Yang, B.; Ai, W.; Lin, J.; Zhang, T.; Tu, Z.; et al. Cytotoxic and antiviral nitrobenzoyl sesquiterpenoids from the marine-derived fungus *aspergillus ochraceus* Jcma1F17. *MedChemComm* **2014**, *5*, 701–705. [CrossRef]
12. Yurchenko, E.A.; Menchinskaya, E.S.; Pislyagin, E.A.; Trinh, P.T.H.; Ivanets, E.V.; Smetanina, O.F.; Yurchenko, A.N. Neuroprotective activity of some marine fungal metabolites in the 6-hydroxydopamin- and paraquat-induced parkinson's disease models. *Mar. Drugs* **2018**, *16*, 457. [CrossRef] [PubMed]
13. Kito, K.; Ookura, R.; Yoshida, S.; Namikoshi, M.; Ooi, T.; Kusumi, T. Pentaketides relating to aspinonene and dihydroaspyrone from a marine-derived fungus, *aspergillus ostianus*. *J. Nat. Prod.* **2007**, *70*, 2022–2025. [CrossRef] [PubMed]
14. Chen, X.W.; Li, C.W.; Cui, C.B.; Hua, W.; Zhu, T.J.; Gu, Q.Q. Nine new and five known polyketides derived from a deep sea-sourced *aspergillus* sp. 16-02-1. *Mar. Drugs* **2014**, *12*, 3116–3137. [CrossRef] [PubMed]
15. Rahbaek, L.; Christophersen, C.; Frisvad, J.; Bengaard, H.S.; Larsen, S.; Rassing, B.R. Insulicolide a: A new nitrobenzoyloxy-substituted sesquiterpene from the marine fungus *aspergillus insulicola*. *J. Nat. Prod.* **1997**, *60*, 811–813. [CrossRef]
16. Zhao, H.Y.; Anbuchezhian, R.; Sun, W.; Shao, C.L.; Zhang, F.L.; Yin, Y.; Yu, Z.S.; Li, Z.Y.; Wang, C.Y. Cytotoxic nitrobenzoyloxy-substituted sesquiterpenes from spongederived endozoic fungus *aspergillus insulicola* md10-2. *Curr. Pharm. Biotechnol.* **2016**, *17*, 271–274. [CrossRef] [PubMed]
17. Smetanina, O.F.; Yurchenko, A.N.; Ivanets, E.V.; Kalinovsky, A.I.; Khudyakova, Y.V.; Dyshlovoy, S.A.; Von Amsberg, G.; Yurchenko, E.A.; Afiyatullov, S.S. Unique prostate cancer-toxic polyketides from marine sediment-derived fungus *isaria felina*. *J. Antibiot.* **2017**, *70*, 856–858. [CrossRef]
18. Yurchenko, A.; Smetanina, O.; Ivanets, E.; Kalinovsky, A.; Khudyakova, Y.; Kirichuk, N.; Popov, R.; Bokemeyer, C.; von Amsberg, G.; Chingizova, E.; et al. Pretrichodermamides d–f from a marine algicolous fungus *penicillium* sp. KMM 4672. *Mar. Drugs* **2016**, *14*, 122. [CrossRef]
19. Gawronski, J.K.; Van Oeveren, A.; Van Der Deen, H.; Leung, C.W.; Feringa, B.L. Simple circular dichroic method for the determination of absolute configuration of 5-substituted 2(5H)-furanones. *J. Org. Chem.* **1996**, *61*, 1513–1515. [CrossRef]
20. Liu, C.; Lou, W.; Zhu, Y.; Nadiminty, N.; Schwartz, C.T.; Evans, C.P.; Gao, A.C. Niclosamide inhibits androgen receptor variants expression and overcomes enzalutamide resistance in castration-resistant prostate cancer. *Clin. Cancer Res.* **2014**, *20*, 3198–3210. [CrossRef]
21. Beekman, A.C.; Woerdenbag, H.J.; Van Uden, W.; Pras, N.; Konings, A.W.T.; Wikström, H.V.; Schmidt, T.J. Structure-cytotoxicity relationships of some helenanolide-type sesquiterpene lactones. *J. Nat. Prod.* **1997**, *60*, 252–257. [CrossRef] [PubMed]

22. Dyshlovoy, S.A.; Menchinskaya, E.S.; Venz, S.; Rast, S.; Amann, K.; Hauschild, J.; Otte, K.; Kalinin, V.I.; Silchenko, A.S.; Avilov, S.A.; et al. The marine triterpene glycoside frondoside a exhibits activity in vitro and in vivo in prostate cancer. *Int. J. Cancer* **2016**, *138*, 2450–2465. [CrossRef] [PubMed]
23. Dyshlovoy, S.A.; Venz, S.; Shubina, L.K.; Fedorov, S.N.; Walther, R.; Jacobsen, C.; Stonik, V.A.; Bokemeyer, C.; Balabanov, S.; Honecker, F. Activity of aaptamine and two derivatives, demethyloxyaaptamine and isoaaptamine, in cisplatin-resistant germ cell cancer. *J. Proteom.* **2014**, *96*, 223–239. [CrossRef] [PubMed]
24. Dyshlovoy, S.A.; Hauschild, J.; Amann, K.; Tabakmakher, K.M.; Venz, S.; Walther, R.; Guzii, A.G.; Makarieva, T.N.; Shubina, L.K.; Fedorov, S.N.; et al. Marine alkaloid monanchocidin a overcomes drug resistance by induction of autophagy and lysosomal membrane permeabilization. *Oncotarget* **2015**, *6*, 17328–17341. [CrossRef] [PubMed]

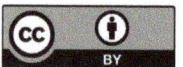

© 2019 by the authors. Licensee MDPI, Basel, Switzerland. This article is an open access article distributed under the terms and conditions of the Creative Commons Attribution (CC BY) license (http://creativecommons.org/licenses/by/4.0/).

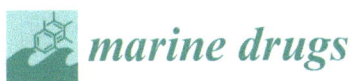

Article

Ubiquitin-Proteasome Modulating Dolabellanes and Secosteroids from Soft Coral *Clavularia flava*

Che-Yen Chiu [1,†], Xue-Hua Ling [1,†], Shang-Kwei Wang [2,*] and Chang-Yih Duh [1,*]

1. Department of Marine Biotechnology and Resources, National Sun Yat-Sen University, Kaohsiung 80441, Taiwan; m025020014@student.nsysu.edu.tw (C.-Y.C.); cooley@mail.nsysu.edu.tw (X.-H.L.)
2. Department of Microbiology and Immunology, Kaohsiung Medical University, Kaohsiung 80708, Taiwan
* Correspondence: skwang@kmu.edu.tw (S.-K.W.); yihduh@mail.nsysu.edu.tw (C.-Y.D.);
Tel.: +886-7-312-1101 (ext. 2150-23) (S.-K.W.); +886-7-525-2000 (ext. 5036) (C.-Y.D.)
† These authors contributed equally to this work.

Received: 10 December 2019; Accepted: 30 December 2019; Published: 3 January 2020

Abstract: We performed a high-content screening (HCS) assay aiming to discover bioactive molecules with proteasome inhibitory activity. By structural elucidation, we identified six compounds purified from soft coral *Clavularia flava*, which potentiates proteasome inhibition. Chemical structure elucidation revealed they are dolabellane- and secosteroid-based compounds including a new dolabellane, clavinflol C (**1**), three known dolabellanes, stolonidiol (**2**), stolonidiol-17-acetate (**3**), and clavinflol B (**4**) as well as two new secosteroids, $3\beta,11$-dihydroxy-24-methyl-9,11-secocholest-5-en-9,23-dione (**5**) and $3\beta,11$-dihydroxy-24-methylene-9,11-secocholest-5-en-9,23-dione (**6**). All six compounds show less cytotoxicity than those of known proteasome inhibitors, bortezomib and MG132. In summary, the high-content measurements of control inhibitors, bortezomib and MG132, manifest the highest ratio >2 in high-content measurement. Of the isolated compounds, **2** and **5** showed higher activity, followed by **3** and **6**, and then **1** and **4** exhibited moderate inhibition.

Keywords: proteasome inhibition; dolabellane; secosteroids; soft coral

1. Introduction

Marine natural products harbor unique chemical structures and exhibit diverse biological activity with potential therapeutic utilities that merit investigation [1]. Synthetic drugs with proteasome inhibition, Velcade (bortezomib), Kyprolis (carfilzomib), and Ninlaro (ixazomib), exemplify therapeutic efficacy for the treatment of multiple myeloma [2,3]. In an effort to develop target-direct drug screening assay, we validated a sensitive and efficient high-content screening assay for discovery of proteasome inhibitor. Our initial efforts identified four natural products of soft corals cembrane-based compounds (sarcophytonin A, sarcophytoxide, sarcophine, and laevigatol A) which potentiate proteasome inhibition [4]. We postulate that proteasome inhibitors may benefit the ecosystem of soft coral reef holobiont. Therefore, we continued the drug screening in an effort to identify marine natural products purified from Formosan soft corals in our laboratory. In this study, we demonstrated the identification of six compounds with proteasome inhibitory activity. Structure elucidation revealed they are dolabellane- and secosteroid-based compounds including a new dolabellane, clavinflol C (**1**), three known dolabellanes, stolonidiol (**2**), stolonidiol-17-acetate (**3**), and clavinflol B (**4**) as well as two new secosteroids, $3\beta,11$-dihydroxy-24-methyl-9,11-secocholest-5-en-9,23-dione (**5**) and $3\beta,11$-dihydroxy-24-methylene-9,11-secocholest-5-en-9,23-dione (**6**) (Figure 1).

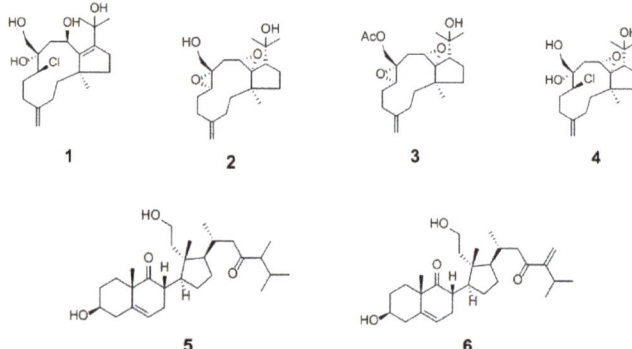

Figure 1. Marine natural products exhibit proteasome inhibition by high-content assays. Dolabellanes are clavinflol C (**1**), stolonidiol (**2**), stolonidiol-17-acetate (**3**), and clavinflol B (**4**). Secosteroids are 3β,11-dihydroxy-24-methyl-9,11-secocholest-5-en-9,23-dione (**5**) and 3β,11-dihydroxy-24-methylene-9,11-secocholest-5-en-9,23-dione (**6**).

2. Results

2.1. Compound Purification and Structure Elucidation

Chromatographic fractionation of ethyl acetate solubles from *C. flava* afforded four dolabellane diterpenes, **1–4**, as well as two secosteroids, **5** and **6**. The three known dolabellane diterpenes, **2–4** were identified by comparison of their spectral data with those of reported literatures [5,6]. The structures of new compounds, **1**, **5**, and **6** were elucidated by analysis of 1D and 2D spectral data (Figures S1–S24).

Clavinflol C (**1**) had a molecular formula of $C_{20}H_{33}O_4Cl$ as deduced from HR-ESI-MS (Figure S1) and NMR data. Its IR bands (Figure S2) indicated the presence of exo-methylene (1,639, 961 cm^{-1}) and hydroxyl (3343 cm^{-1}) groups. The ^{1}H NMR data of **1** (Figure S3) showed a pair of exo-methylene singlets (δ 4.91, 5.00) and an AB quartet for hydroxy-methyl group (δ 3.39, 3.82, J = 11.6 Hz), three methyl singlets (δ 1.03, 1.32, 1.40), an oxygenated methine proton (δ 4.18), and a chlorinated methine proton (δ 4.00). To determine the proton sequence of **1**, a COSY spectrum (Figure S6) revealed the connectivities of H-2/H-3, H-5/H-6/H-7, H-9/H-10, and H-13/H-14. The ^{13}C NMR (Figure S4) and HSQC spectra (Figure S5) of **1** showed signals for three methyl carbons, eight methylene carbons including the exomethylene (δ 113.9, 147.7), two methine carbons, and five quaternary carbons. Detailed analyses of the ^{1}H, ^{13}C NMR, and HSQC spectra revealed that **1** is a dolabellane diterpene with a 5/11 membered ring and a tetrasubstituted olefin at the C-11/C-12 positions. This type of skeleton was further confirmed from the observation of long range correlations of H$_2$-16/C-3, C-5; H$_2$-2/C-4; H$_2$-7/C-8, C-17; H-10/C-1, C-7, C-8, C-9, C-11, H$_3$-15/C-1, C-2, C-11, C-13; H$_2$-13/C-1, C-11, C-12; H$_2$-14/ C-11, C-12; H$_3$-19/C-12, C-18, C-20; H$_3$-20/C-12, C-18, C-19 in the HMBC spectrum (Figure S7). The relative stereochemistry of **1** was determined from NOESY experiments as illustrated in Figure S8. Assuming that H$_3$-15 is α-oriented, key NOESY correlations from H$_3$-15 to H-10 and from H-7 to H-10 suggested that H-10 and H-7 were in the α-orientation. NOESY correlations between H-9a/H-6a and H-9b/H-17b suggested that OH-8 was in the β-orientation.

Compound **5** was isolated as a white amorphous powder, showing a pseudo-molecular ion peak at *m/z* 469.32880 [M + Na]$^+$ in the HR-ESI-MS (Figure S9), consistent with the molecular formula $C_{28}H_{46}$ NaO$_4$ (calculated for 469.32883), requiring six degrees of unsaturation. The presence of an oxymethylene and a keto carbonyl carbon was confirmed by the ^{1}H NMR (Figure S11) (δ$_H$ 3.88 (m, H-11a) and 3.74 (m, H-11b)) and ^{13}C NMR (Figure S12) (δ$_C$ 59.2 (CH$_2$), 212.5 (qC), and 216.2 (qC)) data, as well as from the IR absorption (Figure S10) at 3396 and 1704 cm^{-1}. The diagnostic NMR signals of a 9,11-secosterol were confirmed by the ^{1}H–^{1}H COSY correlation (Figure S14) from H$_2$-11 to H$_2$-12 as well as HMBC correlations (Figure S15) from H3-18 to C-12, C-13, C-14, and

C-17; from H3-19 to C-1, C-5, C-9, and C-10. The NMR features of **5** were analogous to those of 3,11-dihydroxy-24-methyl-9,11-secocholest-5-en-9-one [7], except for the presence of a ketone (δ_C 201.1 (qC)) at C-23. Based on NOESY correlations (Figure S16) of H3-19/H-1, H3-19/H-2, H3-19/H-4, H3-19/H-8, H-3/H-1, H-3/H-2, H-3/H-4, H-8/H3-18, H-8/H-7, H3-18/H-15, H3-18/H-16, H3-18/H-20, and H-14/H-7, the relative stereochemistry at C-3, C-8, C-10, C-13, C-14, C-17, and C-20 in **5** was found to be the same as those of 3β,11-dihydroxy-24-methyl-9,11-secocholest-5-en-9-one [7]. On the basis of the above-mentioned findings, the structure of **5** was consistent with the structure shown as 3β,11-dihydroxy-24-methyl-9,11-secocholest-5-en-9,23-dione.

Compound **6** appeared as a white amorphous powder like **5**. Careful inspection of the 2D NMR spectroscopic data (Figures S21–23) of **6** led to the establishment of the same nucleus as that of **5**. The NMR spectroscopic data (Figures S19 and S20) of **6** were analogous to those of **5**, except for NMR signals due to the conjugated enone in **6**. The location of the conjugated enone was identified by the HMBC correlations (Figure S23) from the methylene protons (H2-22) to the carbonyl carbon (C-23) and from H3-26, 27 to C-24, securing the structure of **6**, which was shown as 3β,11-dihydroxy-24-methylene-9,11-secocholest-5-en-9,23-dione.

2.2. Identification of Marine Compounds Showed High-Content Characteristics of Proteasome Inhibition

The proteasome inhibition assay was performed by following the standard operation protocol of high-content screening (HCS) of EGFP-UL76 aggresome as described previously [4]. A stringent proteasome inhibition was considered as the HCS measurements of marine compounds with an increase greater than 0.2-fold relative to those of the control without treatment. Under this validity criterion, we demonstrated the identification of six compounds with proteasome inhibition and their effects were statistically significant. Four compounds with dolabellane-based structures designated clavinflol C (**1**), stolonidiol (**2**), stolonidiol-17-acetate (**3**), and clavinflol B (**4**) (Figures 2 and 3) [5,8]. Additionally, two unprecedent compounds with secosteroid-based structures designated compound **5** and **6** (Figures 4 and 5). Prior to HCS experiments, the in vitro cell-based MTT (3-(4,5-Dimethylthiazol-2-yl)-2,5-diphenyltetrazolium bromide) cytotoxicity assays were performed against four cell lines: A549 (human lung adenocarcinoma), HT-29 (human colon adenocarcinoma), and P-388 (mouse lymphocytic leukemia). Plasmid pEGFP-UL76 transfected HEK293T (human embryonic kidney large-T antigen-transformed) cell expressing EGFP-UL76 for HCS assay was assessed the ED$_{50}$ using both MTT and high-content nuclear count measurements (Table S1). The ED$_{50}$ values for respective compounds were as follows: compound **1**, >50 µg/mL, >50 µg/mL, >50 µg/mL, >25 µg/mL, and 6.14 µg/mL; stolonidiol (**2**), 3.9 µg/mL, >50 µg/mL, 0.6 µg/mL, >25 µg/mL, and >25 µg/mL; stolonidiol-17-acetate (**3**), >50 µg/mL, >50 µg/mL, >50 µg/mL, >25 µg/mL, and 19.56 µg/mL; clavinflol B (**4**), >50 µg/mL, >50 µg/mL, >50 µg/mL, >25 µg/mL, and 21.33 µg/mL; compound **5**, >50 µg/mL, 3.2 µg/mL, 4.6 µg/mL, 12.28 µg/mL, and 12.13 µg/mL; compound **6**, 5.3 µg/mL, >50 µg/mL, 4.8 µg/mL, >25 µg/mL, and 10.92 µg/mL. Both the MTT assay and high-content nucleus counts were performed to assess the ED$_{50}$ values of HEK293T cells expressing EGFP-UL76 for bortezomib which were 11.95 nM and 24.29 nM and for MG132 were 1.18 µM and 1.91 µM, respectively. Clavinflol B (**4**) showed moderate cytotoxicity in previous reports, which was consistent with our data (Table S1) [6].

Following the HCS assay, the high-content EGFP-UL76 aggresome measurements integrated intensity and average intensity per cell were analyzed and the relative ratios were obtained by normalization to the control. For the ratio of EGFP-UL76 aggresome integrated intensity per cell (Figures 2A and 3A, top panels), the highest ratios for compounds **1, 2, 3, 4, 5,** and **6** were 1.22 ($p = 0.0390$), 2.12 ($p < 0.0010$), 1.74 ($p = 0.0020$), 1.33 ($p < 0.0010$), 2.03 ($p < 0.0010$), and 1.72 ($p < 0.0010$), respectively. The highest ratios of average intensity per cell presented for compounds **1, 2, 3, 4, 5,** and **6** were 1.32 ($p = 0.0371$), 1.75 ($p = 0.0021$), 1.40 ($p < 0.0010$), 1.19 ($p = 0.0117$), 1.85 ($p < 0.0010$), and 1.34 ($p = 0.0089$), respectively (Figures 2A and 3A, bottom panels). Furthermore, all these increases in ratios achieved statistical significance.

Consequently after the assay procedure, we performed Western blotting analysis and q-PCR experiments to examine the levels of EGFP-UL76 protein and mRNA transcript under the same experimental conditions (Figure 2B,C and Figure 3B,C). In these two experiments, cells treated with bortezomib 25 nM and MG132 1 µM were used in parallel as proteasome inhibitory controls. We obtained similar results that the ratios of EGFP-UL76/tubulin under treatment with bortezomib and MG132 showed no difference from the control level, which was consistent with a previous report [4].

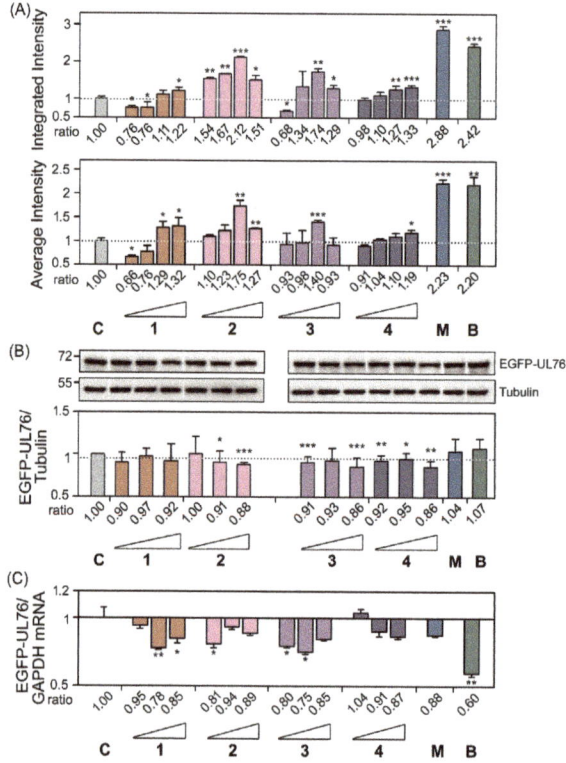

Figure 2. The assessment of proteasome inhibitory activity of marine dolabellanes-based compounds (**1, 2, 3**, and **4**) using a standard operation protocol of high-content EGFP-UL76 aggresomes screening assay. Pure compounds modulated high-content measurements of EGFP-UL76 aggresomes. (**A**) Assessment of the integrated and average intensities of EGFP-UL76 aggresomes (1 to 50 µm) per cell. The tested concentrations were 0.2, 1, 5, and 25 µg/mL for pure compounds **1, 2, 3**, and **4**, respectively. The integrated (top panel) and average (bottom panel) intensities per cell were measured, and the ratios were obtained by normalization to the control without proteasome inhibitor treatment, which is denoted by **C** throughout the text. (**B**) Validation of the EGFP-UL76 protein levels upon the addition of the tested marine compounds. Western blot imaging and densitometric analyses were performed to quantitate the EGFPUL76/tubulin protein ratio with the addition of tested compound treatment at 1, 5, and 25 µg/mL. The molecular mass markers are shown on the left in kDa. (**C**) Quantitative PCR was conducted to assess the transcript ratio of EGFP-UL76/GAPDH in HEK293T cells treated with pure compounds at 1, 5, and 25 µg/mL. The high-content measurements of EGFP-UL76 with the addition of the proteasome inhibitors, bortezomib (25 nM, denoted **B**) and MG132 (1 µM, denoted **M**), were used as positive controls. All data points are the averages of at least three repetitive experiments. The error bars indicate standard deviations. The following symbols are used to indicate statistical significance throughout the text: * $0.01 < p < 0.05$; ** $0.001 < p < 0.01$; *** $p < 0.001$.

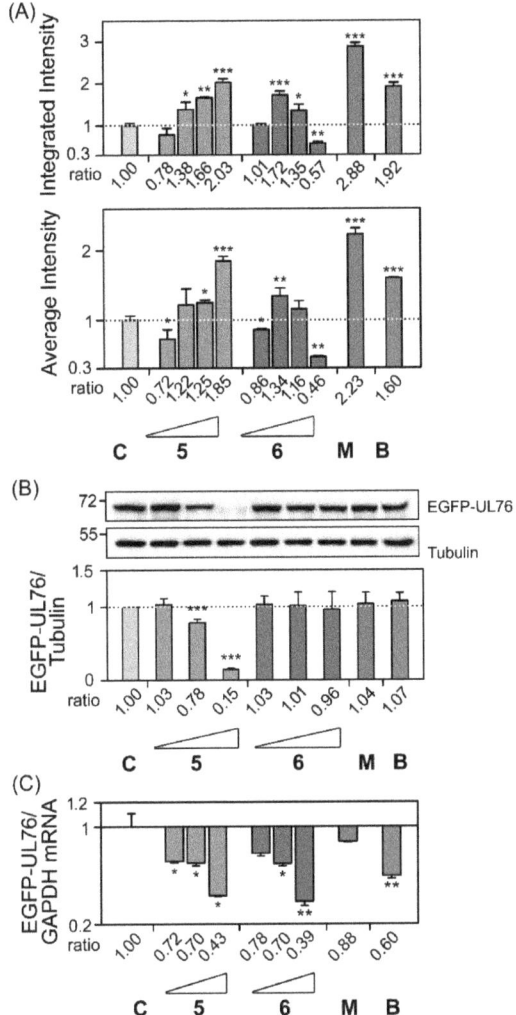

Figure 3. The assessment of proteasome inhibitory activity of marine secosteroid-based compounds (5 and 6) using a standard operation protocol of high-content EGFP-UL76 aggresomes screening assay as described in Figure 2 legend.

Compound **1** did not affect protein ratios of EGFP-UL76/tubulin proteins at 1, 5, and 25 μg/mL of any kind. However, for cells treated with compound **2** at 1, 5, and 25 μg/mL, the ratios were 1.00 ($p = 0.9466$), 0.91 ($p = 0.0359$), and 0.88 ($p < 0.0010$), respectively (Figures 2B and 3B). Nevertheless, the cytotoxic ED_{50} for compound **2** was greater than 25 μg/mL for HEK293T cell in both assays (Table S1). The protein ratios for compound **3** were 0.91 ($p < 0.0010$), 0.96 ($p = 0.1484$), and 0.86 ($p < 0.0010$), respectively. The protein ratios for compound **4** were 0.92 ($p = 0.0045$), 0.95 ($p = 0.0420$), and 0.86 ($p = 0.0014$), respectively. However, HEK293T cells treated with compound **3** and **4** at 25 μg/mL exhibited a lighter toxicity with ED_{50} values of 19.56 and 21.33 μg/mL, respectively. Compound **5** exhibited significant reduction at 5 and 25 μg/mL; the ratios were 0.78 ($p < 0.0010$) and 0.15 ($p < 0.0010$), respectively, which is consistent with cytotoxicity ED_{50} values (Table S1). Compound **6** did not affect protein ratios at any tested concentrations. The results from both the quantitative PCR and

Western blotting analyses revealed that in the tested compound treatment neither the protein nor the mRNA ratios for EGFP-UL76/GADPH were elevated (Figures 2C and 3C). Taking all these results in account, we suggested that the increase in EGFP-UL76 high-content measurement was likely due to the modulation of protein conformation.

After the results, we investigated the phenotypic size of aggresomes and analyzed the high-content data from Figures 2 and 3 by diameter with methods described previously [4]. As shown in the top panels of Figures 4 and 5, compounds **1, 2, 3, 4, 5,** and **6** exhibited the highest ratio increases for count, which were as follows: for pit aggresomes: 1.18 (p = 0.0331), 1.73 (p < 0.0010), 1.76 (p < 0.0010), 1.48 (p < 0.0010), 1.29 (p = 0.0236), and 1.32 (p = 0.0062), respectively; for vesicle aggresomes, 1.43 (p = 0.0028), 1.88 (p < 0.0010), 1.84 (p < 0.0010), 1.54 (p < 0.0010), 1.53 (p < 0.0010), and 1.37 (p = 0.0071), respectively. Similar profiles were observed for the ratios of integrated intensity per cell (Figures 4 and 5, middle panels). Compounds **1, 2, 3, 4, 5,** and **6** showed the highest ratio increases which were as follows: for pit aggresomes, 1.18 (p = 0.0130), 1.48 (p < 0.0010), 1.31 (p = 0.0055), 1.33 (p < 0.0010), 1.41 (p < 0.0010), and 1.21 (p = 0.0097), respectively; for vesicle aggresomes, 1.16 (p = 0.0220), 1.73 (p < 0.0010), 1.76 (p < 0.0010), 1.05 (p = 0.5352), 1.29 (p = 0.0236), and 1.32 (p = 0.0063), respectively. The ratios of average intensity per cell were the same for pit and vesicle aggresomes (Figures 4 and 5, bottom panels). For compounds **1, 2, 3, 4, 5,** and **6** showed the highest increases in ratios observed which were as follows: 1.27 (p = 0.0099), 1.42 (p < 0.0010), 1.25 (p = 0.0034), 1.22 (p = 0.0628), 1.42 (p < 0.0010), and 1.19 (p = 0.0135), respectively.

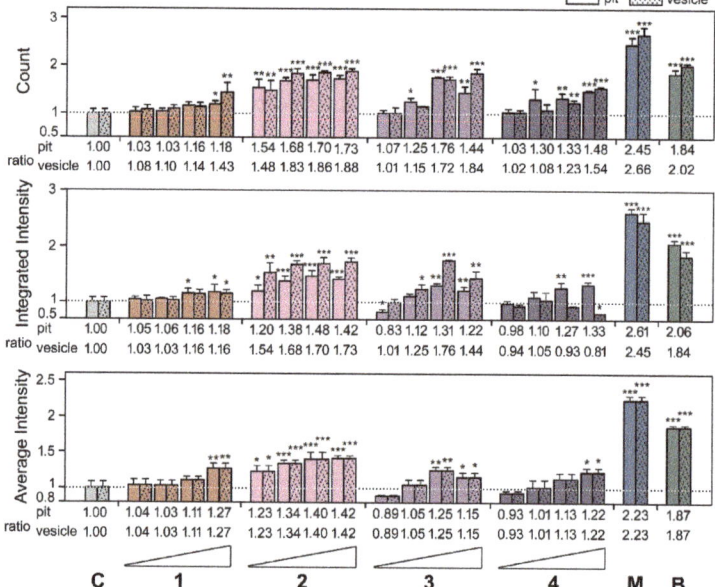

Figure 4. Classification of the high-content measurements of EGFP-UL76 aggresomes by size with marine dolabellanes (**1, 2, 3,** and **4**) at 0.2, 1, 5, and 25 µg/mL treatment. Pit and vesicle denote aggresomes 1 to 5 µm and 5 to 20 µm in diameter, respectively. Measurements of pit and vesicle aggresomes per cell were as follows: count number, integrated intensity, and average intensity. The relative ratio was normalized to control values without pure compound treatment. All data points are the averages of at least three repetitive experiments. The error bars indicate standard deviations. The following symbols are used to indicate statistical significance throughout the text: * 0.01 < p < 0.05; ** 0.001 < p < 0.01; *** p < 0.001.

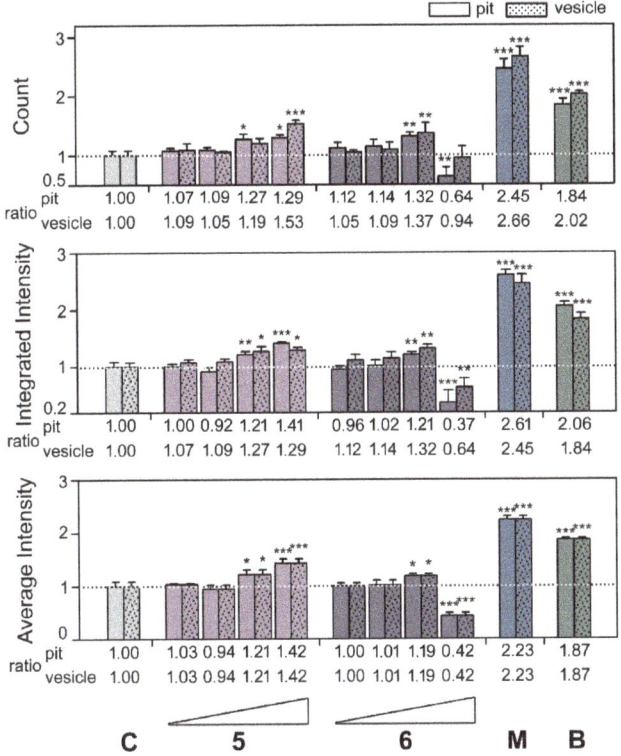

Figure 5. Classification of the high-content measurements of EGFP-UL76 aggresomes by size with marine secosteroid-based compounds (**5** and **6**). Treatment as described in Figure 4 legend.

3. Discussion

During the HCS we assessed dolabellanes-based clavinflol C (**1**), stolonidiol (**2**), and stolonidiol-17-acetate (**3**) and clavinflol B (**4**) with proteasome inhibition activities. Several groups demonstrated that stolonidiol (**2**) and stolonidiol-17-acetate (**3**) enhance the activities of choline acetyl transferase (ChAT) [8], which likely is mediated by protein kinase C [9]. ChAT catalyzes the production of acetylcholine which is an essential neurotransmitter. Moreover, proteasome inhibitor MG132 stabilizes ChAT steady-state protein levels and increases the enzyme activity [10]. Therefore, we reason that stolonidiol may mediate the elevation of ChAT activity via both pathways in the inhibition of proteasome and the activation of protein kinase C [9–11]. Among the four dolabellanes-based compounds with stolonidiol (**2**) 5 µg/mL treatment, the EGFP-UL76 displayed the highest increase ratios of 2.12 and 1.75 of integrated and average intensity, respectively (Figure 2). Consistent to this result, the tolonidiol (**2**) potentiated the highest ratios of aggresome pit and vesicle integrated and average intensities (Figure 4). For the remaining three, increased ratios were moderate, greater than 10% increase, for all the high-content measurements. Compared to compounds **1** and **4**, compound **2** and **3** show a lack of chloride at C-6, which may contribute to a less cytotoxic effect for HEK293T cell and increased efficacy for proteasome inhibition. Acetylation at C-17 of compound **3** may reduce activity in proteasome inhibition.

Overviewing the known proteasome inhibitors with steroid structure were polyhydroxylated sterol-based agosterols [12] and secosteroid-based physalin B and C [13,14]. Endogenous 25-hydroxyvitamin D (25OHDO) was identified to impair sterol regulatory element-binding proteins (SREBPs) activation by inducing proteolytic processing and ubiquitin-mediated degradation of SREBP cleavage-activating protein (SCAP) [15]. In this study, secosteroid-based compound **6** showed the highest inhibitory measurements of EGFP-UL76 integrated and average intensities and at 1 µg/mL (Figure 3), whereas with 5 µg/mL treatment the EGFP-UL76 exhibited the highest increase ratios of pit and vesicle measurements (Figure 5). As for the secosteroid related compound **5**, it showed less potent of proteasome inhibition with 25 µg/mL treatment which exhibited comparable activities to those of compound **6**. Compound **6** with a conjugated double bond may contribute cytotoxicity to HEK293T cells and display a significant reduction of all high-content measurements at 25 µg/mL.

4. Materials and Methods

4.1. Compounds 1–6

In the present study, compounds **1–6** (Figure 1) were isolated from Formosan soft coral *Clavularia flava* (wet weight of 1.1 kg), which was collected at Green Island, Taiwan. Briefly, corals were minced and exhaustively extracted with acetone. The organic extract was partitioned between ethyl acetate and water, and the ethyl acetate layer was separated further over a normal phase silica gel by column chromatography eluted with *n*-hexane, ethyl acetate, and methanol to yield 15 fractions. Fraction 14 (116.5 mg) eluted with *n*-hexane–EtOAc (1:5) was subjected to a RP-18 gravity column (MeOH/H_2O, 70:30 to 100% MeOH) to separate 6 subfractions. Subsequently, a subfraction 14-3 (23 mg) was purified by RP-18 HPLC (50% acetonitrile in H_2O) to obtain **1** (10.2 mg) and **2** (3.2 mg). Fraction 13 (96.7 mg) eluted with *n*-hexane–EtOAc (1:3) was subjected to column chromatography on silica gel using *n*-hexane–EtOAc gradient (10:1 to 1:10) for elution to give 11 subfractions. Subsequently, a subfraction 13-6 (22 mg) was purified by RP-18 HPLC (60% MeOH in H_2O) to obtain **3** (5.2 mg). Fraction 15 (86.5 mg) eluted with *n*-hexane–EtOAc (1:10) was subjected to a RP-18 gravity column (MeOH/H_2O, 70:30 to 100% MeOH) to separate 7 subfractions. Subsequently, a subfraction 15-4 (20 mg) was purified by RP-18 HPLC (50% ACN in H_2O) to obtain **4** (2.4 mg), **5** (3.2 mg), and **6** (3.0 mg).

4.2. High-Content Screening (HCS) Assay for Proteasome Inhibition

We followed the HCS assay routinely conducted in the lab. In brief, the complete assay includes a series of experiments [4]. Experiments were sequentially performed: (1) the DNA transfection into cell culture with compound treatment, (2) cells fixation, (3) image acquisition using an ImageXpress Micro Widefield HCS system (Molecular Device, San Jose, CA, USA), (4) high-content measurements analyzed by modules of MetaExpress, Cell Scoring and Multi-Wavelength Cell Scoring, (5) Western blotting imaging and densitometric analysis, and (6) RNA purification and quantitative PCR.

Supplementary Materials: The following are available online at http://www.mdpi.com/1660-3397/18/1/39/s1, Figure S1. HRESIMS of **1**; Figure S2. IR spectrum of **1**; Figure S3. ^1H NMR spectrum (400 MHz) of **1** in $CDCl_3$; Figure S4. ^{13}C NMR spectrum (100 MHz) of **1** in $CDCl_3$; Figure S5 HSQC spectrum (400 MHz) of **1** in $CDCl_3$; Figure S6 COSY spectrum (400 MHz) of **1** in $CDCl_3$; Figure S7 HMBC spectrum (400 MHz) of **1** in $CDCl_3$; Figure S8 NOESY spectrum (400 MHz) of **1** in $CDCl_3$; Figure S9. HRESIMS of **5** Figure S10. IR spectrum of **5** Figure S11. 1H NMR spectrum (400 MHz) of **5** in C_6D_6; Figure S12. ^{13}C NMR spectrum (100 MHz) of **5** in C_6D_6; Figure S13. HSQC spectrum (400 MHz) of **5** in C_6D_6; Figure S14. COSY spectrum (400 MHz) of **5** in C_6D_6; Figure S15. HMBC spectrum (400 MHz) of **5** in C_6D_6; Figure S16. NOESY spectrum (400 MHz) of **5** in C_6D_6; Figure S17. HRESIMS of **6** Figure S18. IR spectrum of **6** Figure S19. ^1H NMR spectrum (400 MHz) of **6** in C_6D_6; Figure S20. ^{13}C NMR spectrum (100 MHz) of **6** in C_6D_6; Figure S21. HSQC spectrum (400 MHz) of **6** in C_6D_6; Figure S22. COSY spectrum (400 MHz) of **6** in C_6D_6; Figure S23. HMBC spectrum (400 MHz) of **6** in C_6D_6; Figure S24. NOESY spectrum (400 MHz) of **6** in C_6D_6, Table S1: Evaluation of ED_{50} cytotoxicity of tested compounds.

Author Contributions: Conceptualization, S.-K.W. and C.-Y.D.; data curation, S.-K.W.; formal analysis, X.-H.L. and C.-Y.C.; funding acquisition, S.-K.W. and C.-Y.D.; investigation, X.-H.L. and C.-Y.C.; writing—original draft, S.-K.W.; writing—review and editing, C.-Y.D. All authors have read and agreed to the published version of the manuscript.

Funding: This research was supported by grants from the Ministry of Science and Technology, Taiwan, Republic of China (MOST108-2320-B110-005) and from Kaohsiung Medical University (NSYSU-KMU 108-P018) awarded to C.-Y.D. and S.-K.W.

Conflicts of Interest: The authors declare no conflict of interest.

References

1. Abdel-Lateff, A.; Alarif, W.M.; Alburae, N.A.; Algandaby, M.M. Alcyonium octocorals: Potential source of diverse bioactive terpenoids. *Molecules* **2019**, *24*, 1370. [CrossRef] [PubMed]
2. Shirley, M. Ixazomib: First global approval. *Drugs* **2016**, *76*, 405–411. [CrossRef] [PubMed]
3. Sledz, P.; Baumeister, W. Structure-driven developments of 26S proteasome inhibitors. *Annu. Rev. Pharmacol. Toxicol.* **2016**, *56*, 191–209. [CrossRef] [PubMed]
4. Ling, X.H.; Wang, S.K.; Huang, Y.H.; Huang, M.J.; Duh, C.Y. A High-content screening assay for the discovery of novel proteasome inhibitors from Formosan soft corals. *Mar. Drugs* **2018**, *16*, 395. [CrossRef] [PubMed]
5. Mori, K.; Iguchi, K.; Yamada, N.; Yamada, Y.; Inouye, Y. Stolonidiol, a new marine diterpenoid with a strong cytotoxic activity from the Japanese soft coral. *Tetrahedron Lett.* **1987**, *28*, 5673–5676. [CrossRef]
6. Shen, Y.C.; Pan, Y.L.; Ko, C.L.; Kuo, Y.H.; Chen, C.Y. New dolabellanes from the Taiwanese soft coral Clavularia inflata. *J. Chin. Chem. Soc.-Taip.* **2003**, *50*, 471–476. [CrossRef]
7. Kazlauskas, R.; Murphy, P.T. Stolonidiol, a new marine diterpenoid with a strong cytotoxic activity from the Japanese soft coral. *Aust. J. Chem.* **1982**, *35*, 69–75. [CrossRef]
8. Yabe, T.; Yamada, H.; Shimomura, M.; Miyaoka, H.; Yamada, Y. Induction of choline acetyltransferase activity in cholinergic neurons by stolonidiol: Structure-activity relationship. *J. Nat. Prod.* **2000**, *63*, 433–435. [CrossRef] [PubMed]
9. Mason, J.W.; Schmid, C.L.; Bohn, L.M.; Roush, W.R. Stolonidiol: Synthesis, target identification, and mechanism for choline acetyltransferase activation. *J. Am. Chem. Soc.* **2017**, *139*, 5865–5869. [CrossRef] [PubMed]
10. Morey, T.M.; Albers, S.; Shilton, B.H.; Rylett, R.J. Enhanced ubiquitination and proteasomal degradation of catalytically deficient human choline acetyltransferase mutants. *J. Neurochem.* **2016**, *137*, 630–646. [CrossRef] [PubMed]
11. Dobransky, T.; Doherty-Kirby, A.; Kim, A.R.; Brewer, D.; Lajoie, G.; Rylett, R.J. Protein kinase C isoforms differentially phosphorylate human choline acetyltransferase regulating its catalytic activity. *J. Biol. Chem.* **2004**, *279*, 52059–52068. [CrossRef] [PubMed]
12. Tsukamoto, S.; Tatsuno, M.; van Soest, R.W.; Yokosawa, H.; Ohta, T. New polyhydroxy sterols: Proteasome inhibitors from a marine sponge Acanthodendrilla sp. *J. Nat. Prod.* **2003**, *66*, 1181–1185. [CrossRef] [PubMed]
13. Ausseil, F.; Samson, A.; Aussagues, Y.; Vandenberghe, I.; Creancier, L.; Pouny, I.; Kruczynski, A.; Massiot, G.; Bailly, C. High-throughput bioluminescence screening of ubiquitin-proteasome pathway inhibitors from chemical and natural sources. *J. Biomol. Screen* **2007**, *12*, 106–116. [CrossRef] [PubMed]
14. Vandenberghe, I.; Creancier, L.; Vispe, S.; Annereau, J.P.; Barret, J.M.; Pouny, I.; Samson, A.; Aussagues, Y.; Massiot, G.; Ausseil, F.; et al. A novel inhibitor of the ubiquitin-proteasome pathway, triggers NOXA-associated apoptosis. *Biochem. Pharmacol.* **2008**, *76*, 453–562. [CrossRef] [PubMed]
15. Asano, L.; Watanabe, M.; Ryoden, Y.; Usuda, K.; Yamaguchi, T.; Khambu, B.; Takashima, M.; Sato, S.I.; Sakai, J.; Nagasawa, K.; et al. 25-Hydroxyvitamin D, regulates lipid metabolism by inducing degradation of SREBP/SCAP. *Cell Chem. Biol.* **2017**, *24*, 207–217. [CrossRef] [PubMed]

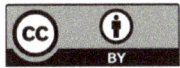

© 2020 by the authors. Licensee MDPI, Basel, Switzerland. This article is an open access article distributed under the terms and conditions of the Creative Commons Attribution (CC BY) license (http://creativecommons.org/licenses/by/4.0/).

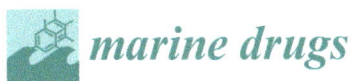

Article

Investigating the Antiparasitic Potential of the Marine Sesquiterpene Avarone, Its Reduced Form Avarol, and the Novel Semisynthetic Thiazinoquinone Analogue Thiazoavarone

Concetta Imperatore [1,2,†], Roberto Gimmelli [3,†], Marco Persico [1,2,†], Marcello Casertano [1,2], Alessandra Guidi [3], Fulvio Saccoccia [3], Giovina Ruberti [3], Paolo Luciano [1], Anna Aiello [1,2], Silvia Parapini [4], Sibel Avunduk [5], Nicoletta Basilico [6], Caterina Fattorusso [1,2,*] and Marialuisa Menna [1,2,*]

[1] The NeaNat Group, Department of Pharmacy, University of Naples "Federico II", Via D. Montesano 49, 80131 Napoli, Italy; cimperat@unina.it (C.I.); marco.persico@unina.it (M.P.); marcello.casertano@unina.it (M.C.); pluciano@unina.it (P.L.); aiello@unina.it (A.A.)

[2] Italian Malaria Network, Centro Interuniversitario di Ricerche Sulla Malaria (CIRM), Department of Pharmacy, University of Naples "Federico II", Via D. Montesano 49, 80131 Napoli, Italy

[3] Institute of Biochemistry and Cell Biology, National Research Council, Campus A. Buzzati-Traverso, Via E. Ramarini, 32, 00015 Monterotondo (Roma), Italy; roberto.gimmelli@ibbc.cnr.it (R.G.); alessandra.guidi@ibbc.cnr.it (A.G.); fulvio.saccoccia@ibbc.cnr.it (F.S.); giovina.ruberti@cnr.it (G.R.)

[4] Dipartimento di Scienze Biomediche per la Salute, Università di Milano, Via Pascal 36, 20133 Milan, Italy; silvia.parapini@unimi.it

[5] Department Vocational School of Medicinal Health Services, Mugla University, 48187 Mugla, Turkey; sibelavunduk@mu.edu.tr

[6] Dipartimento di Scienze Biomediche, Chirurgiche e Odontoiatriche, Università di Milano, Via Pascal 36, 20133 Milan, Italy; nicoletta.basilico@unimi.it

* Correspondence: caterina.fattorusso@unina.it (C.F.); mlmenna@unina.it (M.M.); Tel.: +39081678544 (C.F.); +39081678518 (M.M.)

† These authors equally contributed.

Received: 9 January 2020; Accepted: 11 February 2020; Published: 14 February 2020

Abstract: The chemical analysis of the sponge *Dysidea avara* afforded the known sesquiterpene quinone avarone, along with its reduced form avarol. To further explore the role of the thiazinoquinone scaffold as an antiplasmodial, antileishmanial and antischistosomal agent, we converted the quinone avarone into the thiazinoquinone derivative thiazoavarone. The semisynthetic compound, as well as the natural metabolites avarone and avarol, were pharmacologically investigated in order to assess their antiparasitic properties against sexual and asexual stages of *Plasmodium falciparum*, larval and adult developmental stages of *Schistosoma mansoni* (eggs included), and also against promastigotes and amastigotes of *Leishmania infantum* and *Leishmania tropica*. Furthermore, in depth computational studies including density functional theory (DFT) calculations were performed. A toxic semiquinone radical species which can be produced starting both from quinone- and hydroquinone-based compounds could mediate the anti-parasitic effects of the tested compounds.

Keywords: *Dysidea avara*; avarone/avarol; redox-active compounds; quinones and hydroquinones; dioxothiazinoquinone; *Schistosoma mansoni*; *Plasmodium falciparum*; *Leishmania* spp.; 3D-SAR analysis; DFT studies

1. Introduction

Malaria and neglected tropical diseases (NTDs), a group of parasitic, bacterial, and viral infectious diseases (i.e., *Schistosoma* spp., *Leishmania* spp.), still have high morbidity and/or mortality rates worldwide. They affect more than one billion people and cause chronic illness, physical disability and/or deaths, especially in children and women of childbearing age, mostly in developing countries where they represent a serious hurdle to social and economic growth as well as a health problem [1,2]. Parasites belonging to different species can affect humans and animals concurrently, a phenomenon referred to as multiparasitism, which poses additional diagnostic and therapeutic challenges [3]. The therapeutic strategies for malaria and NTDs are very limited; drug-resistance phenomena, toxicity profiles and drug administration procedures of the few available chemical entities are still challenging. In this view, a research aimed to discover new chemicals active against several parasites is crucial and the marine environment may be an important resource [4,5]. In order to cope with all the reported drawbacks and to limit the costs of the development of brand-new pharmaceutical strategies, several effective antimalarial drugs should be considered for the treatment of other underfunded parasitic diseases. For example, artemisinin and its derivatives, a potent class of antimalarial agents, have been proved to be beneficial for other infectious diseases such as schistosomiasis and leishmaniasis [6]. Furthermore, histone deacetylases (HDAC) inhibitors have been shown to have activity both against some *Plasmodium* species as well as *Leishmania* and *Schistosoma* parasites [7]. Importantly, the blood parasites, *Plasmodium* and *Schistosoma*, both feeding on human hemoglobin, can detoxify the free heme groups through the synthesis of insoluble hemozoin pigments [8]. The interference with hemozoin formation featured an important antischistosomal mechanism of action showed by the antimalarial quinine and quinidine [9].

In the frame of our research for new anti-parasitic chemical entities, we recently identified the thiazinoquinone scaffold as a novel chemotype active against both *Plasmodium falciparum* and *Schistosoma mansoni* [10–14]. We developed this scaffold by creating of a chemical library of thiazinoquinone derivatives designed on the model of aplidinones, natural products isolated from a marine invertebrate (Figure 1). Many compounds exhibited in vitro antiplasmodial activities against the D10 and W2 strains of *P. falciparum* [11,13] with IC_{50} in the low micromolar range. Through an integrated experimental (cyclic voltammetry) and theoretical approach, we demonstrated that the antiplasmodial and anticancer activity of a series of thiazinoquinone compounds was not related to their two electrons redox potential [11,12]. In particular, the antiplasmodial activity was found to depend on the ability of the compound to generate a semiquinone radical species able to form a stable adduct with heme [11]. This was later supported by the design and synthesis of other sets of new thiazinoquinone derivatives, indicating that the activity was related to the ability to form a specific semiquinone radical, and to the ability of this latter to transfer the radical by and hydrogen-radical shift to the R substituent [13]. In addition, several important SARs were obtained. First, the thiazinoquinone moiety was ascertained to be necessary for the antiplasmodial activity, since the corresponding quinone derivatives (e.g., derivatives lacking the 1,1-dioxothiazine moiety) were inactive. Second, the regiochemistry of the heterocyclic ring with respect to the substituents (a methoxyl group and an alkyl chain) on the quinone ring was revealed as crucial for the activity. Third, the nature and shape of the R' substituent were able to affect compound potency and selectivity.

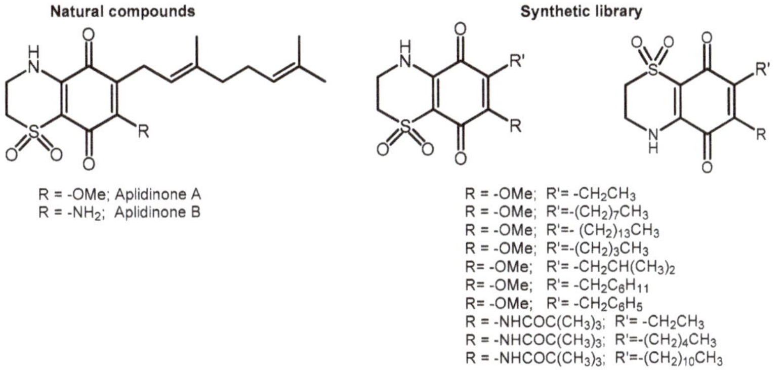

Figure 1. Structures of aplidinones A, B and of thiazinoquinone derivatives.

Successively, we selected both some of the developed methoxy thiazinoquinones, and some ad hoc synthesized new derivatives with the aim of investigating the antischistosomal properties of this chemical scaffold. Compounds were thus tested against larval stage, adult worm couples and eggs of the platyhelminth *S. mansoni* [14]. Many of the tested molecules resulted active and, interestingly, as observed for the antiplasmodial activity, the effects against *S. mansoni* strongly depended on the regiochemistry of the heterocyclic ring, and from the nature and/or steric hindrance of the R′ substituent. Computational studies indicated that semiquinone radical species could be involved also in the mode of action against *S. mansoni* impairing the redox equilibrium within the parasite. Importantly, the R′ properties can affect both the pharmacodynamics and pharmacokinetics of the compounds [14].

In the course of a systematic chemical study of the macroflora and macrofauna of the coastal area of Turkey in the İzmir Bay (Aegean Sea), as a part of our ongoing search for bioactive marine-derived metabolites as leads for drug discovery [15–20], we isolated from the sponge *Dysidea avara* (Schmidt, 1862) the known sesquiterpene quinone avarone (**1**), along with its reduced form avarol (**3**, Figure 2) [21–23]. A wide range of pharmacological properties have been reported for the redox couple avarone (**1**) and avarol (**3**) including anti-tumor [24–26], anti-inflammatory [27–29], anti-mutagenic [30], anti-bacterial [31,32], anti-viral [33,34], anti-oxidant [23,35], anti-platelet [28], anti-psoriatic [36] and anti-biofouling [37,38] activities. Pharmacological studies on synthetic and semisynthetic derivatives of avarone have been previously reported, too [23,39–41]. Based on the above described extensive exploration of the thiazinoquinone scaffold as antiplasmodial and antischistosomal agent [11,13,14], we used the quinone avarone (**1**) as chemical starting point to obtain the semisynthetic thiazinoquinone derivative, thiazoavarone (**2**, Figure 2). Compound **2**, as well as the natural metabolites **1** and **3**, were investigated in order to evaluate their in vitro activity against: (i) asexual stages of D10 and W2 strains and stage V gametocytes of *P. falciparum*, (ii) egg production, larval and adult stages of *S. mansoni*, (iii) promastigote and amastigote stages of *Leishmania infantum* and *Leishmania tropica*. Computational studies, including density functional theory (DFT) calculations, were performed in order to analyze the conformational and redox properties of the two natural metabolites (**1** and **3**), as well as those of the novel semisynthetic analogue **2**.

The obtained results shed light on the putative mechanism of action of the quinone/hydroquinone/thiazinoquinone compounds corroborating the hypothesis that their antiparasitic activity is related to the formation of a toxic semiquinone radical species. Noteworthy, thiazoavarone **2** resulted the most potent antimalarial thiazinoquinone developed by us, highlighting the important role for the activity played by the substituent of the 1,1-dioxo-1,4-thiazine ring.

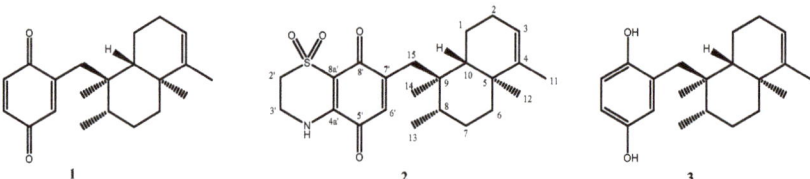

Figure 2. Structure of avarone (**1**), the semisynthetic thiazoavarone (**2**) and avarol (**3**).

2. Results and Discussion

2.1. Chemistry

Avarone (**1**) and avarol (**3**) were isolated from the sponge *D. avara* and purified according to the previously described procedures [21–23]. They were easily identified by comparison of their spectroscopic properties (^{1}H and ^{13}C NMR, HRESI-MS) with those reported in literature [21–23].

Thiazoavarone (**2**) was prepared as reported in Scheme 1. A portion of avarone was dissolved in a solution of $CH_3CN/EtOH$ (1:1) and then hypotaurine and a catalytic amount of salcomine in portion were added. The mixture was stirred for 48 h at room temperature and then was extracted with diethyl ether. The crude material was purified by HPLC on a reverse phase column (Luna 3 µm, 150 × 3.00 mm) ($MeOH/H_2O$ 75:25 v/v%) to afford the pure compound **2**. The nucleophilic addition reaction is regioselective in unsymmetrical quinones but generally leads to the formation of both regioisomers one of which is obtained in large excess with respect to the other. In the case of avarone, a single isomeric product, thiazoavarone **2**, has formed, as determined by MS and NMR spectroscopy; this could be reasonably due to the high steric hindrance of the heavy sesquiterpene moiety.

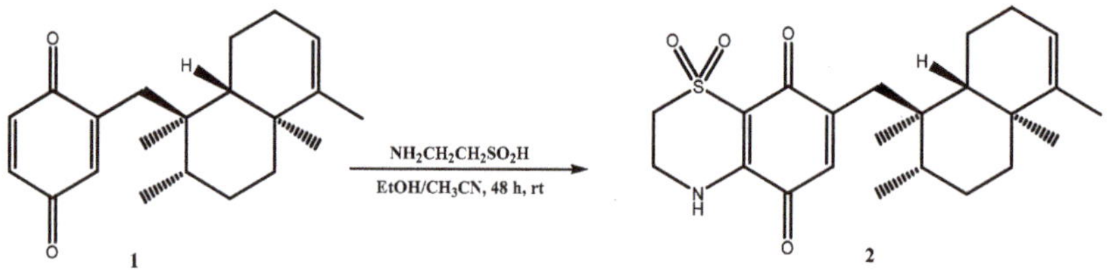

Scheme 1. Coupling of avarone (**1**) with hypotaurine via nucleophilic addition reaction.

Compound **2**, obtained as yellow powder, $[\alpha]_D^{25}$ = +19.2 (c 0.004, MeOH), had a molecular formula of $C_{23}H_{31}NO_4S$ as determined by the HRESI MS ion at m/z $C_{23}H_{31}NO_4SNa$ [M + Na]$^+$ 440.1865 (calculated value: 440.1866). Molecular formula obtained from MS and a first survey of the 1D NMR spectra of **2** ($CDCl_3$) and the comparison with those of the known avarone **1** quickly allowed us to hypothesize that the condensation reaction with hypotaurine has occurred. ^{1}H and ^{13}C NMR data of **2** indicated the same decalin ring system of **1**, and the only difference between the two compounds is in the quinonic portion. Indeed, ^{1}H NMR spectrum of **2** lacked the signals at δ_H 6.51 and 6.71, whereas contained a quite deshielded methylene signals (δ_H 3.30 and 4.05), resonating as two multiplets and each integrating for two protons. Likewise, the ^{13}C spectrum of **2** contained two additional methylene carbon resonances at δ_C 39.8 and at δ_C 48.8 attributable to a nitrogen and sulfoxide-bearing carbons, respectively. The key HMBC cross-peaks (Figure 3) from H-3' to C-2' (δ_C 48.8), C-4a' (δ_C 143.2), and from H-2' to C-3' (δ_C 39.8), C-8a' (δ_C 111.6), from H-6' to C-4a' (δ_C 143.2), and from H-15a and H-15b' to C-8' (δ_C 177.1) indicated the regiochemistry of **2**. It should be noted that only one of possible regioisomer has been obtained.

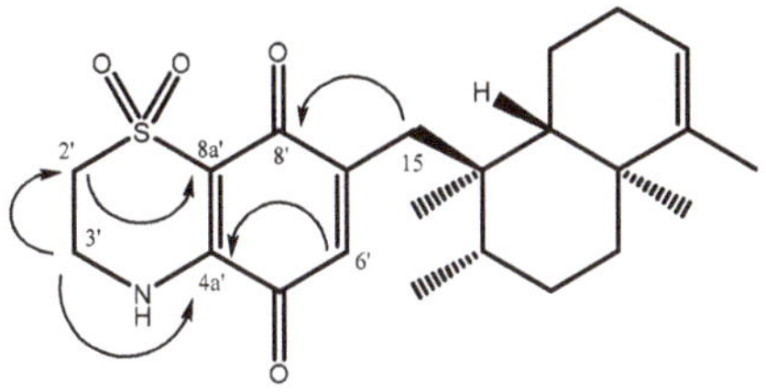

Figure 3. Key ^{1}H-^{13}C HMBC correlations of thiazoavarone (2).

Chemical shifts and coupling patterns of the all signals of **2** were assigned by aid of COSY, HSQC, and HMBC experiments (Table 1). Anyway, a purity higher than 99.8% has been determined by HPLC for compounds **1–3**.

Table 1. ^{1}H (700 MHz) and ^{13}C (125 MHz) NMR data of thiazoavarone (2) in CDCl$_3$.

Pos.	δ_C	δ_H, mult. (J in Hz)	Pos.	δ_C	δ_H, mult. (J in Hz)
1'	-	-	4	143.7	-
2'	48.8	3.30, m	5	38.3	-
3'	39.8	4.05, m	6	35.8	1.03 [a], 1.64 [a]
4'	-	6.41, br s	7	27.3	1.38 [a]
4a'	143.2	-	8	37.1	1.25 [a]
5'	179.3	-	9	43.7	-
6'	131.8	6.50, s	10	47.5	1.03 [a]
7'	152.8	-	11	17.9	1.53, s
8'	177.1	-	12	20.0	0.99, s
8a'	111.6	-	13	16.7	0.96, d, (6.2)
1	19.3	1.50 [a], 1.85, dd, (6.7, 13.2)	14	17.7	0.85, s
2	26.3	1.93 [a], 2.04 [a]	15a	35.6	2.50, d, (13.1)
3	120.9	5.2, br s	15b		2.70, d, (13.1)

[a] Overlapped by other signals.

2.2. In Vitro Activity on P. falciparum and Cytotoxicity

Avarone (**1**) and the semisynthetic 1,1-dioxo-1,4-thiazine analogue (**2**), as well as hydroquinone avarol (**3**) were tested for their in vitro antiplasmodial activity against asexual and sexual (gametocytes stage V) stages of *P. falciparum* (Table 2). A chloroquine-sensitive (CQ-S) D10 and a chloroquine-resistant (CQ-R) W2 strains were used to determine the IC$_{50}$ against asexual stage of parasites. The most potent compound was thiazoavarone (**2**) with an IC$_{50}$ value in the nanomolar range, higher than those exhibited by the previously identified synthetic lead [13]. The high potency of the thiazinoquinone **2**, specifically on the chloroquine-resistant strain W2 and compared with avarone (**1**), lacking the heterocyclic moiety, confirmed once again the high potential of the thiazinoquinone scaffold for development of new antimalarial hits. Interestingly, both natural compounds **1** and **3** also exhibited a remarkable effect against sensitive and resistant *P. falciparum* strains, showing no cross-resistance with chloroquine (see Table 2). In particular, the reduced hydroquinone form (avarol, **3**) resulted significantly more active than the oxidized quinone form (avarone, **1**).

The evaluation of the effects of compounds **1–3** on *Pf* gametocytes stage V, the sexual stage circulating in the bloodstream, was performed in order to evaluate their transmission blocking potential. As evidenced in Table 2, all the three compounds resulted less active against the gametocytes with respect to the parasite asexual stage; this finding is not unexpected since most of the current antimalarial drugs have no effect on the late stage of gametocytes. Avarol (**3**) resulted the most potent in the series against Pf gametocytes stage V with an IC$_{50}$ = 9.30 µM, comparable to that of OZ27, a drug in clinical development (IC$_{50}$ = 6.4 µM) [42].

Table 2. In vitro antimalarial activity against asexual *P. falciparum* parasites from D10 (CQ-sensitive) and W2 (CQ-resistant) strains [a] and against stage V *P. falciparum* gametocytes from a 3D7 transgenic line.

Compounds	D10 (µM) [b]	W2 (µM) [b]	Pf Gametocytes Stage V 3D7elo1-pfs16-CBG99 IC$_{50}$ (µM) [b]
Avarone (1)	2.74 ± 0.51	2.09 ± 0.52	15.53 ± 5.26
Thiazoavarone (2)	0.38 ± 0.15	0.21 ± 0.03	15.01 ± 3.19
Avarol (3)	0.96 ± 0.24	1.10 ± 0.15	9.30 ± 1.90
Methylene blue	-	-	0.155 ± 0.05

[a] Chloroquine (CQ) has been used as positive control (D10 IC$_{50}$ = 0.04 ± 0.01; W2 IC$_{50}$ = 0.54 ± 0.28). [b] The results are the mean ± SD of IC$_{50}$ of three independent experiments performed in duplicate.

Finally, we tested compounds 1–3 for their cytotoxic effects against two different human cell lines, microvascular endothelial (HMEC-1) and acute monocytic leukemia (THP-1) cells differentiated into macrophages; for each compound, we evaluated the selectivity index (SI, Table 2), namely the ratio between the IC$_{50}$ on the human cells HMEC and that on the parasite strains (see Table 3). Thiazoavarone (2) exhibited a high toxicity against both mammalian cell lines, with IC$_{50}$ in the low micromolar concentration range and, consequently, a very low SI. Avarone and avarol (1 and 3) were lowly and moderately cytotoxic, respectively (Table 3) but the hydroquinone 3 exhibited a better SI.

Table 3. IC$_{50}$ against HMEC-1 (human microvascular endothelial cells) and THP-1 (human acute monocytic leukemia cells) and Selectivity Index (SI) of the compounds 1–3.

Compounds	HMEC-1 IC$_{50}$ (µM) [a,b]	THP-1 IC$_{50}$ (µM) [a,c]	SI [d]	
			D10	W2
Avarone (1)	62.19 ± 1.98	>100	22.7	29.8
Thiazoavarone (2)	3.31 ± 1.53	7.41	8.7	15.8
Avarol (3)	36.85 ± 5.79	31.75	38.4	33.5

[a] Camptothecin has been used as positive control (IC$_{50}$ (µM) = 0.018 ± 0.008 on HMEC-1). [b] Data are expressed as mean ± SD of three different experiments performed in duplicate. [c] Data are the mean of two different experiments in duplicate. [d] SI = IC$_{50}$ HMEC-1/IC$_{50}$ *P. falciparum* strain.

2.3. In vitro Activity on Leishmania Parasites

To assess the antileishmanial activity of compounds 1–3 we tested them against promastigote stage of *L. infantum* and *L. tropica* responsible for visceral and cutaneous leishmaniasis, respectively. The results of this study are reported in Table 4 as IC$_{50}$ values with the relevant selectivity indexes (SIs). Considering the couple avarone/avarol, we can notice that, as observed for the antiplasmodial effects, the reduced form (3) is substantially more potent than the oxidized form 1 on both investigated *Leishmania* parasites. This has been reported also for several antileishmanial naphthohydroquinones which resulted more active than the corresponding naphthoquinones [43]. Instead, the hydroquinone metabolite 3 and the thiazinoquinone 2 exhibited similar values of IC$_{50}$ in the range of low micromolar; however, avarol (3) showed a significantly higher SI (see Table 4). Definitely, the above results displayed that introduction of the 1,1-dioxo-1,4-thiazine ring in the structure of avarone (1) to give thiazoavarone (2) meaningfully improves the antileishmanial activity, once again according to the antiplasmodial effects (see Tables 2 and 4).

In addition, compounds 1–3 were also investigated against intracellular amastigotes, the clinically relevant form of *Leishmania*. All compounds resulted from 2 to 4-fold more active against amastigotes than promastigotes; the hydroquinone avarol 3 confirmed itself as a promising agent to be further investigated in efficacy and selectivity, presenting the lowest IC$_{50}$ value in the series and a SI greater than 10 (Table 4) [44].

Table 4. Activity of compounds **1**–**3** against promastigote stage of *L. infantum* and *L. tropica* and against amastigote stage of *L. infantum*.

Compounds	*L. infantum* IC$_{50}$ (µM) [a]	SI$_p$ [c]	*L. tropica* IC$_{50}$ (µM) [a]	SI$_p$ [c]	*L. infantum* Amastigotes IC$_{50}$ (µM) [b]	SI$_a$ [d]
Avarone (**1**)	28.21 ± 0.32	2.2	20.28 ± 3.56	3.1	7.64	8.1
Thiazoavarone (**2**)	8.78 ± 0.26	0.38	9.52 ± 0.32	0.35	4.99	0.67
Avarol (**3**)	7.42 ± 0.27	5.0	7.08 ± 1.91	5.2	3.19	11.6
Amphotericin B	0.20 ± 0.03		0.17 ± 0.04		0.189	

[a] Data are expressed as mean ± SD of three different experiments performed in duplicate. [b] Data are the mean of two different experiments in triplicate. [c] SI$_p$ = IC$_{50}$ HMEC-1/IC$_{50}$ *L. infantum* (*L. tropica*) promastigotes. [d] SI$_a$ = IC$_{50}$ HMEC-1/IC$_{50}$ *L. infantum* amastigotes.

2.4. In Vitro Activity on S. mansoni

Compounds **1**–**3** were tested against larval stage (schistosomula), adult worm couples and eggs of the platyhelminth *S. mansoni*. The most potent compound on schistosomula was thiazoavarone (**2**) with a LC$_{50}$ value in the low micromolar range (Table 5). The natural compounds (**1** and **3**) showed comparable activity, with avarol (**3**) slightly more active than avarone (**1**), both showing a LC$_{50}$ in the high micromolar range (Table 5). Therefore, the presence of a thiazine ring was proved to be very important for activity on schistosomula.

Table 5. Activity of compounds **1**–**3** against *S. mansoni* schistosomula.

Compounds	LC$_{50}$ (µM) [a]
Avarone (**1**)	42.77 ± 1.90
Thiazoavarone (**2**)	5.90 ± 2.59
Avarol (**3**)	33.97 ± 5.52

[a] Data are expressed as mean ± SD of three different experiments.

All three compounds **1**–**3** were also very active on adult worm pairs at 50 µM leading to parasites death 7 days after treatment (Figure 4). However, when used at lower concentration (20 µM), only avarol (**3**) strongly impaired parasites viability (only 20% survival), while thiazoavarone (**2**) was poorly effective against the adult stage (Figure 4), despite its strong lethal effect on the larval stage (Table 5). These results suggest the possibility that the double lipid bilayer coating the adult worms, namely the tegument [45], can interfere with compound **2** uptake by adult parasites.

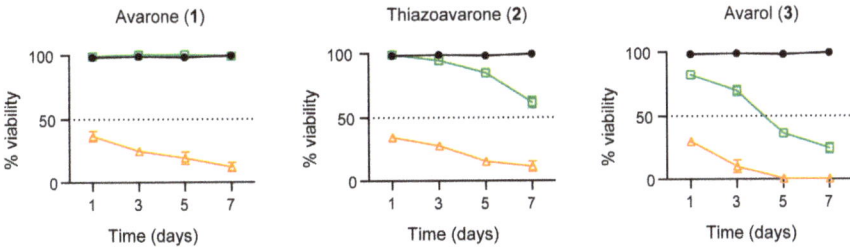

Figure 4. Compounds **1**–**3** impair adult *S. mansoni* viability. Worm pairs were incubated with DMSO (vehicle) (black circle) or the indicated compounds at 50 µM (yellow triangle), or 20 µM (green, square) as described in material and methods. Phenotype analysis was recorded for 7 days and % viability represents the mean ± SEM of three independent experiments.

In the process of drug discovery for schistosomiasis, strategy involving any impairment in egg production and/or development must also be taken into account. In fact, upon mating with males, mature *S. mansoni* adult females, residing in the mesenteric veins of the definitive host, can lay hundreds of eggs each day. The eggs secreted in stool or trapped in the liver respectively cause disease transmission and, as a result of inflammatory granulomas reactions, intestinal and hepato-splenic diseases [46]. Therefore, compounds **1–3** were also assayed against the in vitro laid eggs (IVLEs). The IVLEs produced in the first 48 h by *S. mansoni* pairs and treated for 3 days with vehicle or compounds **1–3** were classified by microscopic observation according to the Vogel and Prata staging system of egg maturation [47]. The thiazoavarone (**2**) resulted the most effective compound, impairing eggs maturation already at 5 µM and resulting in undeveloped and severely damaged eggs at 20 µM (Figure 5). Similar results were obtained with compounds **1** and **3** at 50 µM.

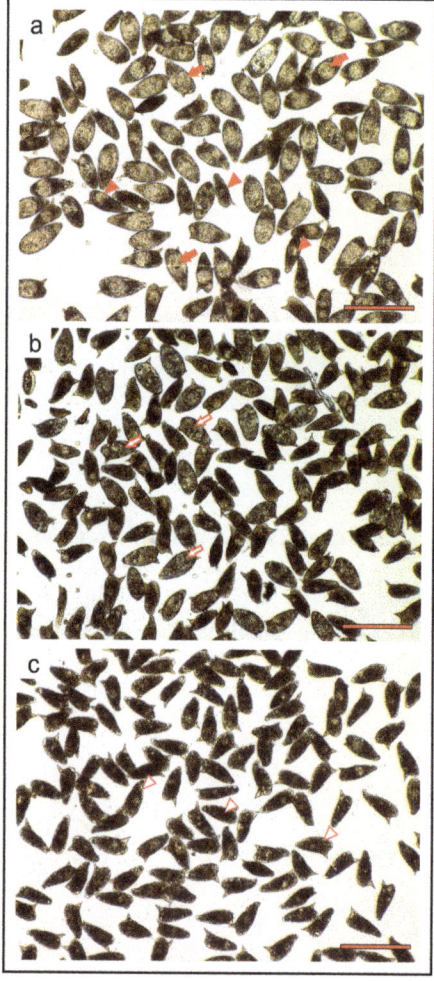

Figure 5. Thiazoavarone (**2**) impairs egg viability and maturation. Representative pictures of IVLEs treated with vehicle (DMSO) (**a**) or compound **2** at 5 µM (**b**) and 20 µM (**c**) for 72 h. Filled red arrows indicate viable eggs at stages III–V (intermediate/developed); filled red triangle indicate viable eggs at stages I–II (immature); red-edged arrows indicate damaged eggs at stages III–V; red-edged triangle indicate damaged eggs at stages I–II. Bar, 200 µm.

2.5. Computational Studies and DFT Calculations

To rationalize the observed SARs, the steric and electronic features of compounds **1–3** were investigated by means of computational studies, including conformational analysis and DFT calculations.

A systematic conformational search considering all rotatable bonds was applied to generate all possible conformations of the compounds, which were, then, subjected to molecular mechanic (MM) geometry optimization using the CFF force field and a distance dependent dielectric constant value of 80 (Discovery Studio 2017, BIOVIA, San Diego USA; see the experimental Section for details) [48]. The global minimum energy conformer (GM) was identified for each compound. All the generated conformers presented an energy difference from the GM (ΔE_{GM}) ≤ 3 kcal/mol. MM conformers were, then, subjected to density functional theory (DFT) calculations. In order to mimic an aqueous environment, all DFT calculations were performed using the conductor-like polarizable continuum model (C-PCM) as solvent model [49]. Moreover, to characterize every structure as minimum, a vibrational analysis was carried out (see the experimental Section for details). Fully optimized DFT conformers were classified into families according to the values of their torsion angles (Tables 6 and 7 and Table S1).

Results evidenced that compounds **1–3** present common conformational features, characterized by the electronic attraction between the hydrogen atoms of the first methylene group of the alkyl substituent and the nearby quinone oxygen, which limits the conformational freedom of R' (Figure 6). Accordingly, the torsional angle τ1 showed just two sets of possible values (~±100°; Tables 6 and 7 and Table S1), and for each of them the rigid sesquiterpene ring could assume three orientations with respect to the thiazinoquinone/quinone/quinol ring (τ2 = ~60°, ~−60° and ~180°; Tables 6 and 7 and Table S1). This determined a total number of six conformers (named I–VI; Figure 6). In the case of the thiazinoquinone derivative **2**, due to the presence of the two opposite flips of the thiazinoquinone ring (τ_{flip} ~ ±60°), we obtained two specular sets of conformers with the same conformational energy (i.e., conformational enantiomers; Figure S10), as previously reported for other thiazinoquinone derivatives [13,14].

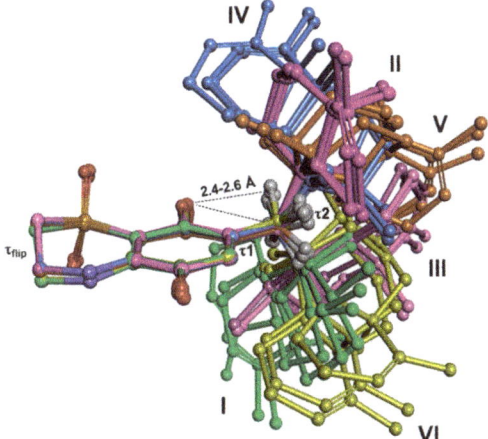

Figure 6. Density functional theory DFT conformers of compounds **1–3** superimposed by the carbon atoms of the quinone/hydroquinone ring. Carbon atoms are colored according to conformer classification (I = green, II = magenta, III = pink, IV = light blue, V = orange, and VI = Yellow); heteroatoms are colored by atom type (H = white, O = red, N = blue, S = orange). Hydrogens are omitted for sake of clarity, with the exception of those of the first methylene group of the R' substituent, whose intramolecular distances from the nearby oxygen atom of the quinone are reported.

Table 6. ΔE_{GM} values (kcal/mol) and torsion angle values (degrees) of the DFT conformers of 2.

Conformer [a]	ΔE_{GM} (kcal/mol)	Torsion Angles (°)	
		τ1 [b]	τ2 [c]
II	0.00	100.38	60.20
I	0.50	−110.21	55.83
IV	1.04	110.37	−72.73
III	1.25	−102.31	179.90
V	2.03	87.13	158.72
VI	3.02	−84.08	−54.03

[a] Only the conformational enantiomers with the value of τ_{flip} ~60° are reported. [b] τ1 torsion angle is defined by e, f, g, and h atoms. [c] τ2 torsion angle is calculated considering f, g, h, and i atoms.

Table 7. ΔE_{GM} values (kcal/mol) and torsion angle values (degrees) of the DFT conformers of 1.

Conformer	ΔE_{GM} (kcal/mol)	Torsion Angles (°)	
		τ1 [a]	τ2 [b]
I	0.00	−91.95	64.65
II	0.01	101.16	60.62
III	1.20	−92.79	169.87
IV	1.25	96.73	−58.29
V	2.33	84.62	173.14
VI	2.64	−81.09	−54.96

[a] τ1 torsion angle is defined by a, b, c, and d atoms. [b] τ2 torsion angle is calculated considering b, c, d, and e atoms.

The fixed position of the methylene group combined with the presence of the rigid sesquiterpene moiety, place in the putative semiquinone radical produced upon one electron reduction/oxidation several hydrogen atoms at a distance (≤3 Å) suitable for an intramolecular radical shift from the oxygen atom to a carbon atom of R′ (see below).

Then, starting from the DFT minima, the redox properties of 1–3 were calculated. At this aim, we considered the two electrons/two protons quinone reduction pathway in a protic solvent (Scheme S1) and all the species involved in the pathway ($Q^{•-}$, $QH^{•}$, QH^{-}, QH_2) were generated and DFT optimized using as starting structures the energetically favored DFT minima I and II.

Two possible protonated semiquinone species may be formed, depending on which of the two quinone oxygen atoms is reduced/oxidized at first. The location of the lowest unoccupied molecular orbital (LUMO) in 1 and 2 and of the highest occupied molecular orbital (HOMO) in 3 indicated the oxygen opposite to the alkyl chain as the most probable site to be reduced and the one close to the alkyl chain as the most probable site to be oxidized, respectively (Figure 7). It is worthy to be mentioned that, regarding the most probable oxidation pathway of 3 to its quinone form, since the deprotonation step is supposed to be the first event in protic solvents (Scheme S1), we calculated the pKa values of the two hydroxyl groups, too. Results indicated the hydroxyl group nearby the alkyl substituent as the first to lose the proton (Figure S11), further supporting the formation of the hydroquinone radical reported in Figure 7.

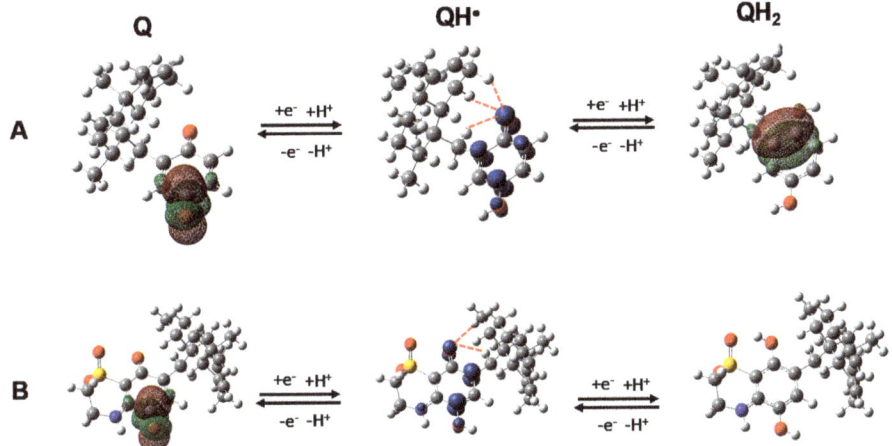

Figure 7. (**A**): DFT global minimum energy conformer (GM) structure of **1** (Q), DFT conformer I of **3** (QH$_2$) and their semiquinone radical (QH$^\bullet$). (**B**) DFT GM structure of **2** (Q) together with its one- and two-electron reduced species QH$^\bullet$ and QH$_2$. Atoms possibly involved in an intramolecular radical shift are evidenced with red dashed lines. The LUMO of **1** and **2**, and the HOMO of **3** are visualized using GaussView with an isosurface value of 0.02 e$^-$/a.u.^{3} The NBO spin density isosurface of the QH$^\bullet$ species is displayed using GaussView with an isosurface value of 0.01 e$^-$/a.u.^{3}. The blue surface (positive spin density) corresponds to an excess of α-electron density.

The standard redox potential (E°) and the standard Gibbs free energy ($\Delta G^0_{red,\,aq}$) of each electron-transfer reaction (see Scheme S1) alongside with the standard Gibbs free energy required for the protonation of the resulting reduced species (ΔG^0_{H+}) of the redox couple **1**, **3** and **2** were calculated (for details see the experimental Section). To further evaluate the propensity of **1** and **2** to undergo a one-electron reduction, the energy of the lowest unoccupied molecular orbital (E$_{LUMO}$) was also taken into account. Similarly, we calculated the ionization potential (IP; i.e., $-E_{HOMO}$) of the radical anion QH$^-$ as indicative of the tendency of the deprotonated species of **3** to undergo a one-electron oxidation. Finally, we considered the energy of the single occupied molecular orbital (E$_{SOMO}$) of the radical species as indicative of the ability to delocalize the unpaired electron. The resulting data are reported in Tables 8 and 9.

Table 8. DFT calculated parameters and standard redox potentials (E°; Q/Q$^{\bullet-}$) of compounds **1**–**3**.

Cmp.	Conf.	E$_{LUMO}$ [a] (Q)	E$_{SOMO}$ [a] (Q$^{\bullet-}$)	E$_{SOMO}$ [a] (QH$^\bullet$)	$\Delta G^0_{red,\,aq}$ [a] (Q/Q$^{\bullet-}$)	E° [b] (Q/Q$^{\bullet-}$)	ΔG^0_{H+} [a] (Q$^{\bullet-}$/QH$^\bullet$)
1, 3	I	−10.62	−143.34	−106.45	−94.58	−328.57	−279.60
1, 3	II	−10.68	−143.42	−106.60	−95.13	−304.65	−279.87
2	I	−17.76	−148.69	−158.60	−95.29	−297.63	−272.91
2	II	−17.83	−148.72	−159.93	−95.66	−281.68	−273.03

[a] kcal/mol. [b] mV.

Table 9. DFT calculated parameters and standard redox potentials (E°; QH•/QH−) of compounds 1–3.

Cmp.	Conf.	$\Delta G°_{red,aq}$ [a] (QH•/QH−)	E° [b] (QH•/QH−)	$\Delta G°_{H+}$ [a] (QH−/QH$_2$)	IP [a] (QH−)	E_{HOMO} [a] (QH$_2$)
1, 3	I	−91.67	−454.64	−295.41	61.09	−158.06
1, 3	II	−89.95	−529.31	−296.77	60.83	−156.34
2	I	−95.22	−300.60	−290.49	130.87	−158.18
2	II	−95.24	−299.70	−289.55	130.94	−159.27

[a] kcal/mol. [b] mV.

A first consideration can be derived comparing the redox properties of the quinone-based compounds **1** and **2**. With respect to **1**, **2** showed either a higher tendency to acquire one electron (lower E_{LUMO} and $\Delta G°_{(red, aq)}$; higher E°; Table 8) and a higher stability of the QH• radical (lower E_{SOMO}; Table 8). While the E_{SOMO} values of the anion radical species showed little difference (E_{SOMO} Q•−; Table 8), on the contrary, the differences became evident after the protonation step (E_{SOMO} QH•). These results, on one hand confirm the key role played by the 1,1-dioxo-1,4-thiazine ring on the electron affinity [11,13,14]; on the other hand, support the hypothesis that the compound activity is related to the formation of the semiquinone radical species. Indeed, the thiazinoquinone derivative **2** resulted overall more potent than the quinone derivative **1**.

A second consideration is that, as evidenced in Figure 7 and Figure S12, all the calculated semiquinone radicals showed a hydrogen atom of the first methylene group together with, at least, another hydrogen atom of the rigid sesquiterpene ring, at a distance suitable for an intra-molecular hydrogen radical shift to the semi- reduced/oxidized oxygen atom (≤3 Å) (Table S2). By consequence, as above mentioned, the presence of the sesquiterpene moiety as alkyl substituent is expected to promote the putative "through space" intramolecular hydrogen radical shift leading to the formation of the toxic radical species. In line with this hypothesis, **2** resulted the most potent thiazinoquinone developed by us against *P. falciparum* D10 and W2 strains as well as against stage V gametocytes. In addition, **1**, although lacking the 1,1-dioxo-1,4-thiazine ring of **2**, resulted still active on *P. falciparum* D10 and W2 strains as well as on schistosomula, contrarily to what previously observed by us for other 1,4-benzoquinone derivatives when compared to the corresponding thiazinoquinone analogues [13,14].

Finally, the hydroquinone **3** showed a higher propensity to be oxidized to the semiquinone radical (i.e., lower E° and IP of the QH− anion) with respect to the corresponding reduced form of **2** (Table 9). Thus, the absence of the 1,1-dioxo-1,4-thiazine ring favors the one-electron oxidation reaction of **3**.

The hydroquinone **3** resulted more active than the corresponding quinone **1** against all considered parasites, while presenting the highest selectivity index with respect to mammalian cells. Both the oxidized and the reduced forms could produce the same putative toxic radical species upon a one-electron transfer reaction. In this view, our results suggest the presence in the parasite cell of a bioactivation reaction partner preferentially binding the hydroquinone (reduced) form (**3**) rather than the quinone (oxidized) form (**1**). This putative bioactivation partner seems not to be present in human cells.

To investigate the role played by molecular pharmacokinetics on the observed SARs, we calculated the distribution coefficient values of **1–3** (clogD, Table S3) (ACD/Percepta 2017). According to Lipinski's rules for drug absorption [50] the thiazinoquinone **2** showed a better cLogD value for cell membrane passive diffusion (cLogD ~ 4) with respect to **1** and **3** (cLogD > 5). However, in specific developmental stages (i.e., *Pf* late gametocytes, promastigote of *L. infantum* and *L. tropica*, amastigote of *L. infantum*, and adult worms of *S. mansoni*) **3** resulted more active than **2** (Tables 2, 4 and 5; Figures 4 and 5). According to what previously reported by us [14], this peculiar activity profile could be due to the significant morphological changes in the parasite during the above-mentioned developmental stages [51–53], which are likely to impair compound ability to penetrate into the parasite by passive diffusion, while it could still penetrate by exploiting the large number of transport proteins expressed on the parasite membrane.

Taken together, the results of our computational investigation indicate that a toxic semiquinone radical species [11,13,14] which can be produced starting both from quinone- and hydroquinone-based compounds could mediate the anti-parasitic effects of the tested compounds 1–3.

3. Materials and Methods

3.1. General Methods

Solvents: Carlo Erba (Pomezia, Rome, Italy). Commercial reagents: Sigma–Aldrich (Saint Louis, MO, USA). TLC: Silica Gel 60 F254, plates 5 × 20, 0.25 mm, Merck (Kenilworth, NJ, USA). Anhydrous solvents: Sigma-Aldrich-Merck. High-resolution ESI-MS analyses were performed on a Thermo LTQ Orbitrap XL mass spectrometer (Thermo-Fisher, San Josè, CA, USA). The spectra were recorded by infusion into the ESI (Thermo-Fisher, San Josè, CA, USA) source dissolving the sample in MeOH. ^{1}H (500 MHz) and ^{13}C (125 MHz) NMR spectra were recorded on an Agilent INOVA spectrometer (Agilent Technology, Cernusco sul Naviglio, Italy) equipped with a ^{13}C enhanced HCN Cold Probe; chemical shifts were referenced to the residual solvent signal (CDCl$_3$: δ_H = 7.26, δ_C = 77.0). For an accurate measurement of the coupling constants, the one-dimensional ^{1}H NMR spectra were transformed at 64 K points (digital resolution: 0.09 Hz). Homonuclear (^{1}H–^{1}H) and heteronuclear (^{1}H–^{13}C) connectivities were determined by COSY and HSQC experiments, respectively. Two and three bond ^{1}H-^{13}C connectivities were determined by gradient 2D HMBC experiments optimized for a $^{2,3}J$ of 8 Hz. $^3J_{H-H}$ values were extracted from 1D ^{1}H NMR. High performance liquid chromatography (HPLC) separations were achieved on a Shimadzu LC-10AT (Shimadzu, Milan, Italy) apparatus equipped with a Knauer K-2301 (LabService Analytica s.r.l., Anzola dell'Emilia, Italy) refractive index.

3.2. Collection, Extraction and Isolation

Several fresh specimens of D. avara were collected along the coast of Narlidere, Bay of Izmir (Turkey, 38°24′45 N 27°8′18 E), in summer of 2017 and immediately frozen and stored at −25 °C until the use. The identification of fresh material was performed by Mr. Arturo Facente while a voucher specimen is deposited at Mugla University, Turkey.

The freshly thawed sponge (21.9 g dry weight after extraction) was homogenized and treated at room temperature with methanol (3 × 1 L) and, subsequently, with dichloromethane (3 × 1 L). The combined extracts were concentrated in vacuo to give an aqueous suspension that was subsequently extracted with BuOH. The butanol soluble material (5.4 g of a dark brown oil), obtained after evaporation of the solvent, was chromatographed on a RP-18 silica gel flash column using a gradient elution (water→methanol→chloroform). The fractions eluted with H$_2$O/MeOH 2:8 (v/v) were chromatographed by HPLC on an RP-18 column (Luna, 3 μm C-18, 150 × 3.00 mm), using MeOH/H$_2$O 95:5 as the eluent (flow 0.5 mL/min). This separation afforded 4.5 mg of pure avarol (3, t_R = 5.4 min) and 26.8 mg of avarone (1, t_R = 9.4 min), identified by comparison of its spectral properties with literature values [21–23].

Avarone (1): yellow powder; [α]$_D^{25}$ = +2.6 (c 0.0014, CH$_3$OH); ^{1}H NMR (CDCl$_3$) spectrum is reported in Supplementary Materials (Figure S6); HRMS (ESI): m/z 313.2156 [M + H]$^+$ (calcd. for C$_{21}$H$_{29}$O$_2$: 313.2162) (Figure S7).

Synthesis of thiazoavarone (2). 20.3 mg of avarone (1, 0.065 mmol) were dissolved in 12 mL of a mixture of CH$_3$CN/EtOH 1: 1 (v/v) and kept under stirring at room temperature; then, a solution of hypotaurine (7 mg, 0.065 mmol) in 2 mL of water was added dropwise together with a catalytic amount of salcomine added in portions. The mixture was stirred for 48 h at room temperature before removing the most of ethanol in vacuo and pouring the residue into water. The orange/yellow mixture was extracted with diethyl ether (60 mL × three times) and the organic phase was washed with brine, dried over sodium sulfate, filtered, and solvent was removed by rotary evaporator. The resulting mixture was chromatographed by HPLC on an RP-18 column (Luna, 3 μm C-18, 150 × 3.00 mm) eluting with MeOH/H$_2$O 75:25 (t_R = 31.6 min) and afforded the pure compound 2 (11 mg, 46%).

Thiazoavarone (2): orange powder; $[\alpha]_D^{25}$ = +19.2 (c 0.0035, CDCl$_3$); ^{1}H and ^{13}C NMR data are reported in Table 1. 1D and 2D NMR data, Figures S2–S5; HRMS (ESI): m/z 440.1865 [M + Na]$^+$ (calcd. for C$_{23}$H$_{31}$NO$_4$SNa: 440.1866) (Figure S1).

Avarol (3): yellow powder; $[\alpha]_D^{25}$ = +12.4 (c 0.0018, CH$_3$OH); ^{1}H NMR (CDCl$_3$) spectrum is reported in Supplementary Materials (Figure S8); HRMS (ESI): m/z 315.2337 [M + H]$^+$ (calcd. for C$_{21}$H$_{31}$O$_2$: 315.2319) (Figure S9).

3.3. P. falciparum Cultures and Drug Susceptibility Assay

P. falciparum cultures were carried out according to Trager and Jensen with slight modifications [13]. The CQ-sensitive strain D10 and the CQ-resistant strain W2 were maintained at 5% hematocrit (human type A-positive red blood cells) in RPMI 1640 (EuroClone, Celbio) medium with the addition of 1% AlbuMax (Invitrogen, Milan, Italy), 0.01% hypoxanthine, 20 mM Hepes, and 2 mM glutamine at 37 °C in a standard gas mixture (1% O$_2$, 5% CO$_2$, and 94% N$_2$). All compounds were dissolved in DMSO and then diluted with medium to achieve the required concentrations (final DMSO concentration <1%, non-toxic to the parasite). Drugs were placed in 96-well flat-bottomed microplates and serial dilutions made. Asynchronous cultures with parasitaemia of 1%–1.5% and 1% final hematocrit were aliquoted into the plates and incubated for 72 h at 37 °C. Parasite growth was determined spectrophotometrically (OD650) by measuring the activity of the parasite lactate dehydrogenase (pLDH), according to a modified version of the method of Makler in control and drug-treated cultures [13]. The antiplasmodial activity is expressed as 50% inhibitory concentrations (IC$_{50}$); each IC$_{50}$ value is the mean ± standard deviation of at least three separate experiments performed in duplicate.

3.4. Gametocytes Cultivation and Susceptibility Assay

The transgenic *P. falciparum* 3D7 strain 3D7elo1-pfs16-CBG99 expressing the *Pyrophorus plagiophthalamus* CBG99 luciferase under a gametocyte specific promoter was used in all the experiments. Parasites were cultured and gametocytes obtained as previously described [54]. Late-stage gametocytes were exposed to compounds at day 11 after N-acetylglucosamine (NAG) addition. Gametocytes stages were counted in Giemsa stained smears and the percentage of stage V gametocytes was higher than 80%. Compounds were prepared by serial dilution, in 96-well plate, in complete medium. Plates were incubated for 72 h at 37 °C under 1% O$_2$, 5% CO$_2$, 94% N$_2$ atmosphere. Luciferase activity was taken as measure of gametocytes viability, as previously described [55]. Briefly, drug-treated gametocyte samples at 2% haematocrit were transferred to 96-well black microplates and D-luciferin (1 mM in citrate buffer 0.1 M, pH 5.5) was added at a 1:1 volume ratio. Luminescence measurements were performed after 10 min with 500 ms integration time using a Sinergy 4 (Biotek) microplate reader. The IC$_{50}$ was extrapolated from the non-linear regression analysis of the concentration–response curve.

3.5. In Vitro Promastigote Susceptibility Assays

Promastigote stage of *L. infantum* strain MHOM/TN/80/IPT1 and *L. tropica* (MHOM/IT/2012/ISS3130) were cultured in Schneider's Drosophila medium (Lonza) supplemented with 10% heat-inactivated fetal calf serum (HyClone) at 24 °C.

The complete medium used for antileishmanial activity assay was RPMI (EuroClone) supplemented with 10% heat-inactivated fetal calf serum (EuroClone), 20 mM Hepes, and 2 mM L-glutamine. To estimate the 50% inhibitory concentration (IC$_{50}$), the MTT (3-[4.5-dimethylthiazol-2-yl]-2.5-diphenyltetrazolium bromide) method was used. Compounds were dissolved in DMSO and then diluted with medium to achieve the required concentrations. Drugs were placed in 96-well round-bottom microplates and seven serial dilutions made. Amphotericin B was used as the reference anti-leishmanial drug. Parasites were diluted in complete medium to 5×10^6 parasites/mL and 100 µL of the suspension was seeded into the plates, incubated at 24 °C for 72 h and then 20 µL of MTT solution (5 mg/mL) was added into each well for 3 h. The plates were then centrifuged, the supernatants discarded and the resulting pellets dissolved in 100 µL of lysing buffer consisting of 20% (*w/v*) of a solution of SDS (Sigma), 40% of *N,N*-dimethylformamide (Merck) in H_2O. The absorbance was measured spectrophotometrically at a test wavelength of 550 nm and a reference wavelength of 650 nm. The results are expressed as IC_{50} which is the dose of compound necessary to inhibit parasite growth by 50%; each IC_{50} value is the mean ± standard deviation of separate experiments performed in duplicate.

3.6. In Vitro Intracellular Amastigote Susceptibility Assays

THP-1 cells (human acute monocytic leukemia cell line) were maintained in RPMI supplemented with 10% FBS (EuroClone), 50 µM 2-mercaptoethanol, 20 mM Hepes, 2 mM glutamine, at 37 °C in 5% CO_2. For *Leishmania* infections, THP-1 cells were plated at 5×10^5 cells/mL in 16-chamber Lab-Tek culture slides (Nunc) and treated with 0.1 µM phorbol myristate acetate (PMA, Sigma) for 48 h to achieve differentiation into macrophages. Cells were washed and infected with metacyclic *L. infantum* promastigotes at a macrophage/promastigote ratio of 1/10 for 24 h. Cell monolayers were then washed and incubated in the presence of test compounds for 72 h. Slides were fixed with methanol and stained with Giemsa. The percentage of infected macrophages in treated and non-treated cells was determined by light microscopy.

3.7. Cytotoxicity Assay

The long-term human microvascular endothelial cell line (HMEC-1) was maintained in MCDB 131 medium (Invitrogen, Milan, Italy) supplemented with 10% fetal calf serum (HyClone, Celbio, Milan, Italy), 10 ng/mL of epidermal growth factor, 1 µg/ml of hydrocortisone, 2 mM glutamine and 20 mM Hepes buffer (EuroClone). For the cytotoxicity assays, HMEC-1 were plated at 10^5 cells/mL in 96-well flat bottom microplates. THP-1 cells were plated at 5×10^5 cells/mL in 96-well flat bottom microplates and treated with 0.1 µM PMA for 48 h to achieve differentiation into macrophages. Cells were then treated with serial dilutions of test compounds and cell proliferation evaluated using the MTT assay described for promastigotes. The results are expressed as IC_{50}, which is the dose of compound necessary to inhibit cell growth by 50%.

3.8. In vitro Effects of Compounds on S. mansoni Parasites and Eggs

Schistosomula were prepared by mechanical transformation of cercariae, as previously described [56]. The ATP-based viability assay with CellTiterGlo (Promega, Italy) on the larval stage of schistosomes was carried out in 96-well, black, tissue culture plates by adaptation of a protocol previously set up in our laboratory [56]. DMSO (vehicle) and gambogic acid (10 µM) were used as the negative and positive controls in each plate and the percentage of viability for each compound was calculated as the ATP reduction against vehicle (0%) and gambogic acid (100%).

All Animal work was approved by the National Research Council, Institute of Cell Biology and Neurobiology animal welfare committee (OPBA) and by the competent authorities of the Italian Ministry of Health, DGSAF, Rome (authorization no. 25/2014-PR and no. 336/2018-PR). All experiments were conducted in respect to the 3R rules according to the ethical and safety rules and guidelines for the use of animals in biomedical research provided by the relevant Italian law and European Union Directive (Italian Legislative Decree 26/2014 and 2010/63/EU) and the International Guiding Principles for Biomedical Research involving animals (Council for the International Organizations of Medical Sciences, Geneva, Switzerland).

A Puerto Rican strain of *S. mansoni* was maintained by passage through albino *Biomphalaria glabrata*, as the intermediate host, and ICR (CD-1) outbred female mice as previously described [56]. Female 4 to 7-week-old mice (Envigo, Udine, Italy) were infected with 200–400 double sex *S. mansoni* cercariae by the tail immersion technique. Adult pairs were harvested from mice 7–8 weeks after infection by reversed perfusion of the hepatic portal system and mesenteric veins. For the viability assays, 5 couples were incubated with the compounds in 3 mL DMEM complete tissue culture medium containing 10% FBS for up to 7 days and phenotypic score was assigned as previously described [57].

For egg-treatment, 5 worm pairs were incubated for 48 h in 3 mL complete tissue culture medium; next the parasites were removed and vehicle (DMSO) or compounds 1–3 were added to each plate containing the eggs previously laid in vitro and observed for 72 h as previously reported [14]. Briefly, images were recorded with a BX41 Olympus microscope and a bright field objective 10× served by a SPOT RT 220-3 Diagnostic Instrument Inc camera. Egg maturation/morphological score was assigned based on the Vogel and Prata' staging system of egg maturation [47].

3.9. Molecular Modelling

Molecular modelling calculations were performed on E4 Server Twin 2× Dual Xeon-5520, equipped with two nodes. Each node: 2× Intel® Xeon® QuadCore E5520-2.26Ghz, 36 GB RAM. The molecular modelling graphics were carried out on a personal computer equipped with Intel(R) Core(TM) i7-4790 processor and SGI Octane 2 workstations.

Conformational property analysis. The apparent pKa and logD values (pH 7.4 and 7.2) of compounds were calculated by using the ACD/Percepta software (ACD/Percepta, Advanced Chemistry Development, Inc., Toronto, ON, Canada, 2017, http://www.acdlabs.com).

The compounds were considered neutral in all calculations performed as a consequence of the estimation of percentage of neutral/ionized forms computed at pH 7.4 (blood pH value) and pH 7.2 (cytoplasm pH value) using the Henderson–Hasselbalch equation. The compounds were built using the Small Molecule tool of Discovery Studio 2017 (Dassault Systèmes BIOVIA, San Diego). Then, the built compounds were subjected to molecular mechanic (MM) energy minimization ($\varepsilon = 80 \times r$) until the maximum RMS derivative was less than 0.001 kcal/Å, using Conjugate Gradient [58] as minimization algorithm. Atomic potentials and charges were assigned using the CFF forcefield [48]. The conformers obtained for each compound were used as starting structure for the subsequent systematic conformational analysis (Search Small Molecule Conformations; Discovery Studio 2017). The conformational space of the compounds was sampled by systematically varying the rotatable bonds sp^3–sp^3 and sp^3–sp^2 with an increment of 60°. The RMSD cutoff for structure selection was set to 0.01 Å. Finally, to ensure a wide variance of the input structures to be successively fully minimized, an energy threshold value of 10^6 kcal/mol was used as selection criteria. The generated structures were then subjected to MM energy minimization (CFF forcefield; $\varepsilon = 80 \times r$) until the maximum RMS derivative was less than 0.001 kcal/Å, using Conjugate Gradient as minimization algorithm. Finally, the resulting conformers were ranked by their potential energy values (i.e., ΔE from the global energy minimum (GM)).

All MM conformers within 5 kcal/mol from GM has been then subjected to DFT calculations. The calculations were carried out using the Gaussian 09 package [59]. All structures were fully optimized at the B3LYP/6-31+G (d,p) level using the conductor-like polarizable continuum model (C-PCM) [49,60,61]. In order to characterize every structure as minimum and to calculate the Gibbs free energy a vibrational analysis was carried out at the same level of theory using the keyword: freq. The RMS force criterion was set to 3×10^{-4} a.u. Partial charges, molecular orbitals and spin density have been calculated using the natural bond orbital (NBO) method [62]. The resulting conformers were ranked by their potential energy values (i.e., ΔE from the global energy minimum (GM)) and classified by their dihedral angle values).

Calculation of redox properties. An appropriate way for calculating the redox potential is by using a thermodynamic cycle. Accordingly, the redox potentials for the compounds was calculated by using the Born–Haber cycle (Scheme 2), which links the Gibbs free energy change of the one-electron transfer reaction in the gas phase with that of the same reaction in aqueous solution [63,64].

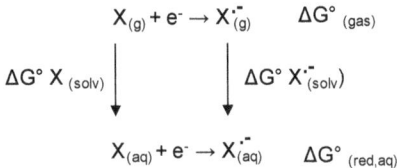

Scheme 2. Born–Haber cycle for a generic one-electron transfer reaction in vacuo and in aqueous solution.

Accordingly, the Born–Haber thermodynamic cycle allows to include the desolvation/solvation effects by calculating the Gibbs free energy values of the reaction in gas phase and in solution. According to this approach, the standard Gibbs free energy of the electron transfer ($\Delta G^0_{red,aq}$), was calculated taking into account the free energy change in the gas phase (ΔG^0_{gas}) and the solvation free energies of the oxidized ($\Delta G^0_{solv}(X)$) and reduced species ($\Delta G^0_{solv}(X^{\bullet-})$) as reported in the following equation:

$$\Delta G^0_{red,aq} = \Delta G^0_{gas} + \left(\Delta G^0_{solv}(X^{\bullet-}) - \Delta G^0_{solv}(X) \right) \tag{1}$$

Accordingly, we, firstly, calculated the Gibbs free energy in gas phase by using the following equation:

$$\Delta G^0_{gas} = G^0_{gas}(X^{\bullet-}) - G^0_{gas}(X) \tag{2}$$

Then, the Gibbs free energy of solvation of both the species X and $X^{\bullet-}$ were calculated according to the following equations:

$$\Delta G^0_{solv}(X) = G^0_{aq}(X) - G^0_{gas}(X) \tag{3}$$

$$\Delta G^0_{solv}(X^-) = G^0_{aq}(X^{\bullet-}) - G^0_{gas}(X^{\bullet-}) \tag{4}$$

The values obtained were used to calculate the standard Gibbs free energy of the overall reaction ($\Delta G^0_{red,aq}$; kcal·mol^{-1}) according to Equation (1). The X and $X^{\bullet-}$ species correspond in our case to Q and $Q^{\bullet-}$, respectively in the first electron transfer, and to $QH^{\bullet}$ and QH^- in the second electron transfer (see Scheme S1).

Finally, the $\Delta G^0_{red,aq}$, were used to calculate the standard reduction potential by the Nernst equation:

$$E^0 = -\frac{\Delta G^0_{red,aq}}{nF} \tag{5}$$

where n is the number of electrons involved in the process (i.e., 1) and F the Faraday constant (23.06 kcal mol^{-1} V^{-1}).

The reduction potential given by the Equation (5) is an absolute value of the parameter and has to be referred to the standard hydrogen electrode (SHE; redox potential of 4.43 V), to obtain the standard redox potential. Accordingly, the value of 4.43 V was subtracted from the values obtained by Equation (5).

On these bases, in order to calculate the redox potential, starting from the structure of the DFT Q GM conformers (i.e., the starting quinone species), the redox states $Q^{\bullet-}$, $QH^{\bullet}$, QH^-, QH_2 were generated. Following the reduction pathway of quinones showed in Scheme S1, each species was generated starting from the DFT optimized species of the previous step and submitted to full DFT optimization both in aqueous solution (using the C-PCM method) and in vacuo using the same parameters above described.

The standard Gibbs free energy for the protonation of the reduced species were calculated by determining ΔG° of the reaction $Y + H^+ \rightarrow YH$ that is $\Delta G^{\circ} = G^{\circ}(YH) - G^{\circ}(Y)$, where Y is $Q^{\bullet-}$ or QH^- DFT conformer. The energy of the frontier molecular orbitals (HOMO, LUMO, and SOMO) were considered for the species Q, $Q^{\bullet-}$, $QH^{\bullet}$ and QH^- fully optimized by DFT calculations performed in the aqueous solution (using the C-PCM method). According to the Koopmans' theorem [65], the ionization potential (IP) is given by the negative of the value of the energy of the HOMO.

4. Conclusions

We investigated the antiparasitic potential of the marine sesquiterpene avarone (**1**), its reduced form avarol (**3**), and thiazoavarone (**2**), a novel semisynthetic thiazinoquinone analogue obtained through a condensation reaction of **1** with hypotaurine, which resulted completely regioselective. Both the natural metabolites **1** and **3**, as well as the semisynthetic derivative **2** resulted active against D10 and W2 strains and late stage gametocytes of *P. falciparum*, against larval and adult developmental stages, and eggs of the platyhelminth *S. mansoni*, and also against promastigote and amastigote forms of *L. infantum* and *L. tropica*. The observed differences in the magnitude of the effects of the three molecules allowed us to draw some interesting conclusions, strongly supported by the results of the DFT analysis. In particular, the thiazinoquinone **2** resulted as significantly more potent than the quinone derivative **1** against D10 and W2 strains of *P. falciparum* as well as on the larval stage of *S. mansoni*. On the other hand, compound **1**, although lacking the 1,1-dioxo-1,4-thiazine ring, resulted still active on *P. falciparum* and on *Schistosoma* larval stage, contrarily to what previously observed for other 1,4-benzoquinone derivatives when compared to the corresponding thiazinoquinone analogues [13,14]. The calculated redox properties of **1** and **2** evidenced for **2** either a higher tendency to acquire one electron and a higher stability of the QH$^\bullet$ radical. Noteworthy, thiazoavarone **2** resulted the most potent antimalarial thiazinoquinone developed by us.

The hydroquinone **3** resulted more active than the corresponding quinone **1** against all considered parasites, with the highest selectivity index with respect to mammalian cells. This led to hypothesize the presence in the studied parasites of a bioactivation reaction partner preferentially binding the reduced form (**3**) rather than the oxidized form (**1**). This putative bioactivation partner seems not to be present in human cells. Finally, comparison of the standard redox potential (E°) and of the ionization potential (IP) of the QH$^-$ anion of **3** with those of the corresponding reduced form of **2**, indicated a higher propensity of **3** to be oxidized to the semiquinone radical and, thus, that the absence of the 1,1-dioxo-1,4-thiazine ring favours the one-electron oxidation reaction of **3**.

These results confirm the key role played by the 1,1-dioxo-1,4-thiazine ring on the electron affinity [11,13,14] and, mainly, corroborate the hypothesis that the compound activity is related to the formation of a toxic semiquinone radical species, which can be produced, upon a one-electron transfer reaction, starting both from quinone- and hydroquinone-based compounds. In the case of the antiplasmodial activity (on the erythrocytic stage of the parasite), our previous results indicated that the bioactivation partner can be represented by free heme (generated during hemoglobin digestion) [11,13]. On the contrary, in the case of *S. mansoni* as well as *Leishmania* parasites, at this stage, we do not know the bioactivation partner of the compounds. However, reactive oxygen species (ROS) generation was found to be involved in the pro-apoptotic mechanism of some natural marine derived thiazinoquinones against Jurkat cells [66]. Thus, it cannot be ruled out that the putative semiquinone radical species reacts with oxygen molecules in cells, generating ROS and future studies will be devoted to clarifying this issue. Moreover, the observed difference between the activity trend of **1**–**3** against the different parasites and their developmental stage may be related to morphological and/or metabolic differences in the targeted organism/stage. Thus, the selective toxicity against the different parasites and their developmental stages can be addressed, taking advantage of the possible bioactivation reaction partners to form the putative toxic radical (i.e., one-electron reduction or oxidation reaction).

Supplementary Materials: The following are available online at http://www.mdpi.com/1660-3397/18/2/112/s1, Figure S1. HRESIMS spectrum of thiazoavarone (**2**), Figure S2. 1H NMR spectrum of thiazoavarone (**2**) in CDCl3, Figure S3. 1H-1H COSY spectrum of thiazoavarone (**2**) in CDCl3, Figure S4. HSQC spectrum of thiazoavarone (**2**) in CDCl3, Figure S5. HMBC spectrum of thiazoavarone (**2**) in CDCl3, Figure S6. HRESIMS spectrum of avarone (**1**), Figure S7. 1H-NMR spectrum of avarone (**1**) in CDCl3, Figure S8. HRESIMS spectrum of avarol (**3**), Figure S9. 1H-NMR spectrum of avarol (**3**) in CDCl3, Figure S10. Conformational enantiomers of thiazoavarone (**2**), Figure S11. Calculated pka values of avarol (**3**) (ACD/Percepta software), Figure S12. DFT conformer of **1**-**3**, and their radical species, Table S1. ΔEGM values and torsion angle values of the DFT conformers of avarol (**3**), Table S2. Hydrogen atoms suitable for an intramolecular radical shift, Table S3. cLogD values of **1**–**3**, Scheme S1. Reduction pathway of quinones in a protic solvent.

Author Contributions: Conceptualization, C.I., C.F. and M.M.; data curation, C.I., R.G., M.P., M.C., A.G., F.S., G.R., P.L., A.A., C.F. and M.M.; formal analysis, C.I., R.G., M.P., M.C., A.G., F.S., G.R., S.P. and S.A.; funding acquisition, G.R., C.F. and M.M.; investigation, C.I., R.G., M.P., M.C., A.G. and F.S.; methodology, C.I., R.G., M.P., M.C., G.R., S.P., N.B., C.F. and M.M.; resources, S.A.; writing—original draft, C.I., R.G., M.P., M.C., G.R., N.B., C.F. and M.M.; writing—review and editing, C.I., R.G., M.P., M.C., A.G., F.S., G.R., P.L., A.A., S.P., S.A., N.B., C.F. and M.M. All authors have read and agree to the published version of the manuscript.

Funding: This research was supported by Ministero dell'Istruzione, dell'Università e della Ricerca (MIUR), PRIN Projects 2010C2LKKJ_006; 20154JRJPP_004, by a grant from Regione Campania-POR Campania FESR 2014/2020 "Combattere la resistenza tumorale: piattaforma integrata multidisciplinare per un approccio tecnologico innovativo alle oncoterapie-Campania Oncoterapie" (*Project N.* B61G18000470007) and by the CNR (National Research Council)-CNCCS (Collezione Nazionale di Composti Chimici e Centro di screening) "Rare, Neglected and Poverty Related Diseases - Schistodiscovery Project" (DSB.AD011.001.003).

Acknowledgments: We wish to thank Asli Kacar and Burcu Omuzbuken for sample collection, and Arturo Facente for identifying the organism.

Conflicts of Interest: The authors declare no conflict of interest.

References

1. World Health Organization. World Malaria Report 2019. Available online: https://www.who.int/publications-detail/world-malaria-report-2019 (accessed on 4 December 2019).
2. World Health Organization. Neglected Tropical Diseases. Program. 2019. Available online: https://www.who.int/neglected_diseases/en/ (accessed on 27 December 2019).
3. Steinmann, P.; Utzinger, J.; Du, Z.W.; Zhou, X.N. Multiparasitism: A neglected reality on global, regional and local scale. *Adv. Parasitol.* **2010**, *73*, 21–50.
4. Newman, D.J.; Cragg, G.M. Natural products as sources of new drugs from 1981 to 2014. *J. Nat. Prod.* **2016**, *79*, 629–661. [CrossRef]
5. Mayer, A.M.S.; Rodríguez, A.D.; Taglialatela-Scafati, O.; Fusetani, N. Marine Pharmacology in 2012–2013: Marine Compounds with Antibacterial, Antidiabetic, Antifungal, Anti-Inflammatory, Antiprotozoal, Antituberculosis, and Antiviral Activities; Affecting the Immune and Nervous Systems, and Other Miscellaneous. *Mar. Drugs* **2017**, *15*, E273. [CrossRef] [PubMed]
6. Loo, C.S.N.; Lam, N.S.K.; Yu, D.; Su, X.-Z.; Lu, F. Artemisinin and its derivatives in treating protozoan infections beyond malaria. *Pharmacol. Res.* **2017**, *117*, 192–217. [CrossRef] [PubMed]
7. Chua, M.J.; Arnold, M.S.J.; Xu, W.; Lancelot, J.; Lamotte, S.; Späth, G.F.; Prina, E.; Pierce, R.J.; Fairlie, D.P.; Skinner-Adams, T.S.; et al. Effect of clinically approved HDAC inhibitors on *Plasmodium*, *Leishmania* and *Schistosoma* parasite growth. *Int. J. Parasitol. Drugs Drug Resist.* **2017**, *7*, 42–50. [CrossRef]
8. Chen, M.M.; Shi, L.; Sullivan, D.J., Jr. Haemoproteus and Schistosoma synthesize heme polymers similar to *Plasmodium* hemozoin and beta-hematin. *Mol. Biochem. Parasitol.* **2001**, *113*, 1–8. [CrossRef]
9. Egan, T.J. Recent advances in understanding the mechanism of hemozoin (malaria pigment) formation. *J. Inorg. Biochem.* **2008**, *102*, 1288–1299. [CrossRef] [PubMed]
10. Aiello, A.; Fattorusso, E.; Luciano, P.; Mangoni, A.; Menna, M. Isolation and structure determination of aplidinones A-C from the Mediterranean ascidian *Aplidium conicum*: A successful regiochemistry assignment by quantum mechanical ^{13}C NMR chemical shift calculations. *Eur. J. Org. Chem.* **2005**, 5024–5030. [CrossRef]
11. Imperatore, C.; Persico, M.; Aiello, A.; Luciano, P.; Guiso, M.; Sanasi, M.F.; Taramelli, D.; Parapini, S.; Cebrián-Torrejón, G.; Doménech-Carbó, A.; et al. Marine inspired antiplasmodial thiazinoquinones: Synthesis, computational studies and electrochemical assays. *RSC Adv.* **2015**, *5*, 70689–70702. [CrossRef]
12. Imperatore, C.; Cimino, P.; Cebrián-Torrejón, G.; Persico, M.; Aiello, A.; Senese, M.; Fattorusso, C.; Menna, M.; Doménech-Carbó, A. Insight into the mechanism of action of marine cytotoxic thiazinoquinones. *Mar. Drugs* **2017**, *15*, 335. [CrossRef]
13. Imperatore, C.; Persico, M.; Senese, M.; Aiello, A.; Casertano, M.; Luciano, P.; Basilico, N.; Parapini, S.; Paladino, A.; Fattorusso, C.; et al. Exploring the antimalarial potential of the methoxy-thiazinoquinone scaffold: Identification of a new lead candidate. *Bioorg. Chem.* **2019**, *85*, 240–252. [CrossRef]

14. Gimmelli, R.; Persico, M.; Imperatore, C.; Saccoccia, F.; Guidi, A.; Casertano, M.; Luciano, P.; Pietrantoni, A.; Bertuccini, L.; Paladino, A.; et al. Thiazinoquinones as New Promising Multistage Schistosomicidal Compounds Impacting *Schistosoma mansoni* and Egg Viability. *ACS Infect. Dis.* **2020**, *6*, 124–137. [CrossRef] [PubMed]
15. Imperatore, C.; Della Sala, G.; Casertano, M.; Luciano, P.; Aiello, A.; Laurenzana, I.; Piccoli, P.; Menna, M. In vitro Antiproliferative Evaluation of Synthetic Meroterpenes Inspired by Marine Natural Products. *Mar. Drugs* **2019**, *17*, 684. [CrossRef] [PubMed]
16. Menna, M.; Aiello, A.; D'Aniello, F.; Fattorusso, E.; Imperatore, C.; Luciano, P.; Vitalone, R. Further investigation of the mediterranean sponge *Axinella polypoides*: Isolation of a new cyclonucleoside and a new betaine. *Mar. Drugs* **2012**, *10*, 2509–2518. [CrossRef] [PubMed]
17. Imperatore, C.; Luciano, P.; Aiello, A.; Vitalone, R.; Irace, C.; Santamaria, R.; Li, J.; Guo, Y.-W.; Menna, M. Structure and Configuration of Phosphoeleganin, a Protein Tyrosine Phosphatase 1B Inhibitor from the Mediterranean Ascidian *Sidnyum elegans*. *J. Nat. Prod.* **2016**, *79*, 1144–1148. [CrossRef] [PubMed]
18. Imperatore, C.; D'Aniello, F.; Aiello, A.; Fiorucci, S.; D'Amore, C.; Sepe, V.; Menna, M. Phallusiasterols A and B: Two new sulfated sterols from the Mediterranean tunicate *Phallusia fumigata* and their effects as modulators of the PXR receptor. *Mar. Drugs* **2014**, *12*, 2066–2078. [CrossRef] [PubMed]
19. Luciano, P.; Imperatore, C.; Senese, M.; Aiello, A.; Casertano, M.; Guo, Y.; Menna, M. Assignment of the Absolute Configuration of Phosphoeleganin via Synthesis of Model Compounds. *J. Nat. Prod.* **2017**, *80*, 2118–2123. [CrossRef]
20. Casertano, M.; Imperatore, C.; Luciano, P.; Aiello, A.; Putra, M.Y.; Gimmelli, R.; Ruberti, R.; Menna, M. Chemical Investigation of the Indonesian Tunicate *Polycarpa aurata* and Evaluation of the Effects Against *Schistosoma mansoni* of the Novel Alkaloids Polyaurines A and B. *Mar. Drugs* **2019**, *17*, 278. [CrossRef]
21. Minale, L.; Riccio, R.; Sodano, G. Avarol, a novel sesquiterpenoid hydroquinone with a rearranged drimane skeleton from the sponge *Dysidea avara*. *Tetrahedron Lett.* **1974**, *38*, 3401–3404. [CrossRef]
22. De Rosa, S.; Minale, L.; Riccio, R.; Sodano, G. The absolute configuration of avarol, a rearranged sesquiterpenoid hydroquinone from a marine sponge. *J. Chem. Soc. Perkins Trans. 1* **1976**, *13*, 1408–1414. [CrossRef]
23. Cozzolino, R.; De Giulio, A.; De Rosa, S.; Strazzullo, G.; Gašić, M.J.; Sladić, D.; Zlatović, M. Biological Activities of Avarol Derivatives, 1. Amino Derivatives. *J. Nat. Prod.* **1990**, *53*, 699–702. [CrossRef]
24. Müller, W.E.G.; Zahn, R.K.; Gašić, M.J.; Dogović, N.; Maidhof, A.; Becker, C.; Diehl-Seifert, B.; Eich, E. Avarol, a cytostatically active compound from the marine sponge *Dysidea avara*. *Comp. Biochem. Physiol.* **1985**, *80C*, 47–52. [CrossRef]
25. Müller, W.E.G.; Maidhof, A.; Zahn, R.K.; Schröder, H.C.; Gašić, M.J.; Heidemann, D.; Bernd, A.; Kurelec, B.; Eich, E.; Seibert, G. Potent antileukemic activity of the novel cytostatic agent avarone and its analogues in vitro and in vivo. *Cancer Res.* **1985**, *45*, 4822–4826. [PubMed]
26. Müller, W.E.G.; Sladić, D.; Zahn, R.K.; Bässler, K.H.; Dogović, N.; Gerner, H.; Gašić, M.J.; Schröder, H.C. Avarol-induced DNA Strand Breakage in vitro and in Friend Erythroleukemia Cells. *Cancer Res.* **1987**, *47*, 6565–6571.
27. Ferrándiz, M.L.; Sanz, M.J.; Bustos, G.; Payá, M.; Alcaraz, M.J.; De Rosa, S. Avarol and avarone, two new anti-inflammatory agents of marine origin. *Eur. J. Pharmacol.* **1994**, *253*, 75–82. [CrossRef]
28. Belisario, M.A.; Maturo, M.; Avagnale, G.; De Rosa, S.; Scopacasa, F.; De Caterina, M. In vitro effect of avarone and avarol, a quinone/hydroquinone couple of marine origin, on platelet aggregation. *Pharmacol. Toxicol.* **1996**, *79*, 300–304. [CrossRef]
29. Lucas, R.; Giannini, C.; D'Auria, M.V.; Payá, M. Modulatory effect of bolinaquinone, a marine sesquiterpenoid, on acute and chronic inflammatory processes. *J. Pharmacol. Exp. Ther.* **2003**, *304*, 1172–1180. [CrossRef]
30. Kurelec, B.; Zahn, R.K.; Gašić, M.J.; Britvić, S.; Lucić, D.; Müller, W.E. Antimutagenic activity of the novel antileukemic agents, avarone and avarol. *Mutat. Res.* **1985**, *144*, 63–66. [CrossRef]
31. Seibert, G.; Raether, W.; Dogović, N.; Gašić, M.J.; Zahn, R.K.; Müller, W.E.G. Antibacterial and antifungal activity of avarone and avarol. *Zent. Bakteriol. Hyg.* **1985**, *260A*, 379–386. [CrossRef]
32. Sarin, P.S.; Sun, D.; Thornton, A.; Müller, W.E.G. Inhibition of replication of the etiological agent of acquired immune deficiency syndrome (human T-lymphotropic retrovirus/lymphadenopathy-associated virus) by avarol and avarone. *J. Natl. Cancer Inst.* **1987**, *78*, 663–666.

33. Loya, S.; Hizi, A. The inhibition of human immunodeficiency virus type 1 reverse transcriptase by avarol and avarone derivatives. *FEBS Lett.* **1990**, *269*, 131–134. [CrossRef]
34. De Rosa, S. Marine Natural Products: Analysis, Structure Elucidation, Bio-Activity and Potential Use as Drug. In *Natural Products in the New Millenium: Prospects and Industrial Applications*; Rauter, A.P., Palma, F.B., Justino, J., Araújo, M.E., Dos Santos, S.P., Eds.; Kluwer: Dordrecht, The Netherlands, 2002; pp. 441–461.
35. Belisario, M.A.; Maturo, M.; Pecce, R.; De Rosa, S.; Villani, G.R. Effect of avarol and avarone on in vitro-induced microsomal lipid peroxidation. *Toxicology* **1992**, *72*, 221–233. [CrossRef]
36. Amigó, M.; Payá, M.; Braza-Boïls, A.; De Rosa, S.; Terencio, M.C. Avarol inhibits TNF-alpha generation and NF-kB activation in human cells and in animal models. *Life Sci.* **2008**, *82*, 256–264. [CrossRef]
37. Tsoukatou, M.; Maréchal, J.P.; Hellio, C.; Novaković, I.; Tufegdzic, S.; Sladić, D.; Gašić, M.J.; Clare, A.S.; Vagias, C.; Roussis, V. Evaluation of the Activity of the Sponge Metabolites Avarol and Avarone and their Synthetic Derivatives Against Fouling Micro- and Macroorganisms. *Molecules* **2007**, *12*, 1022–1034. [CrossRef] [PubMed]
38. Vilipic, J.; Novakovic, I.; Stanojkovic, T.; Matic, I.; Segan, D.; Kljajic, Z.; Sladic, D. Synthesis and biological activity of amino acid derivatives of avarone and its model compound. *Bioorg. Med. Chem.* **2015**, *23*, 6930–6942. [CrossRef]
39. Bozic, T.; Novakovic, I.; Gasic, M.J.; Juranic, Z.; Stanojkovic, T.; Tufegdzic, S.; Kljajic, Z.; Sladic, D. Synthesis and biological activity of derivatives of the marine quinone avarone. *Eur. J. Med.Chem.* **2010**, *5*, 923–929. [CrossRef]
40. Diaz-Marrero, A.R.; Austin, P.; Van Soest, R.; Matainaho, T.; Roskelley, C.D.; Roberge, M.; Andersen, R.J. Avinosol, a meroterpenoid-nucleoside conjugate with antiinvasion activity isolated from the marine sponge Dysidea sp. *Org. Lett.* **2006**, *8*, 3749–3752. [CrossRef]
41. De Giulio, A.; De Rosa, S.; Strazzullo, G.; Diliberto, L.; Obino, P.; Marongiu, M.E.; Pani, A.; La Colla, P. Synthesis and evaluation of cytostatic and antiviral activities of 3′ and 4′-avarone derivatives. *Antivir. Chem. Chemother.* **1991**, *2*, 223–227. [CrossRef]
42. Butterworth, A.S.; Skinner-Adams, T.S.; Gardiner, D.L.; Trenholme, K.R. *Plasmodium falciparum* gametocytes: With a view to a kill. *Parasitology* **2013**, *140*, 1718–1734. [CrossRef]
43. Pérez-Pertejo, Y.; Escudero-Martínez, J.M.; Reguera, R.M.; Balaña-Fouce, R.; García, P.A.; Jambrina, P.G.; San Feliciano, A.; Castro, M.-Á. Antileishmanial activity of terpenylquinones on *Leishmania infantum* and their effects on *Leishmania* topoisomerase IB. *Int. J. Parasitol. Drugs Drug Resist.* **2019**, *11*, 70–79. [CrossRef]
44. Katsuno, K.; Burrows, J.N.; Duncan, K.; van Huijsduijnen, R.H.; Kaneko, T.; Kita, K.; Slingsby, B.T. Hit and lead criteria in drug discovery for infectious diseases of the developing world. *Nat. Rev. Drug Discov.* **2015**, *14*, 751–758. [CrossRef] [PubMed]
45. Skelly, P.J.; Shoemaker, C.B. Induction cues for tegument formation during the transformation of *Schistosoma mansoni* cercariae. *Int. J. Parasitol.* **2000**, *30*, 625–631. [CrossRef]
46. McManus, D.P.; Dunne, D.W.; Sacko, M.; Utzinger, J.; Vennervald, B.J.; Zhou, X.-N. Schistosomiasis. *Nat. Rev. Dis. Primers* **2018**, *4*, 13. [CrossRef] [PubMed]
47. Michaels, R.M.; Prata, A. Evolution and characteristics of *Schistosoma mansoni* eggs laid in vitro. *J. Parasitol.* **1968**, *54*, 921–930. [CrossRef]
48. Ewig, C.S.; Berry, R.; Dinur, U.; Hill, J.R.; Hwang, M.J.; Li, H.; Liang, C.; Maple, J.; Peng, Z.; Stockfisch, T.P.; et al. Derivation of class II force fields. VIII. Derivation of a general quantum mechanical force field for organic compounds. *J. Comput. Chem.* **2001**, *22*, 1782–1800. [CrossRef]
49. Cossi, M.; Rega, N.; Scalmani, G.; Barone, V. Energies, structures, and electronic properties of molecules in solution with the C-PCM solvation model. *J. Comp. Chem.* **2003**, *24*, 669–681. [CrossRef]
50. Lipinski, C.A.; Lombardo, F.; Dominy, B.W.; Feeney, P.J. Experimental and computational approaches to estimate solubility and permeability in drug discovery and development settings. *Adv. Drug Deliv. Rev.* **2001**, *46*, 3–26. [CrossRef]
51. Van Hellemond, J.J.; Retra, K.; Brouwers, J.F.; van Balkom, B.W.; Yazdanbakhsh, M.; Shoemaker, C.B.; Tielens, A.G. Functions of the tegument of schistosomes: Clues from the proteome and lipidome. *Int. J. Parasitol.* **2006**, *236*, 691–699. [CrossRef]
52. Skelly, P.J.; Wilson, R.A. Making sense of the schistosome surface. *Adv. Parasitol.* **2006**, *65*, 185–284.
53. Sunter, J.; Gull, K. Shape, form, function and *Leishmania* pathogenicity: From textbook descriptions to biological understanding. *Open Biol.* **2017**, *7*, 170165. [CrossRef]

54. D'Alessandro, S.; Silvestrini, F.; Dechering, K.; Corbett, Y.; Parapini, S.; Timmerman, M.; Galastri, L.; Basilico, N.; Sauerwein, R.; Alano, P.; et al. A *Plasmodium falciparum* screening assay for anti-gametocyte drugs based on parasite lactate dehydrogenase detection. *J. Antimicrob. Chemother.* **2013**, *68*, 2048–2058. [CrossRef] [PubMed]
55. D'Alessandro, S.; Camarda, G.; Corbett, Y.; Siciliano, G.; Parapini, S.; Cevenini, L.; Michelini, E.; Roda, A.; Leroy, D.; Taramelli, D.; et al. A chemical susceptibility profile of the *Plasmodium falciparum* transmission stages by complementary cell-based gametocyte assays. *J. Antimicrob. Chemother.* **2016**, *71*, 1148–1158. [CrossRef] [PubMed]
56. Lalli, C.; Guidi, A.; Gennari, N.; Altamura, S.; Bresciani, A.; Ruberti, G. Development and validation of a luminescence-based, medium-throughput assay for drug screening in *Schistosoma mansoni*. *PLoS Negl. Trop. Dis.* **2015**, *9*, e0003484. [CrossRef] [PubMed]
57. Guidi, A.; Lalli, C.; Gimmelli, R.; Nizi, E.; Andreini, M.; Gennari, N.; Saccoccia, F.; Harper, S.; Bresciani, A.; Ruberti, G. Discovery by organism based high-throughput screening of new multi-stage compounds affecting *Schistosoma mansoni* viability, egg formation and production. *PLoS Negl. Trop. Dis.* **2017**, *11*, e0005994. [CrossRef]
58. Fletcher, R. Unconstrained optimization. In *Practical Methods of Optimization*, 1st ed.; John Wiley & Sons Ltd.: New York, NY, USA, 1980; Volume 1, pp. 1–128. ISBN 978-0471277118.
59. Gaussian 09 Citation. Available online: https://gaussian.com/g09citation/ (accessed on 13 February 2020).
60. Becke, D. Density-functional thermochemistry. III. The role of exact exchange. *J. Chem. Phys.* **1993**, *98*, 5648–5652. [CrossRef]
61. Lee, C.; Yang, W.; Parr, R.G. Development of the Colle-Salvetti correlation-energy formula into a functional of the electron density. *Phys. Rev. B Condens. Matter Mater. Phys.* **1988**, *37*, 785–789. [CrossRef]
62. Reed, E.; Weinstock, R.B.; Weinhold, F. Natural Population Analysis. *J. Chem. Phys.* **1985**, *83*, 735–746. [CrossRef]
63. Li, J.; Fisher, C.L.; Chen, J.L.; Bashford, D.; Noodleman, L. Calculation of Redox Potentials and pKa Values of Hydrated Transition Metal Cations by a Combined Density Functional and Continuum Dielectric Theory. *Inorg. Chem.* **1996**, *35*, 4694–4702. [CrossRef]
64. Moens, J.; Geerlings, P.; Roos, G. A Conceptual DFT Approach for the Evaluation and Interpretation of Redox Potentials. *Chem. Eur. J.* **2007**, *13*, 8174–8184. [CrossRef]
65. Koopmans, T. Ordering of Wave Functions and Eigenenergies to the Individual Electrons of an Atom. *Physica* **1933**, *1*, 104–113. [CrossRef]
66. Aiello, A.; Fattorusso, E.; Luciano, P.; Macho, A.; Menna, M.; Muñoz, E. Antitumor effects of two novel naturally occurring terpene quinones isolated from the mediterranean ascidian *Aplidium conicum*. *J. Med. Chem.* **2005**, *48*, 3410–3416. [CrossRef] [PubMed]

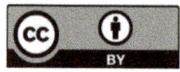

© 2020 by the authors. Licensee MDPI, Basel, Switzerland. This article is an open access article distributed under the terms and conditions of the Creative Commons Attribution (CC BY) license (http://creativecommons.org/licenses/by/4.0/).

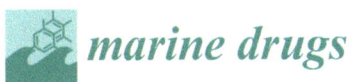

Article

Antifouling Napyradiomycins from Marine-Derived Actinomycetes *Streptomyces aculeolatus* †

Florbela Pereira [1], Joana R. Almeida [2], Marisa Paulino [3], Inês R. Grilo [4], Helena Macedo [3,4], Isabel Cunha [2], Rita G. Sobral [4], Vitor Vasconcelos [2,5] and Susana P. Gaudêncio [1,3,*]

[1] LAQV, Chemistry Department, Faculty for Sciences and Technology, NOVA University of Lisbon, 2829-516 Caparica, Portugal; florbela.pereira@fct.unl.pt
[2] CIIMAR/CIMAR—Interdisciplinary Centre of Marine and Environmental Research, University of Porto, Terminal de Cruzeiros do Porto de Leixões, Avenida General Norton de Matos, 4450-208 Matosinhos, Portugal; joana.reis.almeida@gmail.com (J.R.A.); isabel.cunha@ciimar.up.pt (I.C.); vmvascon@fc.up.pt (V.V.)
[3] UCIBIO, Chemistry Department, Blue Biotechnology and Biomedicine Lab, Faculty for Sciences and Technology, NOVA University of Lisbon, 2829-516 Caparica, Portugal; m.paulino@campus.fct.unl.pt (M.P.); h.macedo@campus.fct.unl.pt (H.M.)
[4] UCIBIO, Life Sciences Department, MOLMICRO of Bacterial Pathogens Lab, Faculty for Sciences and Technology, NOVA University of Lisbon, 2829-516 Caparica, Portugal; inesgrilo@fct.unl.pt (I.R.G.); rgs@fct.unl.pt (R.G.S.)
[5] Biology Department, Faculty of Sciences, Porto University, Rua do Campo Alegre, 4069-007 Porto, Portugal
* Correspondence: s.gaudencio@fct.unl.pt
† Dedicated to the memory of our friend and colleague Ilda Santos-Sanches.

Received: 6 December 2019; Accepted: 16 January 2020; Published: 18 January 2020

Abstract: The undesired attachment of micro and macroorganisms on water-immersed surfaces, known as marine biofouling, results in severe prevention and maintenance costs (billions €/year) for aquaculture, shipping and other industries that rely on coastal and off-shore infrastructures. To date, there are no sustainable, cost-effective and environmentally safe solutions to address this challenging phenomenon. Therefore, we investigated the antifouling activity of napyradiomycin derivatives that were isolated from actinomycetes from ocean sediments collected off the Madeira Archipelago. Our results revealed that napyradiomycins inhibited ≥80% of the marine biofilm-forming bacteria assayed, as well as the settlement of *Mytilus galloprovincialis* larvae (EC$_{50}$ < 5 µg/ml and LC$_{50}$/EC$_{50}$ >15), without viability impairment. In silico prediction of toxicity end points are of the same order of magnitude of standard approved drugs and biocides. Altogether, napyradiomycins disclosed bioactivity against marine micro and macrofouling organisms, and non-toxic effects towards the studied species, displaying potential to be used in the development of antifouling products.

Keywords: marine natural products; actinomycetes; biofouling; antifouling; antibiofilm; napyradiomycins; meroterpenoids; hybrid isoprenoids; drug discovery; bioprospection

1. Introduction

Marine biofouling is the undesired accumulation of micro and macroorganisms on submerged surfaces, including bacteria, algae, larvae, and adults of various phyla, and their by-products, in a dynamic process that begins immediately after water-submersion and takes hours to months to develop [1]. Biofouling formation is divided into four distinct phases: soon after the physical adherence of macromolecules, the process becomes biological, designated as the microfouling phase, in which a bacterial biofilm is responsible for the establishment of an appropriate surface for the subsequent macrofouling organisms to settle, first as spores and larvae which then develop into adults [2,3].

Marine biofouling creates risk to several industries such as aquaculture, power plants, and shipping, amongst others [4,5]. Settlement on the vessel´s hull damages the rudder and propulsion systems [4,6], and leads to an increasing drag of up to 60%, requiring up to 40% higher fuel consumption, in addition to increased CO_2 and SO_2 emissions [7]. Moreover, hull biofouling and ballast water transfer are the main causes for the introduction and spread of nonindigenous marine species into ecosystems worldwide leading to environmental imbalances [8–12]. Antifouling (AF) methods are estimated to save the shipping industry around €60 billion/year in fuel [4]. The most effective AF coatings contain biocides, such as tributyltin (TBT) and tributyltin oxide (TBTO), which were proven to be harmful to non-target organisms and the environment [13]. In fact, the International Maritime Organization banned TBT from ship surfaces in 2008, sparking the demand for new generations of nontoxic or environmentally benign AF solutions [14–16].

In the last years, several reviews reported studies on natural products (NP) isolated from marine organisms with AF activity [17–25]. The quest for AF agents from marine sources started with 2-furanone bromine derivatives extracted from red algae that were reported to prevent fouling [26]. Oroidin, a bromopyrrole alkaloid with AF activity isolated from sponges, inspired the design of 50-synthetic analogs [27,28]. An interesting approach to create AF "living" paints was developed [29] using marine bacteria that were directly encapsulated into polyurethane coatings [30] and hydrogels [31]. Regarding actinomycetes as AF sources, lobocompactol, a diterpene from *Streptomyces cinnabarinus*, was active against the macroalgae *Ulva pertusa*, the diatom *Navicula annexa*, and the bacterium *Pseudomonas aeruginosa* [32,33]. The 6-benzyl and 6-isobutyl 2,5-diketopiperazine derivatives from *S. praecox* were also active against *U. pertusa* and *N. annexa* [34]. 2,5-Diketopiperazines from *S. fungicidicus* and a branched-chain fatty acid, 12-methyltetradecanoid acid, from *Streptomyces* sp. inhibited the barnacle *Balanus amphitrite* and the polychaeta *Hydroides elegans* larval attachment, respectively [35–37]. Quercetin, a flavonoid obtained from *S. fradiae* revealed activity against the cyanobacteria *Anabena sp.* and *Nostoc sp.*, and mussel *Perna indica* larvae [38]. To the best of our knowledge, ivermectin, a chemically modified form of avermectin, a macrolide isolated from *S. avermitilis*, commonly used to treat parasitic worms and as insecticide, is the only marketed AF agent obtained from actinomycetes, although terrestrial, which is used in paints for macrofouling inhibition.

We focused on bioprospecting marine-derived actinomycetes as producers of biofouling inhibitors for the potential development of marine-derived sustainable antifouling products. Napyradiomycins are a class of hybrid isoprenoids and/or meroterpenoids known for their antimicrobial and anticancer activities [39,40]. The napyradiomycins reported herein were isolated from a marine-derived actinomycete collection obtained from ocean sediments collected off the Madeira Archipelago [41]. The napyradiomycin molecular network with antibiofilm statistical bioactivity prediction was reported in a recent study by our group [42]. Here, we describe the capacity of napyradiomycins isolated from *S. aculeolatus* to inhibit micro and macrofouling species, and evaluate their ecotoxicity using an in silico approach. Targeting the primary attachment phases of the fouling process would allow preventing accumulation of other marine species. We recently patented the use of napyradiomycin derivatives for marine antifouling paints and coatings [43].

2. Results and Discussion

2.1. Napyradiomycin Derivatives Description

Ethyl acetate (EtOAc) extracts of *Streptomyces aculeolatus* PTM-029 and PTM-420 [41,42] were subjected to micro and macro antifouling bioassay-directed fractionation and isolation, first by silica flash chromatography and subsequently by C_{18} reversed-phase HPLC to yield nine samples comprising twelve napyradiomycin derivatives (**1–12**) (Figure 1). The structures of all compounds were established by HR-MS and interpretation of NMR spectroscopic data, especially 2D NMR (i.e., COSY, HSQC, HMBC, TOCSY experiments), and by comparing the data with those previously reported for napyradiomycins [39,44–49]. All isolated napyradiomycins (**1–12**) were previously reported and their structural characterization is described in the Supplementary Materials. Napyradiomycins SF2415B3 (**3**), 4-dehydro-4a-dechloro- napyradiomycin SF2415B3 (**7**), A80915A (**9**), A80915C (**10**),

4-dehydro-4a-dechloro- napyradiomycin A80915A (**12**) and A1 (**1**), 18-hydroxynapyradiomycin A1 (**2**), A2 (**4**), 16-oxonapyradiomycin A2 (**5**), 4-dehydro-4a-dechloro-16-oxonapyradiomycin A2 (**6**), B3 (**8**), 4-dehydro-4a-dechloro-napyradiomycin B3 (**11**) were isolated from strains PTM-029 and PTM-420, respectively. Interestingly, there was a marked difference in these two sets of napyradiomycins: all the napyradiomycins isolated from PTM-029 (**3**), (**7**), (**9**), (**10**), and (**12**) have a methyl group in the core structure at position 7, while the ones obtained from strain PTM-420 (**1**), (**2**), (**4–6**), (**8**), and (**11**) have a hydrogen atom in that position (Figure 1).

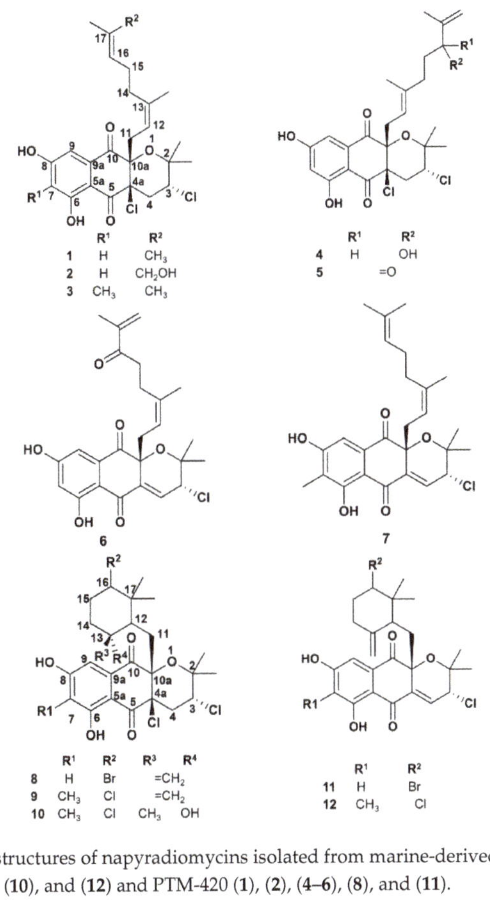

	R^1	R^2
1	H	CH_3
2	H	CH_2OH
3	CH_3	CH_3

	R^1	R^2
4	H	OH
5		=O

	R^1	R^2	R^3	R^4
8	H	Br		$=CH_2$
9	CH_3	Cl		$=CH_2$
10	CH_3	Cl		CH_3 OH

	R^1	R^2
11	H	Br
12	CH_3	Cl

Figure 1. Chemical structures of napyradiomycins isolated from marine-derived *S. aculeolatus* strains PTM-029 (**3**), (**7**), (**9**), (**10**), and (**12**) and PTM-420 (**1**), (**2**), (**4–6**), (**8**), and (**11**).

Despite some of the napyradiomycins were isolated as a mixture (**3** and **7**), (**5** and **6**), (**8** and **11**), and (**9** and **12**) no further purification efforts were performed, since antifouling agents are commonly used as mixture of compounds. For example, ivermectin antifouling product is commercialized as a mixture of two homologous compounds, ~80% of ivermectin B1a, with an ethyl group at position C-26 and ~20% of ivermectin B1b, with a methyl group at C-26 [50].

2.2. Assessment of Napyradiomycin Derivatives Micro and Macrofouling Inhibitory Activity

The antimicrofouling activity of napyradiomycins (**1–12**) was evaluated by testing their inhibitory activity on bacterial propagation and bacterial biofilm formation. Five species of marine bacteria, which are biofilm prolific and described as fouling effectors, including dominant primary colonizers of submerged surfaces [51], were chosen as models for our bioactivity assays, namely *Marinobacter* *hydrocarbonoclasticus* (DSM 8798), *Cobetia marina* (DSM 4741), *Micrococcus luteus* (DSM 20030, ATCC 4698), *Pseudooceanicola batsensis* (DSM 15984) and *Phaeobacter inhibens* (DSM 17395) [52–58].

2.2.1. Antibacterial Activity

As a first screening approach, liquid cultures of *M. hydrocarbonoclasticus*, and *C. marina* in a 96-well format were analyzed for bacterial growth inhibition by percent decrease in OD_{600} after incubation with napyradiomycins (**1–12**) at 31.25 µg/mL.

No PTM-029 napyradiomycins had activity against *M. hydrocarbonoclasticus* or *C. marina*, while PTM-420 napyradiomycins (**1**) and (**8 and 11**) revealed antibacterial activity against *C. marina*. Therefore, PTM-420 napyradiomycins were further tested against three other marine bacterial species, *M. luteus*, *P. batsensis*, and *P. inhibens*.

Napyradiomycin (**1**) inhibited the growth of *M. luteus*, *P. batsensis*, and *C. marina* (96.1 ± 0.5%, 53.9 ± 0.3%, and 19.8 ± 0.6%, respectively), while (**8 and 11**) inhibited the growth of the same three species in addition to *P. inhibens* (95.9 ± 0.1%, 25.3 ± 0.6%, 20.8 ± 1.3%, and 13.0 ± 3.7%, respectively). Napyradiomycin (**4**) only inhibited the growth of *M. luteus* (72.5 ± 7.7%), at this concentration (Figure 2). The remaining napyradiomycins (**2**) and (**5 and 6**) had no effect on bacterial growth of these marine bacterial species, at a concentration of 31.25 µg/mL.

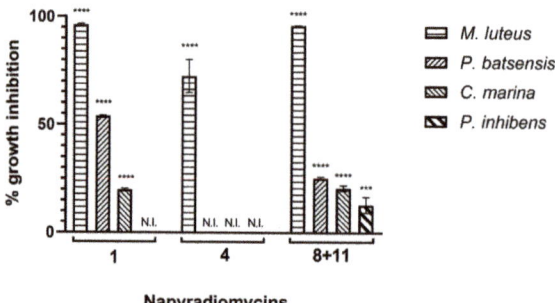

Figure 2. Growth inhibition assay performed for napyradiomycins (**1–12**), at a concentration of 31.25 µg/mL. After incubation for 18 h, bacterial growth was assayed by measuring OD_{600nm}. The growth of *M. hydrocarbonoclasticus* was not inhibited by any of the napyradiomycins tested at this concentration, while (**2**), (**3 and 7**), (**5 and 6**), (**9 and 12**), (**10**), and (**12**) did not inhibit growth of any of the bacteria tested. Percentage of growth inhibition refers to the percentage of growth that was inhibited in the presence of napyradiomycins, when compared to growth with only DMSO. Shown are the average results of three replicates and error bars represent the standard error of the mean (SEM). N.I.—not inhibited; results were statistically significant (**** $p < 0.0001$, *** $p < 0.001$, Dunnett's test).

Napyradiomycins (**1**), (**4**) and (**8 and 11**) were further assayed at lower concentrations (serial 2-fold dilutions, 15.60 µg/mL to 0.98 µg/mL), against the bacterial species for which they showed antibacterial activity at a concentration of 31.25 µg/mL (Figure 3 and Table 1).

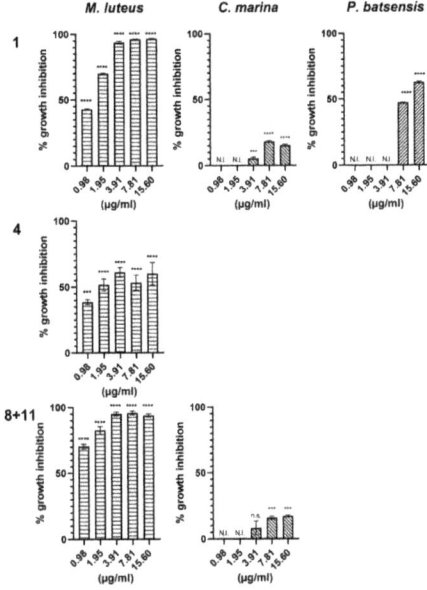

Figure 3. Bacterial growth inhibition of *M. luteus*, *C. marina*, and *P. batsensis* by napyradiomycins (**1**), (**4**), and (**8 and 11**). Napyradiomycins were added to the growth medium of the different bacteria and after 18 h incubation, bacterial growth was assayed by measuring OD_{600nm}. Percentage of growth inhibition refers to the percentage of growth that was inhibited in the presence of the napyradiomycins, when compared to growth with only DMSO. Shown are the average results of three replicates and error bars represent the standard error of the mean (SEM). N.I. not inhibited; results were statistically significant (**** $p < 0.0001$, *** $p < 0.001$, n.s. $p > 0.05$, Dunnett's test).

Table 1. Percentage of growth inhibition of different marine bacteria with the addition of napyradiomycins (**1**), (**4**), and (**8 and 11**). Shown are the average values of the percentage of growth inhibition of three replicates with the standard error of the mean (SEM). N.I.—not inhibited.

Napyradiomycin	(1)			(4)	(8 and 11)	
Concentration (µg/mL)	*M. luteus*	*C. marina*	*P. batsensis*	*M. luteus*	*M. luteus*	*C. marina*
15.60	96.5 ± 0.2	15.3 ± 0.7	62.7 ± 0.6	60.1 ± 8.5	93.9 ± 1.3	17.4 ± 0.5
7.81	96.0 ± 0.3	18.2 ± 0.7	47.4 ± 0.3	53.3 ± 5.7	96.8 ± 1.4	16.0 ± 1.2
3.91	93.6 ± 1.1	5.5 ± 0.8	N.I.	61.2 ± 3.7	95.1 ± 1.5	8.3 ± 5.1
1.95	69.8 ± 0.5	N.I.	N.I.	51.7 ± 4.5	82.7 ± 2.9	N.I.
0.98	42.9 ± 0.4	N.I.	N.I.	38.7 ± 1.9	70.5 ± 1.9	N.I.

Napyradiomycin (**1**) drastically inhibited (>90%) the growth of *M. luteus* at a concentration of 3.91 µg/mL. At the lowest tested concentration, 0.98 µg/mL, (**1**) significantly inhibited the growth of *M. luteus* (42.9 ± 0.4%). For *C. marina*, (**1**) was active at higher concentrations, albeit with a lower growth inhibition percentage (5.5 ± 0.9% for 3.91 µg/mL; 18.2 ± 0.7% for 7.81 µg/mL, and 15.3 ± 0.7% for 15.60 µg/mL). The growth of *P. batsensis* was also significantly inhibited by this napyradiomycin at the concentration of 7.81 µg/mL (47.4 ± 0.3%) and 15.60 µg/mL (62.7 ± 0.6%).

Napyradiomycin (**4**) was able to significantly inhibit approximately 50% of the growth of *M. luteus* at all tested concentrations.

Napyradiomycins (**8 and 11**) drastically inhibited (>90%) the growth of *M. luteus* at a concentration of 3.91 µg/mL. At the lowest concentration, 0.98 µg/mL, (**8 and 11**) still inhibited bacterial growth significantly (70.5 ± 1.9%). The growth of *C. marina* was also significantly inhibited by (**8 and 11**) at concentrations of 7.81 µg/mL (16.0 ± 1.2%), and 15.60 µg/mL (17.4 ± 0.5%). Although (**8 and 11**) inhibited the bacterial growth of P. inhibens and P. batsensis at a concentration of 31.25 µg/mL their growth was not inhibited at the lower tested concentrations (15.60 µg/mL to 0.98 µg/mL).

CuSO$_4$ (5 µM), a potent antifouling agent used in antifouling paints, was used as reference. The growth of P. inhibens, P. batsensis, and M. hydrocarbonoclasticus was inhibited by CuSO$_4$ (66.2 ± 5.6%, 44.8 ± 6.3%, and 35.8 ± 0.8%). M. luteus and C. marina growth was not inhibited.

2.2.2. Antibiofilm Activity

In a 96-well plate, biofilm grown cultures of M. hydrocarbonoclasticus and C. marina were incubated with napyradiomycins (1–12) at a concentration of 31.25 µg/mL. After discarding the media, biofilm inhibition was determined from OD$_{600}$ measurements of crystal violet stained cells resuspended from the plate bottom with acetic acid. All napyradiomycins extracted from the actinomycete strain PTM-029 (3 and 7), (9 and 12), (10), and (12) showed significant biofilm inhibition towards M. hydrocarbonoclasticus that ranged from 25.1 ± 10.2% for (10) to 48.2 ± 1.9% for (9 and 12). Additionally, napyradiomycins (3 and 7) also showed significant biofilm inhibition towards C. marina (23.4 ± 4.9%) (Figure 4 and Table 2).

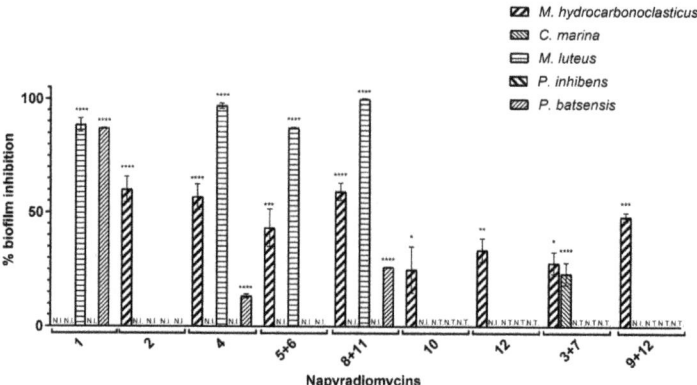

Figure 4. Biofilm inhibition assay performed using napyradiomycins (1–12), at a concentration of 31.25 µg/mL. After incubation for 18 h, planktonic cells were washed, and biofilm was stained using crystal violet and measured at OD$_{600nm}$. The biofilm formation of P. inhibens was not inhibited by any of the napyradiomycins tested at this concentration. Percentage of biofilm inhibition refers to the percentage of biofilm that was inhibited in the presence of the napyradiomycins, when compared to biofilm formation with only DMSO. Shown are the average results of three replicates and error bars represent the standard error of the mean (SEM). N.I.—not inhibited; N.T.—not tested, results were statistically significant (**** $p < 0.0001$, *** $p < 0.001$, ** $p < 0.01$, * $p < 0.05$; Dunnett's test).

Table 2. Results from the biofilm inhibition assay performed using napyradiomycins (1–12) at a concentration of 31.25 µg/mL. Shown are the average values of the percentage of biofilm inhibition of three replicates with the standard error of the mean (SEM). N.I.—not inhibited, N.T.—not tested.

Napyradiomycin	% Biofilm Inhibition ± SEM				
	M. hydrocarbonoclasticus	C. marina	M. luteus	P. batsensis	P. inhibens
(1)	N.I.	N.I.	88.6 ± 2.9	87.2 ± 0.1	N.I.
(2)	60.2 ± 5.7	N.I.	N.I.	N.I.	N.I.
(4)	56.9 ± 5.7	N.I.	97.0 ± 1.2	13.4 ± 0.8	N.I.
(5 and 6)	43.4 ± 8.2	N.I.	87.3 ± 0.3	N.I.	N.I.
(8 and 11)	59.3 ± 3.8	N.I.	100 ± 0.3	26.2 ± 0.0	N.I.
(10)	25.1 ± 10.2	N.I.	N.T.	N.T.	N.T.
(12)	33.7 ± 5.1	N.I.	N.T.	N.T.	N.T.
(3 and 7)	28.0 ± 4.8	23.4 ± 4.9	N.T.	N.T.	N.T.
(9 and 12)	48.2 ± 1.9	N.I.	N.T.	N.T.	N.T.

All PTM-420 napyradiomycins, except (1) showed significant antibiofilm activity against *M. hydrocarbonoclasticus* (4, 56.9 ± 5.7%; 8 and 11, 59.3 ± 3.8%; 5 and 6, 43.4 ± 8.2%; 2, 60.2 ± 5.7%).

As for the bacterial growth inhibition assays, compounds isolated from PTM-420 were tested against three other marine bacterial species, *M. hydrocarbonoclasticus*, *C. marina*, *M. luteus*, *P. batsensis*, and *P. inhibens* (Figure 4 and Table 2).

Napyradiomycin (4) showed significant antibiofilm activity against *M. luteus* and *P. batsensis* (97.0 ± 1.2%, and 13.4 ± 0.8%, respectively). Likewise, (8 and 11) also showed significant antibiofilm activity against *M. luteus* and *P. batsensis* (100.0 ± 0.3% and 26.2 ± 0.0%, respectively). Napyradiomycin (1) had high antibiofilm activity against *M. luteus* and *P. batsensis* (88.6 ± 2.9% and 87.2 ± 0.1%, respectively), while (5 and 6) inhibited the biofilm formation of *M. luteus* (87.3 ± 0.3%) (Figure 4 and Table 2).

PTM-420 napyradiomycins, were assayed at lower concentrations (serial 2-fold dilutions, 15.60 μg/mL to 0.98 μg/mL), against the bacterial species for which they showed antibiofilm activity at a concentration of 31.25 μg/mL (Table 3 and Figure 5).

Table 3. Percentage of inhibition of biofilm formation for different marine bacteria in the presence of different concentrations of napyradiomycins (1), (2), (4), (5 and 6), and (8 and 11). Shown are the average values of the percentage of biofilm inhibition of three replicates with the standard error of the mean (SEM). N.I.—not inhibited.

Napyradiomycin	(1)		(2)	(4)		(5 and 6)		(8 and 11)		
Concentration (μg/mL)	*M. luteus*	*P. batsensis*	*M. hydro.*	*M. hydro.*	*M. luteus*	*M. hydro.*	*M. luteus*	*M. hydro.*	*M. luteus*	*P. batsensis*
15.6	95.4 ± 0.9	86.9 ± 1.0	56.6 ± 0.9	82.3 ± 1.5	88.8 ± 4.2	38.8 ± 8.4	80.1 ± 6.5	62.8 ± 4.0	100 ± 0.3	37.8 ± 0.7
7.81	96.7 ± 0.5	28.4 ± 2.8	51.7 ± 2.0	67.0 ± 5.5	86.7 ± 3.0	53.2 ± 8.2	65.9 ± 12.3	64.9 ± 3.0	100 ± 0.8	23.1 ± 0.2
3.91	95.8 ± 2.9	38.1 ± 0.6	67.7 ± 1.2	84.5 ± 2.0	100 ± 0.4	43.8 ± 9.4	82.5 ± 5.1	72.5 ± 2.3	100 ± 0.6	7.1 ± 4.2
1.95	90.3 ± 3.8	17.7 ± 0.8	56.5 ± 5.7	78.1 ± 3.0	91.7 ± 0.9	44.1 ± 9.6	32.2 ± 13.9	52.7 ± 10.2	100 ± 0.3	7.9 ± 1.0
0.98	59.0 ± 7.4	4.3 ± 4.3	24.6 ± 9.8	56.1 ± 5.6	93.8 ± 4.1	48.2 ± 6.4	33.3 ± 7.4	66.3 ± 6.9	100 ± 0.9	N.I.

Napyradiomycins (8 and 11) completely abolished (100%) biofilm formation of *M. luteus* at all tested concentrations. Biofilm formation by this species was nearly completely inhibited (>90%) by (1) at concentrations higher than 1.95 μg/mL, and at the lowest concentration of 0.98 μg/mL inhibition was of 59.0 ± 7.4%. At this concentration, biofilm formation was also nearly eliminated by (4) (>90%). Napyradiomycins (5 and 6) significantly inhibited the biofilm formation (~80%) of *M. luteus*, at a concentration of 3.91 μg/mL and higher. Biofilm formation of *M. hydrocarbonoclasticus* was inhibited by (2), (4), (5 and 6), and (8 and 11) by at least 50% at all tested concentrations and 80% in the case of (4).

P. batsensis biofilm formation was inhibited by (8 and 11) at a concentration of 1.95 μg/mL and higher. Napyradiomycin (1) also efficiently inhibited biofilm formation of *P. batsensis* (86.9 ± 1.0%) at a concentration of 15.60 μg/mL, and was moderately active at lower concentrations (Table 3).

The most promising compounds for antimicrofouling are those that inhibit biofilm formation without killing the bacteria. Compounds (4), (5 and 6), (8 and 11), and (3 and 7) have potential in this respect, as all inhibit biofilm formation of at least two of the marine bacterial species assayed without inhibiting their growth at the same concentration.

Specifically, (4) inhibited the growth of only *M. luteus* but was able to inhibit biofilm formation of *M. luteus* and *M. hydrocarbonoclasticus* (Figure 4 and Table 2). In addition, at the lowest tested concentration (0.98 μg/mL), the antibacterial activity against *M. luteus* was 38.7 ± 7.7%, while biofilm inhibition was over 90%. Therefore, (4) showed antimicrofouling effectiveness at low concentrations.

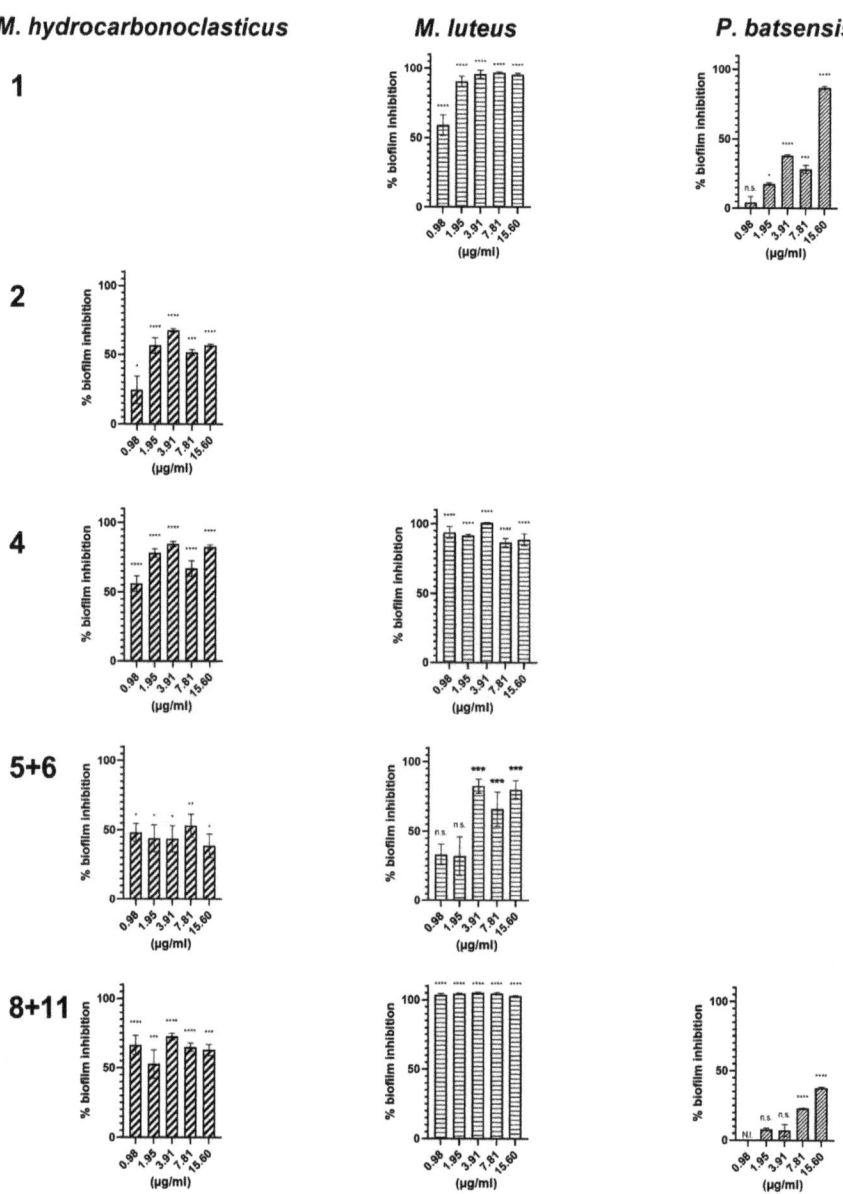

Figure 5. Inhibition of biofilm formation of *M. hydrocarbonoclasticus*, *M. luteus*, and *P. batsensis* by napyradiomycins (**1**), (**2**), (**4**), (**5** and **6**), and (**8** and **11**). Napyradiomycins were added to the biofilm growth medium of the different bacteria and after 18 h incubation planktonic cells were washed, and biofilm was stained using crystal violet and measured at OD_{600nm}. Percentage of biofilm inhibition refers to the percentage of biofilm that was inhibited in the presence of the napyradiomycins, when compared to biofilm formation with only DMSO. Shown are the average results of three replicates and error bars represent the standard error of the mean (SEM). N.I.—not inhibited; results were statistically significant (**** $p < 0.0001$, *** $p < 0.001$, ** $p < 0.01$, * $p < 0.05$, n.s. $p > 0.05$, Dunnett's test).

Napyradiomycins (**5** and **6**) showed no antibacterial activity, but high biofilm inhibition of *M. luteus* and *M. hydrocarbonoclasticus* (e.g., for a concentration of 3.91 µg/mL, biofilm formation of *M. luteus* was inhibited by 82.5 ± 5.1%, while biofilm formation by *M. hydrocarbonoclasticus* was inhibited by 43.8 ± 9.4%).

Napyradiomycins (**8** and **11**) showed inhibitory activity of biofilm formation and a variable degree of antibacterial activity against three of the five tested marine bacteria. For *M. hydrocarbonoclasticus*, (**8** and **11**) did not inhibit growth but significantly inhibited biofilm formation (~60%) for all tested concentration. For *M. luteus*, growth inhibition and complete biofilm abolishment (100%) was observed for all tested concentrations, however for the lowest concentration, growth inhibition was lower (70.5 ± 1.9%), indicating selective antibiofilm activity. For *P. batsensis*, growth inhibition (25.3 ± 0.6%) was observed only for the highest tested concentration (31.25 µg/mL), but significant inhibition of biofilm formation was observed at lower concentrations (37.8 ± 0.7% at a concentration of 15.60 µg/mL), with no detected antibacterial activity).

Finally, napyradiomycins (**3** and **7**) significantly inhibited (>20%) biofilm formation of *M. luteus* and *C. marina*, at a concentration of 31.25 µg/mL, while not showing any antibacterial effect on these marine bacterial species.

The antibiofilm activity of these napyradiomycins is not dependent on their antibacterial activity, which means that these compounds could be used as AF agents that will not contribute to antibiotic/biocide resistance.

The biofilm formation of *P. inhibens* and *P. batsensis* was inhibited by $CuSO_4$ (12.9 ± 6.4% and 41.4 ± 0.9%). *M. luteus*, *M. hydrocarbonoclasticus*, and *C. marina* biofilm formation was not inhibited.

2.3. Antifouling Evaluation against Mytilus Galloprovincialis Larval Settlement

Napyradiomycins (**1–12**) were screened against *M. galloprovincialis* plantigrade larval settlement to assess antimacrofouling activity. Most reports use tropical species and only a few involve temperate or cold-water species [59,60], we recognized the need to use European fouling species able to grow in temperate climate in bioassays.

The compounds revealed EC_{50} values ranging from 0.10 to 6.34 µg/mL (Table 4).

Table 4. Response of *M. galloprovincialis* plantigrade larvae settlement following incubation with napyradiomycins (**1–12**), after a 15 h acute exposure assay. Pearson goodness-of-fit (Chi-Square-χ^2) significance was considered at $p < 0.05$ and 95% lower and upper confidence limits (95% LCL; UCL) were presented. Therapeutic ratio (LC_{50}/EC_{50}) was used to evaluate the effectiveness of each compound vs. its toxicity. Negative control: dimethylsulphoxide (DMSO) = 100% settlement; Positive control: $CuSO_4$ 0.16 µg/mL (5 µM) = 0% settlement.

Napyradiomycin	EC_{50} [Conf. limits] (µg/mL)	Chi-Square Test	LC_{50} (µg/mL)	LC_{50}/EC_{50}
(1)	0.655 [0.300; 0.906]	$\chi^2 = 217.986; df = 18; p < 0.001$	>12	18.32
(2)	1.999 [1.581; 2.547]	$\chi^2 = 414.500; df = 18; p < 0.001$	>12	6.00
(3 and 7)	1.092 [0.225; 2.933]	$\chi^2 = 555.409; df = 18; p < 0.001$	>12	10.99
(4)	6.339 [5.602; 7.181]	$\chi^2 = 144.409; df = 18; p < 0.001$	>12	1.89
(5 and 6)	4.331 [2.911; 7.091]	$\chi^2 = 617.072; df = 18; p < 0.001$	>12	2.77
(8 and 11)	0.727 [0.065; 1.406]	$\chi^2 = 458.713; df = 18; p < 0.001$	>12	16.51
(9 and 12)	0.451 [0.192; 0.760]	$\chi^2 = 770.695; df = 22; p < 0.001$	>12	26.58
(10)	0.102 [0.072; 0.140]	$\chi^2 = 844.065; df = 42; p < 0.001$	>12	117.28
(12)	0.947 [0.586; 1.473]	$\chi^2 = 729.107; df = 22; p < 0.001$	>12	12.67

All compounds revealed a good level of effectiveness, which is defined by an EC_{50} value < 25 µg/mL [61]. The most effective napyradiomycins, showing an EC_{50} below 1 µg/mL were (**1**) (EC_{50} 0.66 µg/mL), (**8** and **11**) (EC_{50} = 0.73 µg/mL), (**9** and **12**) (EC_{50} = 0.45 µg/mL), (**10**) (EC_{50} = 0.10 µg/mL), and (**12**) (EC_{50} = 0.95 µg/mL) (Table 4). Interestingly, the EC_{50} of (**10**) was better than the commercial agent ivermectin (EC_{50} = 0.4 µg/mL value against *M. edulis*) [62].

Regarding toxicity, none of the tested compounds caused mortality of *M. galloprovincialis* larvae at the highest tested concentration (12 µg/mL). Thus, LC_{50} values were considered higher than 12 µg/mL.

The EC_{50} and LC_{50} values were used to calculate the therapeutic ratios (LC_{50}/EC_{50}). To meet the standard requirement for efficacy level of natural antifouling agents the US Navy program established a cut-off above 15 for the therapeutic ratio [21]. Therefore, the most promising antifouling agents towards *M. galloprovincialis* larvae are napyradiomycins (**1**) (LC_{50}/EC_{50} = 18.3), (**8 and 11**) (LC_{50}/EC_{50} = 16.5), (**9 and 12**) (LC_{50}/EC_{50} = 26.6), and (**10**) (LC_{50}/EC_{50} = 117.3) (Table 4).

2.4. Napyradiomycins in Silico Ecotoxicity Evaluation

The ecotoxicity of diverse pharmaceuticals, biocides and chemical compounds have forced regulatory authorities to recommend the application of in silico risk assessment to predict the fate of these molecules and their potential ecological and indirect human health effects. Using the Toxicity Estimation Software Tool (T.E.S.T.) [63], napyradiomycins (**1–12**) were evaluated for potential ecotoxicity, the prediction results are in Table 5.

Table 5. Toxicity end point predictions for napyradiomycins **1–12**.

#	Toxicity End Points for Consensus Models						
	Fathead Minnow [1]	Daphnia magna [2]	Tetrahymena pyriformis [3]	Oral Rat [4]	Bioconcentration Factor	Developmental Toxicity [5]	Ames Mutagenicity [6]
1	0.27	0.76	3.01	495.72	22.17	0.88; DT	0.23; MN
2	0.22	0.45	1.22	291.93	10.25	0.72; DT	0.17; MN
3	0.05	0.17	310	505.42	42.17	0.71; DT	0.31; MN
4	0.13	1.64	1.22	491.94	5.31	0.51; DT	0.36; MN
5	0.05	3.23	3.09	478.12	26.41	0.73; DT	0.15; MN
6	0.09	2.28	2.87	1246.67	10.36	0.92; DT	0.18; MN
7	0.06	1.23	2.87	895.08	26.62	0.96; DT	0.17; MN
8	0.04	0.41	1.65	1055.66	18.59	0.95; DT	0.27; MN
9	0.04	0.98	1.56	1516.88	22.55	0.91; DT	0.25; MN
10	0.63	0.91	1.62	390.57	36.37	0.74; DT	0.29; MN
11	0.02	0.38	5.61	1414.33	31.86	0.93; DT	0.19; MN
12	0.05	0.45	5.29	687.01	68.24	0.90; DT	0.19; MN

[1] 96 hour LC_{50} (mg/L). [2] 48 hour LC_{50} (mg/L). [3] 48 hour IGC_{50} (mg/L), the Nearest Neighbor model, the other models are unable to predict this end point. [4] LD_{50} (mg/kg). [5] DT: developmental toxicant. [6] MN: mutagenicity negative.

In accordance with the European Union Directive 2001/59/EC and the Regulation on the Classification, Labelling and Packaging of Substances and Mixtures (CLP) 1272/2008, the in silico TEST results classified compounds **1–12**, with the danger symbol N ("dangerous for the environment"), risk phrase 50 ("very toxic to aquatic organisms" to "toxic to aquatic organisms"), acute toxicity estimate (ATE) category 4 ("practically non-toxic and not an irritant"), and as developmental toxicants with low bioaccumulation factor and mutagenicity negative [64–67].

In comparison, predictions of toxicity were performed for seven approved drugs: bimatoprost (**S1**), a topical medication used for controlling the progression of glaucoma or ocular hypertension; alfuzosin (**S2**), a nonselective alpha-1 adrenergic antagonist used in the therapy of benign prostatic hypertrophy; lovastatin (**S3**), a fungal metabolite isolated from cultures of *Aspergillus terreus* and a potent anticholesteremic agent; antimycin A (**S4**), an antibiotic produced by *Streptomyces* sp.; oxethazaine (**S5**), an anesthetic; calcipotriene (**S6**), a synthetic derivative of calcitriol or Vitamin D used for the treatment of moderate plaque psoriasis in adults; and latanoprost (**S7**), a prostaglandin F2alpha analogue and a prostanoid selective FP receptor agonist with an ocular hypertensive effect, (Supplementary Table S1), two antifouling agents (ivermectin B1b (**S8**) and ivermectin B1a (**S9**), (Supplementary Table S2), and arsenic and copper substances used in marine paints (Supplementary Table S3).

The predicted values related with environmental toxicity for (**1–12**) (Table 5) are in the same order of magnitude and have the same classification than those obtained for the Prestwick approved drugs (**S1–S7**) (Supplementary Table S1) and the two antifouling approved biocides **S8**, **S9** (Supplementary Table S2). Except for ATE, in which our napyradiomycins showed lower toxicity than **S1–S9** (category ≤ 4).

Comparing the toxicity predictions for (**1–12**) (Table 5) with the values for copper (Supplementary Table S3), we may predict that these MNP are less toxic than copper, which is widely used in antifouling paints and coatings [64,65]. Arsenic showed lower aquatic toxicity values than (1–12) but higher acute toxicity. Overall, the in silico results suggest napyradiomycins as a suitable model to test for Naval Sea Systems Command (NAVSEA) standards and proceed in the antifouling coatings development roadmap (http://www.nstcenter.biz/navy-product-approval-process/navy-community-coatings-roadmap/, accessed on 6th January 2020).

2.5. SAR Analysis

To date, 61 napyradiomycin derivatives have been discovered and elucidated [42]. In general, the chemical structure of the napyradiomycins consists of a semi-napthoquinone core, a prenyl unit attached at C-4a that is cyclized to form a tetrahydropyran ring in all the napyradiomycins reported here (Figure 1), and a monoterpenoid substituent attached at C-10a. The variation of the chemical structure of napyradiomycins is mainly due from the monoterpenoid subunit (10-carbon), which can be linear (as the napyradiomycins **1–7**) or cyclized to a 6-membered ring (as napyradiomycins **8–12**). As mentioned above, napyradiomycins from the strains PTM-029 and PTM-420 differ by a methyl group at position 7 instead of hydrogen, respectively (Figure 1). Overall, the antifouling activities of (**1–12**) ranked in descending order are summarized as: (**1**) > (**8 and 11**) > (**4**) for antibacterial activity, (**4**) > (**5 and 6**) > (**8 and 11**) > (**3 and 7**) for antimicrofouling, and (**10**) > (**9 and 12**) > (**1**) > (**8 and 11**) > (**12**) > (**3 and 7**) for antimacrofouling activity. Interestingly, all the napyradiomycins with antibacterial activity and the three napyradiomycins with highest antimicrofouling activity were isolated from the strain PTM-420 with a hydrogen atom at position 7. Conversely, the methyl containing napyradiomycins from PTM-029 generally had higher antimacrofouling activity.

Based on the biosynthetic scheme for napyradiomycins reported by Moore and co-workers [68], (**1**), (**2**), (**4–6**), (**8**), (**11**) lack the methylation of flaviolin by the methyltransferase NapB5. Similar behavior occurs with the 10-carbon monoterpenoid subunit, which is linear in almost all of the napyradiomycins with more potent antibacterial and antimicrofouling activities, with the exception of napyradiomycins (**8 and 11**), and cyclized to a 6-membered ring in most of the most active antimacrofouling napyradiomycins, except for napyradiomycins (**1**) and (**3 and 7**). Therefore, our antifouling results (micro and macro) suggest a correlation with this biosynthetic feature. Napyradiomycins (**8 and 11**) stand out as having the ability to inhibit both micro and macrofouling, this feature appears to be related with the presence of a bromine substitute at C-16 (Figure 1). MNP bromide derivatives seem to play an important role as antifouling agents, as 2-furanone bromine derivatives [26] and bromopyrrole alkaloids from oroidin family [27,28].

3. Materials and Methods

3.1. General Experimental Procedures

The optical rotations were measured using a Bellingham+Stanley (Berlin, Germany), model ADP410 Polarimeter with a 5 dm cell. UV/VIS spectra were recorded using an Ultraspect 3100 Pro Amersham Biosciences spectrophotometer (Champaign, IL, USA) with a path length of 1 cm, and IR spectra were recorded on a Perkin Elmer Spectrum Two FT-IR Spectrometer (Santa Clara, CA, USA). ^{1}H and 2D NMR spectral data were recorded at 400 or 600 MHz in CDCl$_3$ containing Me$_4$Si as internal standard on Bruker Advance and Bruker BioSpin spectrometers respectively (Ettlingen, Germany). ^{13}C NMR spectra were acquired at 100 MHz on a Bruker Advance spectrometer. High resolution ESI-TOF mass spectra were obtained through acquired services using an Agilent 6230 Accurate-Mass TOFMS spectrometer (Santa Clara, CA, USA) by the mass spectrometry facility at the Department of Chemistry and Biochemistry at the University of California, San Diego, La Jolla, CA. Low-resolution LC/MS data were measured through acquired services at MARINOVA, CIIMAR, Portugal, using a Thermo Finnigan Surveyor HPLC System (Thermo Fisher Scientific, Needham, MA, USA), coupled with Mass Spectrometry LCQ Fleet™ Ion Trap Mass Spectrometer (Thermo Fisher Scientific, Needham,

MA, USA), with reversed-phase C_{18} column (Phenomenex Luna, 100 mm × 1.0 mm, 5 µm), ACN:H_2O 10–100% gradient, with 0.1% formic acid, at a flow rate of 0.7 mL/min.

3.2. Collection and Isolation of Marine-Derived Actinomycetes

Sediment samples were collected in June 2012 off shore of the Madeira Archipelago of Portugal. Strain PTM-029 was isolated from samples collect near Madeira Island at 728 m using a dredge, while PTM-420 was isolated from samples collected from Desertas Island at 15 m on SCUBA. The sediments were inoculated using a heat-shock method: wet sediment (c. 0.5 g) was diluted with 2 mL of sterile seawater (SSW). After mixing, the diluted samples were allowed to settle for few minutes, heated to 55 °C for 6 min. 50 µL of the top layer was spread on an agar plate, with seawater based medium SWA (18 g agar per L) with the antifungal cycloheximide (100 µl/L).

Inoculated Petri dishes were incubated at RT (c. 25–28 °C) and monitored periodically over 6 months for actinomycete growth. The PTM-029 and PTM-420 colonies were successively transferred onto new seawater based A1 medium (10 g starch, 4 g yeast extract, 2 g peptone per L) until the attaining of pure strain. PTM-029 and PTM-420 were grown in liquid culture (without agar) and cryopreserved in 10% (v/v) glycerol at −80 °C.

3.3. Phylogenetic Analysis of Strains PTM-029 and PTM-420

Strains PTM-029 and PTM-420 were cultured in 4mL of A1 medium, with agitation (200 rpm) at 25 °C for 7 days. Genomic DNA was isolated using the Wizard® Genomic DNA Purification Kit (Promega, Madison, WI, USA) protocol for Gram positive bacteria. The manufacturer recommendations were followed, though with longer incubation periods of the lytic enzyme (i.e., lysozyme) and the RNase solution to obtain sufficient amounts of genomic DNA. The 16S rRNA gene was amplified using the primers 27F (5'-AGAGTTTGATCCTGGCTCAG-3') and 1492R (5'-TACGGCTA CCTTGTTACGACTT-3') [41,69] and purified using SureClean PCR cleanup kit (BioLine, London, UK), using the protocol provided by the manufacturer. Purified PCR reactions were cycle- sequenced with the primers listed above at STABVIDA, Lda (www.stabvida.net), using ABI BigDye® Terminator v3.1 Cycle Sequencing Kit (Needham, MA, USA). Purified products were run on an ABI PRISM® 3730xl Genetic Analyzer (Needham, MA, USA) and sequence traces were edited using Sequencing Analysis 5.3.1 from Applied Biosystems™ (Needham, MA, USA). The sequence was compared to the GenBank database by the blastn algorithm.

PTM-029 and PTM-420 sequences have been deposited in GenBank under accession numbers KP869059 and KP869064 respectively, available at www.ncbi.nlm.nih.gov/genbank.

3.4. Growth Conditions and Crude Extract Production

The actinomycetes (strains PTM-029 and PTM-420) were grown in 20 Erlenmeyer flasks with 2L capacity, each containing 1 L of seawater based A1 medium with agitation (200 rpm) at 30 °C. After seven days of incubation, the culture was extracted thrice with half volume of EtOAc and evaporated to dryness in vacuum to yield ~1.0 g of crude extracts.

3.5. Isolation of Napyradiomycins

The PTM-029 (~1.0 g) and PTM-420 crude extracts (~1.0 g) were fractionated by silica flash chromatography, eluted with step gradients of isooctane/EtOAc followed by EtOAc/MeOH. A mixture of five napyradiomycins from PTM-029 and seven from PTM-420 eluted with the 8:2 and 6:4 fractions of isooctane/EtOAc, respectively, and further isolated by reversed phase HPLC (Phenomenex Luna, 250 mm × 4.6 mm, 5 µm, 100 Å, 1.5 mL/min, UV 210, 250 and 360 nm) using a gradient solvent system from 70% to 100% CH_3CN in water (0.1% TFA) over 90 min to yield napyradiomycins (**1**, 12.86 mg), (**2**, 5.04 mg), (**3** and **7**, 6.80 mg), (**4**, 11.36 mg), (**5** and **6**, 1.67 mg), (**8** and **11**, 5.21 mg), (**9** and **12**, 7.40 mg), and (**10**, 13.20 mg) as orange oils. The data for structural characterization is described in the Supplementary Materials.

3.6. Antimicrofouling Evaluation

3.6.1. Bacterial Growth Conditions

Five marine bacterial species were used as models to assess antimicrofouling activity. The biofilm-forming marine bacteria *Marinobacter hydrocarbonoclasticus* DSM 8798 (ATCC 49840), *Cobetia marina* DSM 4741, *Phaeobacter inhibens* DSM 17,395, and *Pseusooceanicola batsensis* DSM 15,984 were obtained from DSMZ (Leibniz Institute DSMZ—German collection of Microorganisms and Cell Cultures) and *Micrococcus luteus* [55]. Cultures were routinely grown in liquid marine broth (Carl Roth GmbH, Karlsruhe, Germany) with agitation (180 rpm) or on agar-supplemented marine broth, at 28 °C (*M. hydrocarbonoclasticus* and *C. marina*) or 30 °C (*P. inhibens* and *P. batsensis*). *M. luteus* was maintained in Brain Heart Infusion broth (BHI, Becton Dickinson, GmbH, Heidelberg, Germany) with agitation (180 rpm) or on agar-supplemented BHI, at 37 °C.

3.6.2. Antibacterial Activity Evaluation Assays

The antibacterial activity of the napyradiomycins (**1–12**) was assessed in 96-well polystyrene flat bottom microplates (Nunclon Delta Surface, Thermo Scientific, Roskilde, Denmark) following previously reported procedures [42]. For initial screening, bacterial overnight cultures were diluted to an optical density (OD_{600nm}) of 0.2 and incubated statically at 28 °C (*M. hydrocarbonoclasticus*, *C. marina*), 30 °C (*P. inhibens*, *P. batsensis*) or 37 °C (*M. luteus*) in a 96-well microplate in the presence or absence of 31.25 µg/mL of the napyradiomycins, solubilized in DMSO. After 24 h (*M. hydrocarbonoclasticus*, *C. marina*) or 48 h (*P. batsensis*, *P. inhibens*, *M. luteus*) incubation, the OD_{600nm} was determined (Molecular Devices, Spectra Max 190). The napyradiomycins which showed antibacterial activity at a concentration of 31.25 µg/mL were then tested at lower concentrations (2-fold serial dilutions: 15.60, 7.81, 3.91, 1.95, and 0.98 µg/mL), and the protocol was repeated as described above. The percentage of growth inhibition was calculated as the amount of growth relative to that of the bacterial species without added compounds (with the same amount of DMSO added). $CuSO_4$ (5 µM), a potent antifouling agent used in antifouling paints, was used as reference.

All assays were performed in triplicate, and results are representative of the average and standard error of the mean (SEM). Statistical analysis was performed in GraphPad Prism 8.0.2 (San Diego, CA, USA), using one-way ANOVA followed by a Dunnett's multiple comparisons test against the control (species grown with the same amount of DMSO added).

3.6.3. Antibiofilm Activity Evaluation Assays

The antibiofilm activity of napyradiomycins (**1–12**) against the five marine bacterial species was assessed in 96-well polystyrene flat bottom microplates (Nunclon Delta Surface, Thermo Scientific, Roskilde, Denmark) as previously reported [42]. For initial screening, bacterial overnight cultures were diluted to an optical density (OD_{600nm}) value of 0.2 and incubated statically at 28 °C (*M. hydrocarbonoclasticus*, *C. marina*), 30 °C (*P. inhibens*, *P. batsensis*) or 37 °C (*M. luteus*) in the 96-well microplate in the presence or absence of 31.25 µg/mL of napyradiomycins, solubilized in DMSO. After 24 h (*M. hydrocarbonoclasticus*, *C. marina*) or 48 h (*P. batsensis*, *P. inhibens*, *M. luteus*) incubation, the OD_{600nm} was determined. The planktonic cells and media were discarded, and the wells were washed twice with deionized water. The biofilm was fixed for 1 h at 60 °C and stained with crystal violet 0.06% for 10 min. The dye was discarded, and the wells were again washed twice with deionized water. The stained biofilm was solubilized with 30% acetic acid and the OD_{600nm} was determined. The napyradiomycins which showed antibiofilm activity at a concentration of 31.25 µg/mL were then tested at lower concentrations (2-fold serial dilutions: 15.60, 7.81, 3.91, 1.95, 0.98 µg/mL), and the protocol was repeated as described above. The percentage of biofilm inhibition was calculated as the amount of biofilm relative to that of the bacterial species without added compounds (with the same amount of DMSO added). $CuSO_4$ (5 µM), a potent antifouling agent used in antifouling paints, was used as reference.

All assays were performed in triplicate, and results are representative of the average and standard error of the mean (SEM). Statistical analysis was performed in GraphPad Prism 8.0.2, using one-way ANOVA followed by a Dunnett's multiple comparisons test against the control (species grown with the same amount of DMSO added).

3.7. Antimacrofouling Evaluation: Mussel Larvae Mytilus Galloprovincialis Acute Toxicity Assay

Mussel (*M. galloprovincialis*) adhesive larvae (plantigrades) were used to assess in vivo the antifouling activity of napyradiomycins (**1–12**) towards macrofouling. Juvenile mussel aggregates were collected at the intertidal rocky shore during low spring tides, at Memória beach, Matosinhos, Portugal (41°13′59″ N; 8°43′28″ W). At the laboratory, immediately before the bioassays, mussel plantigrade larvae were screened and isolated from the juvenile aggregates using a binocular microscope (Olympus SZX2-ILLT, Hamburg, Germany) and washed with filtered seawater to remove organic debris. Only competent plantigrade larvae (those showing foot exploratory behavior) were selected and used in the exposure bioassays following previously validated procedures [70,71]. Plantigrades were exposed in 24-well polystyrene plates for 15 h in the darkness at 18 °C. DMSO was used as solvent for crude extracts, fractions and pure compounds stock and working solutions. Working solutions were prepared by successive dilutions of stock solutions in DMSO and then diluted in filtered seawater to obtain the test solutions. DMSO concentration in test solutions was always 0.1%. Four well replicates were used per condition with five larvae per well. Two negative controls, one with ultra-pure water and the other with DMSO 0.1% were included in all bioassays, as well as a positive control with 5 µM $CuSO_4$ (a potent antifouling agent). Anti-settlement bioactivity was determined by the presence/absence of fixed byssal threads produced by each individual larvae for all the conditions tested. Napyradiomycins were tested at 5 µg/mL and those showing anti-settlement activity were tested at higher and lower successive concentrations (12, 6, 3, 1.5, 0.75, and 0.375 µg/mL) for the determination of the semi-maximum response concentrations (EC_{50}) that had an anti-settlement effect in mussel larvae. Chi-square Pearsons goodness-of-fit test was applied to data in order to determine EC_{50}. Significance was considered at $p < 0.01$ for all analyses, and 95% lower and upper confidence limits [95% LCL; UCL] were presented. Therapeutic ratio (LC_{50}/EC_{50}) was used to evaluate the effectiveness vs. toxicity of compounds [19,21].

3.8. In Silico Environmental Toxicity Assessment

The in silico toxicity evaluation was done using the Toxicity Estimation Software Tool (T.E.S.T.) [63], https://www.epa.gov/chemical-research/toxicity-estimation-software-tool-test, that was developed to allow users to easily estimate toxicity using a variety of QSAR methodologies. In accordance with the European Union Directive 2001/59/EC and the Regulation on the Classification, Labelling and Packaging of Substances and Mixtures (CLP) 1272/2008, a substance can be classified as "harmful", "toxic", and "very toxic" to aquatic organisms depending on the 96-hour LC_{50} for fish (e.g., fathead minnow), 48 hour LC_{50} for daphnids (e.g., *Daphnia magna*), and others assays such as 72-hour IC_{50} for algae or 40 hour IGC_{50} for protozoans (e.g., *Tetrahymena pyriformis*). If IC_{50} or LC_{50} or IGC_{50} are below 1 mg/L, a substance is classified as "very toxic to aquatic organisms" (danger symbol N, risk phrase R50). If the values obtained for toxicity are between 1 and 10 mg/L, a substance is classified as "toxic to aquatic organisms" (danger symbol N, risk phrase R51). A substance is classified as "harmful to aquatic organisms" if the end points obtained are between 10 and 100 mg/L (risk phrase R52). Classification is also based on the assessment of ready biodegradability or bioaccumulation potential (i.e., bioconcentration factor, BCF). If BCF ≥ 100, a compound is classified as "may cause long-term adverse effects in the aquatic environment" (risk phrase R53) [64,65]. The acute toxicity estimate (ATE) categories, identified by the CLP regulation, depend on the Oral rat LD_{50} [66]. The four ATE thresholds are; a) category 1, ATE ≤ 5 mg/Kg, a substance is classified as "Fatal if swallowed", b) category 2, $5 <$ ATE ≤ 50 mg/Kg, a substance is classified as "Fatal if swallowed", c) category 3, $50 <$ ATE ≤ 300 mg/Kg, a substance is classified as "Toxic if swallowed", d) category 4, $300 <$ ATE ≤ 2000 mg/Kg, a compound is classified as "Harmful if swallowed" and e) category 5, ATE > 2000 mg/Kg, a substance is classified as "may be Harmful if swallowed". Mutagenicity, carcinogenicity and reproductive toxicity are some of the most important endpoints to evaluate toxicity towards humans. Mutagenic toxicity can be experimentally assessed by various test systems; the most common is the Ames test, which makes use of a genetically engineered *Salmonella typhimurium* and *Escherichia coli* bacterial strains [67].

4. Conclusions

The bioprospection of marine-derived actinomycetes revealed napyradiomycins as potential antifouling agents. Given their potent antibacterial, antibiofilm, and antisettlement activities, they revealed the capacity to prevent growth or the primary adhesion of marine bacterial species to submersed abiotic surfaces as well as other subsequent fouling steps. Napyradiomycin (**1**) exhibited the higher antibacterial activity, (**4**) the higher microfouling inhibitory activity, and (**10**) the most potent antimacrofouling activity. However, napyradiomycins (**8** and **11**) would be our first choice for the development of antifouling paints, as they were active against all the assayed marine organisms. This broad spectrum activity is a clear advantage towards the commercialized products, including ivermictin and $CuSO_4$, which are more limited, as they are directed for macrofouling inhibition only. Overall, in silico toxicity predictions of napyradiomycins suggest toxicity similar to marketed drugs and antifouling biocides, low bioaccumulation factor, and no mutagenicity. Taken together with the absence of toxic effects against the assayed species, napyradiomycins could be considered for further investigation as active ingredients for the marine antifouling paints and coatings development pipeline. In particular, the 3-chloro-napyradiomycin scaffold is indicated to be a key functional moiety for micro and macrofouling activities, especially having a bromine substitute at position C-16, such as (**8** and **11**). The correlation between napyradiomycin's biosynthetic features and antifouling activities (micro and macro) opens prospects for their engineered biosynthetic enhanced yield production and future commercialization.

Supplementary Materials: The following are available online at http://www.mdpi.com/1660-3397/18/1/63/s1, napyradiomycins (**1–12**) structural characterization description; Table S1. Toxicity end point predictions for seven Prestwick approved drugs; Table S2. Toxicity end point predictions for two antifouling approved drugs; Table S3. Aquatic toxicity, environmental fate data and classification of copper and arsenic, experimental data.

Author Contributions: Bioresources: actinomycetes isolation and characterization, S.P.G.; fouling bacteria, R.G.S.; mussel larvae I.C. and J.R.A.; crude extract preparation, fractionation, compound isolation, and structure elucidation S.P.G., F.P., and M.P.; SAR analysis, S.P.G. and F.P.; in silico model, F.P.; in silico data analysis, S.P.G. and F.P.; antibacterial and antibiofilm screening R.G.S., I.R.G., and H.M.; antifouling screening V.V., I.C., and J.R.A.; writing—original draft preparation, S.P.G., F.P., R.G.S., I.R.G., I.C., and J.R.A.; writing—review and editing, S.P.G., F.P., R.G.S., I.R.G., I.C., and J.R.A.; supervision, S.P.G., R.G.S., and V.V.; project administration, S.P.G., R.G.S., V.V., I.C. and J.R.A.; funding acquisition, S.P.G., R.G.S., V.V., I.C. and J.R.A. All authors have read and agreed to the published version of the manuscript.

Funding: This work was supported by the Applied Molecular Biosciences Unit-UCIBIO which is financed by national funds from FCT/MCTES (UID/Multi/04378/2019). It was also supported by CIIMAR which is financed by national funds from FCT/MCTES (UID/Multi/04423/2019). Funding from the 7th Framework Programme (FP7/2007–2013) under grant agreement PCOFUND-GA-2009-246542, DFRH/WIIA/102/2011 and SFRH/BI/52130/2013. Financial support provided by FCT/MCTES through grants IF/00700/2014 and SFRH/BPD/110020/2015. Funding also provided by the projects PTDC/QUI-QUI/119116/2010, PTDC/BIA-MIC/31645/2017, PTDC/BTA-GES/32359/2017, and PTDC/BTA-BTA/31422/2017 (POCI-01-0145-FEDER-031422), financed by FCT/MCTES, COMPETE2020 and PORTUGAL2020. The NMR spectrometers are part of The National NMR Facility, supported by FCT (RECI/BBB-BQB/0230/2012).

Acknowledgments: SPG is indebted to W. Fenical, P. R. Jensen, and C. A. Kauffman from Scripps Institution of Oceanography, San Diego, USA, for the sustenance given to perform the sediment sample collection. P. Castilho from Madeira University and M. Freitas from Funchal Marine Biology Station are acknowledged for their hospitality and logistic support during the field expedition. To M. Wilson for English revision.

Conflicts of Interest: The authors declare no conflicts of interest.

References

1. Magin, C.M.; Cooper, S.P.; Brennan, A.B. Non-toxic antifouling strategies. *Mater. Today* **2010**, *13*, 36–44. [CrossRef]

2. Abarzua, S.; Jakubowski, S. Biotechnological Investigation for the Prevention of Biofouling. 1. Biological and Biochemical Principles for the Prevention of Biofouling. *Mar. Ecol. Prog. Ser.* **1995**, *123*, 301–312. [CrossRef]
3. Conrad, J.C.; Poling-Skutvik, R. Confined Flow: Consequences and Implications for Bacteria and Biofilms. *Annu. Rev. Chem. Biomol. Eng.* **2018**, *9*, 175–200. [CrossRef] [PubMed]
4. Schultz, M.P.; Bendick, J.A.; Holm, E.R.; Hertel, W.M. Economic impact of biofouling on a naval surface ship. *Biofouling* **2011**, *27*, 87–98. [CrossRef] [PubMed]
5. Schultz, M.P. Effects of coating roughness and biofouling on ship resistance and powering. *Biofouling* **2007**, *23*, 331–341. [CrossRef] [PubMed]
6. Schultz, M.P.; Walker, J.M.; Steppe, C.N.; Flack, K.A. Impact of diatomaceous biofilms on the frictional drag of fouling-release coatings. *Biofouling* **2015**, *31*, 759–773. [CrossRef] [PubMed]
7. Bhushan, B. Biomimetics: Lessons from nature—An overview. *Philos. Trans. A Math Phys. Eng. Sci.* **2009**, *367*, 1445–1486. [CrossRef] [PubMed]
8. Ware, C.; Berge, J.; Sundet, J.H.; Kirkpatrick, J.B.; Coutts, A.D.M.; Jelmert, A.; Olsen, S.M.; Floerl, O.; Wisz, M.S.; Alsos, I.G. Climate change, non-indigenous species and shipping: Assessing the risk of species introduction to a high-Arctic archipelago. *Divers. Distrib.* **2014**, *20*, 10–19. [CrossRef]
9. Ashton, G.V.; Davidson, I.C.; Geller, J.; Ruiz, G.M. Disentangling the biogeography of ship biofouling: Barnacles in the Northeast Pacific. *Glob. Ecol. Biogeogr.* **2016**, *25*, 739–750. [CrossRef]
10. Pettengill, J.B.; Wendt, D.E.; Schug, M.D.; Hadfield, M.G. Biofouling likely serves as a major mode of dispersal for the polychaete tubeworm Hydroides elegans as inferred from microsatellite loci. *Biofouling* **2007**, *23*, 161–169. [CrossRef]
11. Piola, R.F.; Johnston, E.L. The potential for translocation of marine species via small-scale disruptions to antifouling surfaces. *Biofouling* **2008**, *24*, 145–155. [CrossRef] [PubMed]
12. Yamaguchi, T.; Prabowo, R.E.; Ohshiro, Y.; Shimono, T.; Jones, D.; Kawai, H.; Otani, M.; Oshino, A.; Inagawa, S.; Akaya, T.; et al. The introduction to Japan of the Titan barnacle, Megabalanus coccopoma (Darwin, 1854) (Cirripedia: Balanomorpha) and the role of shipping in its translocation. *Biofouling* **2009**, *25*, 325–333. [CrossRef] [PubMed]
13. Sonak, S.; Pangam, P.; Giriyan, A.; Hawaldar, K. Implications of the ban on organotins for protection of global coastal and marine ecology. *J. Environ. Manag.* **2009**, *90*, S96–S108. [CrossRef] [PubMed]
14. Callow, J.A.; Callow, M.E. Trends in the development of environmentally friendly fouling-resistant marine coatings. *Nat. Commun.* **2011**, *2*. [CrossRef] [PubMed]
15. Kirschner, C.M.; Brennan, A.B. Bio-Inspired Antifouling Strategies. *Annu. Rev. Mater. Res.* **2012**, *42*, 211–229. [CrossRef]
16. Chambers, L.D.; Stokes, K.R.; Walsh, F.C.; Wood, R.J.K. Modern approaches to marine antifouling coatings. *Surf. Coat. Technol.* **2006**, *201*, 3642–3652. [CrossRef]
17. Othmani, A.; Bunet, R.; Bonnefont, J.L.; Briand, J.F.; Culioli, G. Settlement inhibition of marine biofilm bacteria and barnacle larvae by compounds isolated from the Mediterranean brown alga Taonia atomaria. *J. Appl. Phycol.* **2016**, *28*, 1975–1986. [CrossRef]
18. Satheesh, S.; Ba-akdah, M.A.; Al-Sofyani, A.A. Natural antifouling compound production by microbes associated with marine macroorganisms—A review. *Electron. J. Biotechnol.* **2016**, *21*, 26–35. [CrossRef]
19. Almeida, J.R.; Vasconcelos, V. Natural antifouling compounds: Effectiveness in preventing invertebrate settlement and adhesion. *Biotechnol. Adv.* **2015**, *33*, 343–357. [CrossRef]
20. Qian, P.Y.; Li, Z.R.; Xu, Y.; Li, Y.X.; Fusetani, N. Mini-review: Marine natural products and their synthetic analogs as antifouling compounds: 2009–2014. *Biofouling* **2015**, *31*, 101–122. [CrossRef]
21. Qian, P.Y.; Xu, Y.; Fusetani, N. Natural products as antifouling compounds: Recent progress and future perspectives. *Biofouling* **2010**, *26*, 223–234. [CrossRef] [PubMed]
22. Dobretsov, S.; Dahms, H.U.; Qian, P.Y. Inhibition of biofouling by marine microorganisms and their metabolites. *Biofouling* **2006**, *22*, 43–54. [CrossRef] [PubMed]
23. Wang, K.-L.; Wu, Z.-H.; Wang, Y.; Wang, C.-Y.; Xu, Y. Mini-Review: Antifouling Natural Products from Marine Microorganisms and Their Synthetic Analogs. *Mar. Drugs* **2017**, *15*, 266. [CrossRef] [PubMed]
24. Qi, S.-H.; Ma, X. Antifouling Compounds from Marine Invertebrates. *Mar. Drugs* **2017**, *15*, 263. [CrossRef]
25. Dahms, H.U.; Dobretsov, S. Antifouling Compounds from Marine Macroalgae. *Mar. Drugs* **2017**, *15*, 265. [CrossRef]

26. Dworjanyn, S.A.; de Nys, R.; Steinberg, P.D. Chemically mediated antifouling in the red alga Delisea pulchra. *Mar. Ecol. Prog. Ser.* **2006**, *318*, 153–163. [CrossRef]
27. Richards, J.J.; Ballard, T.E.; Huigens, R.W.; Melander, C. Synthesis and screening of an oroidin library against Pseudomonas aeruginosa biofilms. *Chembiochem* **2008**, *9*, 1267–1279. [CrossRef]
28. Melander, C.; Moeller, P.D.R.; Ballard, T.E.; Richards, J.J.; Huigens, R.W.; Cavanagh, J. Evaluation of dihydrooroidin as an antifouling additive in marine paint. *Inter. Biodeterior. Biodegrad.* **2009**, *63*, 529–532. [CrossRef]
29. Yee, L.H.; Holmstrom, C.; Fuary, E.T.; Lewin, N.C.; Kjelleberg, S.; Steinberg, P.D. Inhibition of fouling by marine bacteria immobilised in kappa-carrageenan beads. *Biofouling* **2007**, *23*, 287–294. [CrossRef]
30. Perry, T.D.; Zinn, M.; Mitchell, R. Settlement inhibition of fouling invertebrate larvae by metabolites of the marine bacterium Halomonas marina within a polyurethane coating. *Biofouling* **2001**, *17*, 147–153. [CrossRef]
31. Gatenholm, P.; Holmstrom, C.; Maki, J.S.; Kjelleberg, S. Toward Biological Antifouling Surface-Coatings—Marine -Bacteria Immobilized in Hydrogel Inhibit Barnacle Larvae. *Biofouling* **1995**, *8*, 293–301. [CrossRef]
32. Bavya, M.; Mohanapriya, P.; Pazhanimurugan, R.; Balagurunathan, R. Potential bioactive compound from marine actinomycetes against biofouling bacteria. *Indian J. Geo-Mar. Sci.* **2011**, *40*, 578–582.
33. Cho, J.Y.; Kim, M.S. Induction of Antifouling Diterpene Production by Streptomyces cinnabarinus PK209 in Co-Culture with Marine-Derived Alteromonas sp KNS-16. *Biosci. Biotechnol. Biochem.* **2012**, *76*, 1849–1854. [CrossRef] [PubMed]
34. Cho, J.Y.; Kang, J.Y.; Hong, Y.K.; Baek, H.H.; Shin, H.W.; Kim, M.S. Isolation and Structural Determination of the Antifouling Diketopiperazines from Marine-Derived Streptomyces praecox 291-11. *Biosci. Biotechnol. Biochem.* **2012**, *76*, 1116–1121. [CrossRef] [PubMed]
35. Li, X.; Dobretsov, S.; Xu, Y.; Xiao, X.; Hung, O.S.; Qian, P.-Y. Antifouling diketopiperazines produced by a deep-sea bacterium, Streptomyces fungicidicus. *Biofouling* **2006**, *22*, 201–208. [CrossRef]
36. Xu, Y.; He, H.P.; Schulz, S.; Liu, X.; Fusetani, N.; Xiong, H.R.; Xiao, X.; Qian, P.Y. Potent antifouling compounds produced by marine Streptomyces. *Bioresour. Technol.* **2010**, *101*, 1331–1336. [CrossRef]
37. Xu, Y.; Li, H.L.; Li, X.C.; Xiao, X.; Qian, P.Y. Inhibitory Effects of a Branched-Chain Fatty Acid on Larval Settlement of the Polychaete Hydroides elegans. *Mar. Biotechnol.* **2009**, *11*, 495–504. [CrossRef]
38. Gopikrishnan, V.; Radhakrishnan, M.; Shanmugasundaram, T.; Pazhanimurugan, R.; Balagurunathan, R. Antibiofouling potential of quercetin compound from marine-derived actinobacterium, Streptomyces fradiae PE7 and its characterization. *Environ. Sci. Pollut. Res.* **2016**, *23*, 13832–13842. [CrossRef]
39. Cheng, Y.B.; Jensen, P.R.; Fenical, W. Cytotoxic and Antimicrobial Napyradiomycins from Two Marine-Derived Streptomyces Strains. *Eur. J. Organ. Chem.* **2013**, 3751–3757. [CrossRef]
40. Farnaes, L.; Coufal, N.G.; Kauffman, C.A.; Rheingold, A.L.; DiPasquale, A.G.; Jensen, P.R.; Fenical, W. Napyradiomycin Derivatives, Produced by a Marine-Derived Actinomycete, Illustrate Cytotoxicity by Induction of Apoptosis. *J. Nat. Prod.* **2014**, *77*, 15–21. [CrossRef]
41. Prieto-Davo, A.; Dias, T.; Gomes, S.E.; Rodrigues, S.; Parera-Valadezl, Y.; Borralho, P.M.; Pereira, F.; Rodrigues, C.M.P.; Santos-Sanches, I.; Gaudencio, S.P. The Madeira Archipelago As a Significant Source of Marine-Derived Actinomycete Diversity with Anticancer and Antimicrobial Potential. *Front. Microbiol.* **2016**, *7*. [CrossRef] [PubMed]
42. Bauermeister, A.; Pereira, F.; Grilo, I.R.; Godinho, C.C.; Paulino, M.; Almeida, V.; Gobbo-Neto, L.; Prieto-Davo, A.; Sobral, R.G.; Lopes, N.P.; et al. Intra-clade metabolomic profiling of MAR4 Streptomyces from the Macaronesia Atlantic region reveals a source of anti-biofilm metabolites. *Environ. Microbial.* **2019**. [CrossRef] [PubMed]
43. Gaudêncio, S.P.; Sobral, R.G.; Pereira, F.; Santos-Sanches, I.; Gonçalves, S.P.; Cunha, I.; Almeida, J.R.; Vasconcelos, V. Utilização de napiradiomicinas com atividade anti-incrustante e suas composições. Portuguese Patent PT115055, 4 October 2018.
44. Shiomi, K.; Nakamura, H.; Iinuma, H.; Naganawa, H.; Isshiki, K.; Takeuchi, T.; Umezawa, H. Structures of New Antibiotics Napyradiomycins. *J. Antibiot.* **1986**, *39*, 494–501. [CrossRef] [PubMed]
45. Motohashi, K.; Sue, M.; Furihata, K.; Ito, S.; Seto, H. Terpenoids produced by actinomycetes: Napyradiomycins from Streptomyces antimycoticus NT17. *J. Nat. Prod.* **2008**, *71*, 595–601. [CrossRef]

46. Wu, Z.C.; Li, S.M.; Li, J.; Chen, Y.C.; Saurav, K.; Zhang, Q.B.; Zhang, H.B.; Zhang, W.J.; Zhang, W.M.; Zhang, S.; et al. Antibacterial and Cytotoxic New Napyradiomycins from the Marine-Derived Streptomyces sp SCSIO 10428. *Mar. Drugs* **2013**, *11*, 2113–2125. [CrossRef]
47. Fukuda, D.S.; Mynderse, J.S.; Baker, P.J.; Berry, D.M.; Boeck, L.D.; Yao, R.C.; Mertz, F.P.; Nakatsukasa, W.M.; Mabe, J.; Ott, J.; et al. A80915, A New Antibiotic Complex Produced By Streptomyces aculeolatus—Discovery, Taxonomy, Fermentation, Isolation, Caharacterization, and Antibacterial Evaluation. *J. Antibiot.* **1990**, *43*, 623–633. [CrossRef]
48. Soria-Mercado, I.E.; Prieto-Davo, A.; Jensen, P.R.; Fenical, W. Antibiotic terpenoid chloro-dihydroquinones from a new marine actinomycete. *J. Nat. Prod.* **2005**, *68*, 904–910. [CrossRef]
49. Gomi, S.; Ohuchi, S.; Sasaki, T.; Itoh, J.; Sezaki, M. Studies on New Antibiotics-SF2415. 2. The Structure Elucidation. *J. Nat. Prod.* **1987**, *40*, 740–749. [CrossRef]
50. Pinori, E.; Berglin, M.; Brive, L.M.; Hulander, M.; Dahlstrom, M.; Elwing, H. Multi-seasonal barnacle (Balanus improvisus) protection achieved by trace amounts of a macrocyclic lactone (ivermectin) included in rosin-based coatings. *Biofouling* **2011**, *27*, 941–953. [CrossRef]
51. Dang, H.; Li, T.; Chen, M.; Huang, G. Cross-ocean distribution of Rhodobacterales bacteria as primary surface colonizers in temperate coastal marine waters. *Appl. Environ. Microbiol.* **2008**, *74*, 52–60. [CrossRef]
52. Ekblad, T.; Bergstroem, G.; Ederth, T.; Conlan, S.L.; Mutton, R.; Clare, A.S.; Wang, S.; Liu, Y.L.; Zhao, Q.; D'Souza, F.; et al. Poly(ethylene glycol)-Containing Hydrogel Surfaces for Antifouling Applications in Marine and Freshwater Environments. *Biomacromolecules* **2008**, *9*, 2775–2783. [CrossRef] [PubMed]
53. Akesso, L.; Pettitt, M.; Callow, J.; Callow, M.; Stallard, J.; Teer, D.; Liu, C.; Wang, S.; Zhao, Q.; D'Souza, F.; et al. The potential of nano-structured silicon oxide type coatings deposited by PACVD for control of aquatic biofouling. *Biofouling* **2009**, *25*, 55–67. [CrossRef]
54. D'Souza, F.; Bruin, A.; Biersteker, R.; Donnelly, G.; Klijnstra, J.; Rentrop, C.; Willemsen, P. Bacterial assay for the rapid assessment of antifouling and fouling release properties of coatings and materials. *J. Ind. Microbiol. Biotechnol.* **2010**, *37*, 363–370. [CrossRef] [PubMed]
55. Michael, V.; Frank, O.; Bartling, P.; Scheuner, C.; Göker, M.; Brinkmann, H.; Petersen, J. Biofilm plasmids with a rhamnose operon are widely distributed determinants of the 'swim-or-stick' lifestyle in roseobacters. *ISME J.* **2016**, *10*, 2498–2513. [CrossRef] [PubMed]
56. Majzoub, M.E.; McElroy, K.; Maczka, M.; Thomas, T.; Egan, S. Causes and Consequences of a Variant Strain of. *Front. Microbiol.* **2018**, *9*, 2601. [CrossRef] [PubMed]
57. Inbakandan, D.; Murthy, P.S.; Venkatesan, R.; Khan, S.A. 16S rDNA sequence analysis of culturable marine biofilm forming bacteria from a ship's hull. *Biofouling* **2010**, *26*, 893–899. [CrossRef]
58. El-Masry, M.H.; Hassouna, M.S.; El-Rakshy, N.; Mousa, I.E. Bacterial populations in the biofilm and non-biofilm components of a sand filter used in water treatment. *FEMS Microbiol. Lett.* **1995**, *131*, 263–269. [CrossRef]
59. Hellio, C.; Marechal, J.P.; Veron, B.; Bremer, G.; Clare, A.S.; Le Gal, Y. Seasonal variation of antifouling activities of marine algae from the Brittany coast (France). *Mar. Biotechnol.* **2004**, *6*, 67–82. [CrossRef]
60. Briand, J.F. Marine antifouling laboratory bioassays: An overview of their diversity. *Biofouling* **2009**, *25*, 297–311. [CrossRef]
61. Che, Q.; Zhu, T.; Qi, X.; Mandi, A.; Kurtan, T.; Mo, X.; Li, J.; Gu, Q.; Li, D. Hybrid Isoprenoids from a Reeds Rhizosphere Soil Derived Actinomycete Streptomyces sp CHQ-64. *Org. Lett.* **2012**, *14*, 3438–3441. [CrossRef]
62. Davies, I.M.; McHenery, J.G.; Rae, G.H. Environmental risk from dissolved ivermectin to marine organisms. *Aquaculture* **1997**, *158*, 263–275. [CrossRef]
63. Young, D.M. *The Toxicity Estimation Software Tool (T.E.S.T.)*; New England Green Chemistry Networking Forum: Boston, MA, USA, 2010.
64. Tisler, T.; Zagorc-Koncan, J. Aquatic toxicity of selected chemicals as a basic criterion for environmental classification. *Arh. Hig. Rada. Toksikol.* **2003**, *54*, 207–213. [PubMed]
65. Schipper, C.A.; Rietjens, I.M.C.M.; Burgess, R.M.; Murk, A.J. Application of bioassays in toxicological hazard, risk and impact assessments of dredged sediments. *Mar. Pollut. Bull.* **2010**, *60*, 2026–2042. [CrossRef] [PubMed]
66. Diaza, R.G.; Manganelli, S.; Esposito, A.; Roncaglioni, A.; Manganaro, A.; Benfenati, E. Comparison of in silico tools for evaluating rat oral acute toxicity. *SAR QSAR Environ. Res.* **2015**, *26*, 1–27. [CrossRef]

67. Gini, G.; Franchi, A.M.; Manganaro, A.; Golbamaki, A.; Benfenati, E. ToxRead: A tool to assist in read across and its use to assess mutagenicity of chemicals. *SAR QSAR Environ. Res.* **2014**, *25*, 999–1011. [CrossRef]
68. Winter, J.M.; Moffitt, M.C.; Zazopoulos, E.; McAlpine, J.B.; Dorrestein, P.C.; Moore, B.S. Molecular basis for chloronium-mediated meroterpene cyclization—Cloning, sequencing, and heterologous expression of the napyradiomycin biosynthetic gene cluster. *J. Biol. Chem.* **2007**, *282*, 16362–16368. [CrossRef]
69. Gontang, E.A.; Fenical, W.; Jensen, P.R. Phylogenetic diversity of gram-positive bacteria cultured from marine sediments. *Appl. Environ. Microbiol.* **2007**, *73*, 3272–3282. [CrossRef]
70. Almeida, J.R.; Correia-da-Silva, M.; Sousa, E.; Antunes, J.; Pinto, M.; Vasconcelos, V.; Cunha, I. Antifouling potential of Nature-inspired sulfated compounds. *Sci. Rep.* **2017**, *7*, 42424. [CrossRef]
71. Antunes, J.; Pereira, S.; Ribeiro, T.; Plowman, J.E.; Thomas, A.; Clerens, S.; Campos, A.; Vasconcelos, V.; Almeida, J.R. A Multi-Bioassay Integrated Approach to Assess the Antifouling Potential of the Cyanobacterial Metabolites Portoamides. *Mar. drugs* **2019**, *17*, 111. [CrossRef]

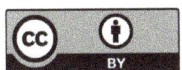

© 2020 by the authors. Licensee MDPI, Basel, Switzerland. This article is an open access article distributed under the terms and conditions of the Creative Commons Attribution (CC BY) license (http://creativecommons.org/licenses/by/4.0/).

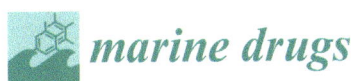

Article

Amentadione from the Alga *Cystoseira usneoides* as a Novel Osteoarthritis Protective Agent in an Ex Vivo Co-Culture OA Model

Nuna Araújo [1], Carla S. B. Viegas [1,2], Eva Zubía [3], Joana Magalhães [4,5,6], Acácio Ramos [7], Maria M. Carvalho [7], Henrique Cruz [7], João Paulo Sousa [7], Francisco J. Blanco [4,5], Cees Vermeer [8] and Dina C. Simes [1,2,*]

1. Centre of Marine Sciences (CCMAR), University of Algarve, 8005-139 Faro, Portugal; naraujo@ualg.pt (N.A.); caviegas@ualg.pt (C.S.B.V.)
2. GenoGla Diagnostics, Centre of Marine Sciences (CCMAR), University of Algarve, 8005-139 Faro, Portugal
3. Department of Organic Chemistry, Faculty of Marine and Environmental Sciences, University of Cadiz, 11510 Puerto Real (Cádiz), Spain; eva.zubia@uca.es
4. Unidad de Medicina Regenerativa, Grupo de Investigación en Reumatología (GIR), Instituto de Investigación Biomédica de A Coruña (INIBIC), Complejo Hospitalario Universitario de A Coruña (CHUAC), Sergas, 15006 A Coruña, Spain; joana.cristina.silva.magalhaes@sergas.es (J.M.); fblagar@sergas.es (F.J.B.)
5. Agrupación Estratégica CICA-INIBIC, Universidade da Coruña (UDC), 15006 A Coruña, Spain
6. Centro de Investigación Biomédica en Red (CIBER), 28029 Madrid, Spain
7. Department of Orthopedics and Traumatology, Hospital Particular do Algarve (HPA), 8005-226 Gambelas-Faro, Portugal; acacioramos@gmail.com (A.R.); mariamiguelfc@gmail.com (M.M.C.); cruzhenrique@hotmail.com (H.C.); jprsous@gmail.com (J.P.S.)
8. Cardiovascular Research Institute CARIM, Maastricht University, 6229 EV Maastricht, The Netherlands; cees.vermeer@outlook.com
* Correspondence: dsimes@ualg.pt

Received: 12 November 2020; Accepted: 3 December 2020; Published: 7 December 2020

Abstract: Osteoarthritis (OA) remains a prevalent chronic disease without effective prevention and treatment. Amentadione (YP), a meroditerpenoid purified from the alga *Cystoseira usneoides*, has demonstrated anti-inflammatory activity. Here, we investigated the YP anti-osteoarthritic potential, by using a novel OA preclinical drug development pipeline designed to evaluate the anti-inflammatory and anti-mineralizing activities of potential OA-protective compounds. The workflow was based on in vitro primary cell cultures followed by human cartilage explants assays and a new OA co-culture model, combining cartilage explants with synoviocytes under interleukin-1β (IL-1β) or hydroxyapatite (HAP) stimulation. A combination of gene expression analysis and measurement of inflammatory mediators showed that the proposed model mimicked early disease stages, while YP counteracted inflammatory responses by downregulation of COX-2 and IL-6, improved cartilage homeostasis by downregulation of MMP3 and the chondrocytes hypertrophic differentiation factors Col10 and Runx2. Importantly, YP downregulated NF-κB gene expression and decreased phosphorylated IkBα/total IkBα ratio in chondrocytes. These results indicate the co-culture as a relevant pre-clinical OA model, and strongly suggest YP as a cartilage protective factor by inhibiting inflammatory, mineralizing, catabolic and differentiation processes during OA development, through inhibition of NF-κB signaling pathways, with high therapeutic potential.

Keywords: osteoarthritis; amentadione; preclinical osteoarthritis models; marine compounds; *Cystoseira usneoides*; inflammation; mineralization; chondrocytes; synoviocytes; cartilage explants

1. Introduction

Osteoarthritis (OA) is a prevalent degenerative arthritic disease, a chronic condition that causes pain and disability among elderly patients [1,2]. An estimated 10% to 15% of all adults aged over 60 have some degree of OA [3], with prevalence doubling since the mid-20th century [4]. OA has been defined as a "whole joint" and multifactorial disease, characterized by synovial inflammation, progressive loss of articular cartilage and remodeling of the underlying bone [5,6].

Although OA physiopathology is still not completely understood, chronic inflammation is known to play a critical role in disease development and progression, with accumulating evidence supporting the association between OA pathology and different markers of inflammation [7]. OA cartilage and synovium overexpress cytokines and pro-inflammatory mediators that stimulate the accumulation of proteolytic enzymes, aggrecanases and matrix metalloproteinases (MMPs) responsible for the extracellular matrix (ECM) degradation, and for mediating detrimental effects through innate immunity signals [8,9]. In particular, MMP3 is known to mediate the integrity of various constituents of the ECM, such as collagens (types II, III, IV, V, VII, IX, X), fibronectin, elastin, proteoglycans, directly or through the activation of other pro-MMPs and pro-TNFα, in OA [10]. This molecular condition together with chondrocyte differentiation into a hypertrophic phenotype, result in loss of the ability to restore the ECM with consequent cartilage degradation. Basic calcium phosphate (BCP) deposition in the cartilage and synovial membrane is closely associated with OA inflammation, and contributes to local tissue damage and failed tissue repair, further intensifying hyaline articular cartilage loss and progressive joint deterioration [11–13].

Current osteoarthritis prevention and treatment are still very limited and unsatisfactory, with therapeutics focused mainly in drugs which improve pain or symptoms, such as topic and oral nonsteroidal anti-inflammatory drugs, acetaminophen, and opioids [14]. Although there are some advances in the design of new molecules to target cartilage repair and bone, or to treat inflammation and pain, at present, no effective OA drugs have yet been approved [15], making the search for new potential molecules a priority to overcome the growing burden of OA.

In addition, the lack of reliable models able to simulate the physiologic OA scenario, contributes to slow down the discovery of novel preventive or therapeutic agents. Monolayer (2D) cell culture approaches are limited by the lack of a physiologic context, while three-dimensional human tissue systems, although taking into consideration cell–cell and cell–extracellular matrix interactions, are still not demonstrative of the OA heterogeneity [16,17]. Preclinical animal models represent a more complex system, but are not totally representative of the human physiopathology, frequently leading to the failure of therapeutic responses in a later stage of the drug validation process.

In the search of effective drugs that might prevent or slow down the development of the disease, natural products derived from plants and marine organisms, remain a source of new molecular entities for the treatment of chronic inflammatory related diseases, including osteoarthritis [18,19]. Dietary supplements, of natural and synthetic origin, representing a nutritional and health benefit, were already associated with OA in human clinical trials. Although most were associated with OA pain relief, some were shown to modify the inflammatory OA process, by balancing anabolic and catabolic joint events, and promoting the synthesis of structural articulation precursors [20–22].

Among natural products, those containing phenolic rings, such as the flavonoids and some meroterpenoids, are usually provided of interesting biological activities, and have been shown to modulate cytokines such as tumor necrosis factor-α (TNFα), interleukin-1β (IL-1β) and interleukin-6 (IL-6), with a crucial role in chronic inflammatory and autoimmune diseases [23]. Some terpenoids based drugs are already available in the pharmaceutical market such as artemisinin and paclitaxel (Taxol®), acting as antimalarial and anticancer drugs, respectively [24].

In recent years, a series of meroterpenoids isolated from the brown alga *Cystoseira usneoides* have been shown to exhibit anti-inflammatory and antioxidant activities, by reducing the secretion of pro-inflammatory cytokines and downregulating the expressions of COX-2 and iNOS enzymes in THP-1 activated macrophages [25–28]. Among those, amentadione (YP) (Figure S1) showed radical-scavenging activity and demonstrated a significant role in reducing the production of TNFα in LPS-stimulated THP-1 human macrophages [26]. These results led us to further investigate the anti-inflammatory action of this pure marine compound and its potential as a novel cartilage protective agent in an OA context. For this purpose, we designed an OA preclinical pipeline consisting of an in vitro 2D-cell based system followed by an ex vivo explant-based and co-culture OA models. Our aim is to evaluate the potential protective effect of YP in the interplay between mineralization and inflammatory processes involved in OA development and progression.

2. Results

2.1. YP Acts as an Anti-Inflammatory Agent in the Articular OA Cell System Model

To evaluate the anti-inflammatory potential of YP in the mineralization and inflammatory processes involved in OA development and progression, a first screening was performed on THP-1 macrophages (THP-1 MOM). The inflammatory response of lipopolysaccharide (LPS)-induced THP-1 MOM was significantly reduced by pre-treatment with YP in a dose dependent manner (Figure S2a), as previously reported [25,26]. Additionally, the increased levels of TNFα production in calcium/phosphate (Ca/P) hydroxyapatite (HAP)-treated THP-1 MOM, confirmed the induction of a pro-inflammatory response [29], which was reduced by YP pre-treatment (Figure S2b). Cell proliferation assays were performed to confirm that tested HAP and YP did not affect THP-1 MOM cell viability (Figure S3). Based on these results, YP was further tested on a previously established articular OA cell system, consisting of human chondrocytes and synoviocytes primary cell cultures [30].

Human synoviocytes and chondrocytes primary cells were pre-treated with YP for 24 h followed by IL-1β (Figure 1) and HAP (Figure 2) stimulation. The effect of YP was determined by measuring gene expression of the inflammatory marker cyclo-oxygenase-2 (COX-2) and levels of IL-6 released into the cell culture media. Pre-treatment with YP followed by IL-1β stimulation resulted in a significant downregulation of COX-2 and decreased levels of IL-6 in both type of cells, relative to non-treated cells (Figure 1a,b). No cytotoxicity was observed in chondrocytes and synoviocytes, when treated with different YP concentrations (Figure S4).

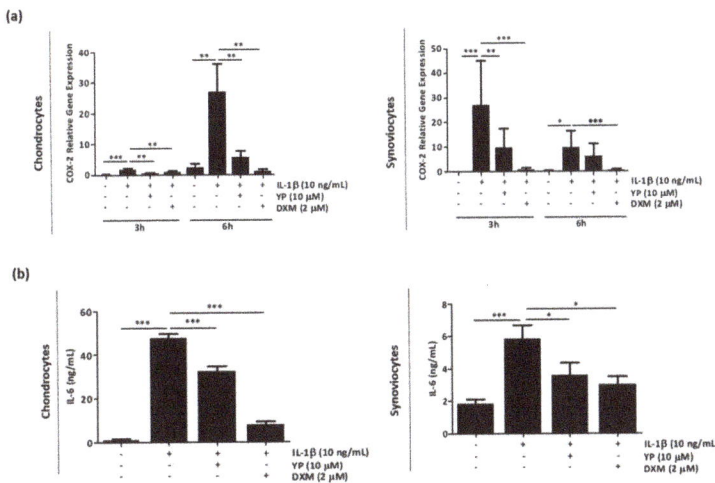

Figure 1. Amentadione (YP) reduces the levels of inflammatory markers in articular-derived cells stimulated with IL-1β (**a**,**b**). Primary chondrocytes and synoviocytes were pre-treated with 10 μM YP for 24 h, followed by stimulation with 10 ng/mL IL-1β during different time points. (**a**) Relative gene

expression of the inflammatory marker COX-2 was determined by qPCR, at 3 h and 6h post IL-1β stimulation in chondrocytes and synoviocytes. (**b**) Levels of IL-6 in cell culture media 6 h post IL-1β stimulation, determined by ELISA. Cells treated with 2 μM dexamethasone (DXM) were used as a positive anti-inflammatory control. Data are presented as means of at least three independent experiments. All graphs show mean ± SD. One-way ANOVA and multiple comparisons were achieved with the Dunnett's test. Statistical significance was defined as $p \leq 0.05$ (*), $p \leq 0.005$ (**) and $p \leq 0.0005$ (***).

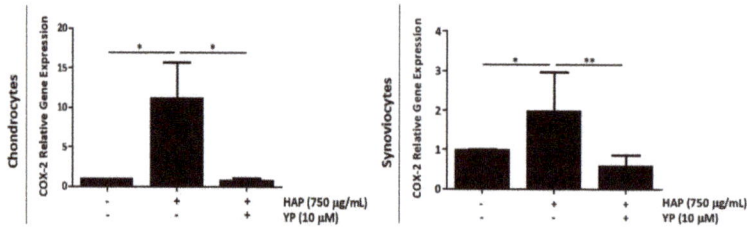

Figure 2. YP downregulates the inflammatory marker COX-2 in articular-derived cells stimulated with hydroxyapatite (HAP). Primary chondrocytes and synoviocytes were pre-treated with 10 μM YP for 24 h, followed by stimulation with 750 μg/mL HAP during 6 h. Relative gene expression of COX-2 was determined by qPCR, at 6 h post HAP stimulation in chondrocytes and synoviocytes. Data are presented as means of two independent experiments, with duplicates. All graphs show mean ± SD. One-way ANOVA and multiple comparisons were achieved with the Dunnett's test. Statistical significance was defined as $p \leq 0.05$ (*) and $p \leq 0.005$ (**).

Interestingly, a similar upregulation of the inflammatory marker COX-2 was observed in chondrocytes and synoviocytes treated with HAP, which was reduced by YP pre-treatment (Figure 2). No cytotoxicity was observed in chondrocytes and synoviocytes, when treated with different HAP concentrations (Figure S5).

These results demonstrate a promising anti-inflammatory effect of YP in the articular OA cell system model, through downregulation of inflammatory genes either when stimulated with IL-1β or treated with the mineralizing agent HAP.

2.2. YP Modulates Cartilage Homeostasis under Mineralizing Conditions in an Ex-Vivo Cartilage Explant Model

Since cartilage is the main affected tissue in OA, and ectopic mineralization is a known trigger of several joint alterations, including inflammation and cell differentiation, ultimately leading to cartilage degradation, cartilage tissue explants were first selected as an experimental model to evaluate ex vivo the effect of YP in response to HAP stimulation. Cartilage explants used in all experimental conditions were classified as normal- to early-OA tissues through the modified Mankin score [31]. Histological analysis revealed a smooth surface, a normal and uniform structural organization, and a normal to slight reduction in matrix staining, with Mankin total score ranging from 1 to 4 in the 1/13 modified Mankin scale (Table S1). The results showed that HAP treatment significantly upregulated collagen-10 (Col10), runt-related transcription factor-2 (Runx2) and matrix metalloproteinase-3 (MMP3) relative to control explants (Figure 3a), with simultaneous increased accumulation of MMP3 and the inflammatory marker IL-6 (Figure 3b). Pre-treatment of human cartilage explants with YP and further HAP stimulation, resulted not only in a significant down-regulation of the referred differentiation and ECM-related genes (Figure 3a), but also in decreased levels of the inflammatory marker IL-6 and the catabolic OA marker MMP3, responsible for ECM degradation (Figure 3b).

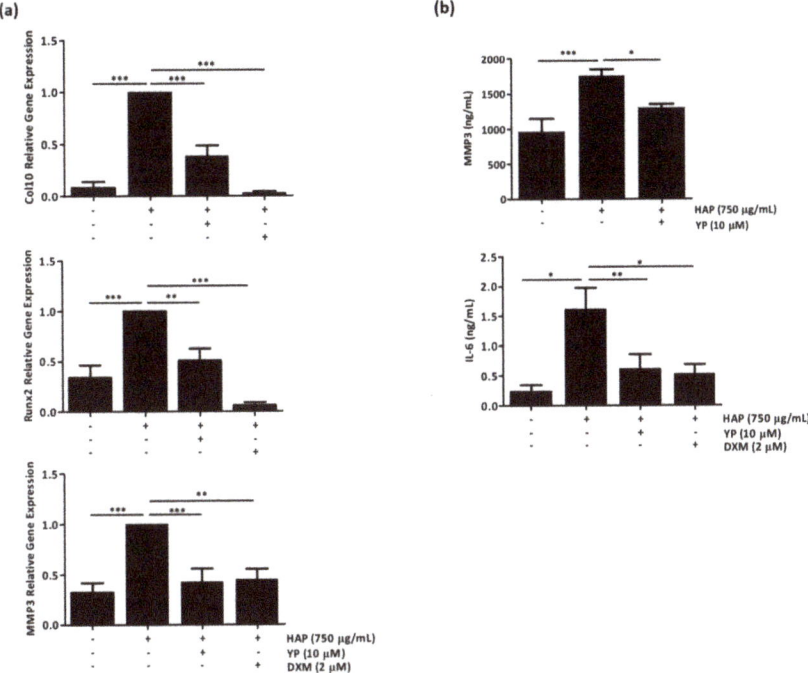

Figure 3. YP downregulates cell differentiation, extracellular matrix degradation and pro-inflammatory markers associated with osteoarthritis (OA) in the ex vivo cartilage explant model under HAP stimulation. Human cartilage explants were pre-treated with 10 µM YP for 24 h, followed by 72 h of 750 µg/mL HAP stimulation. Relative gene expression of Col10, Runx2 and MMP3 was determined by qPCR (**a**), and levels of MMP3 and IL-6 accumulation in the culture media were determined by ELISA (**b**). DXM indicates treatments with 2 µM dexamethasone. Data are presented as means of at least three independent experiments. All graphs show mean ±SD. One-way ANOVA and multiple comparisons were achieved with the Dunnett's test. Statistical significance was defined as $p \leq 0.05$ (*), $p \leq 0.005$ (**) and $p \leq 0.0005$ (***).

2.3. YP Function as a Protective Agent against Cartilage Deterioration under OA Promoting Conditions in an Explant-Based Co-Culture OA Model

Since in the joint environment cartilage and synovial membrane are known to be involved in an interrelated and complex crosstalk affecting cartilage integrity and driving OA progression, an ex vivo explant-based co-culture OA model was developed and used to study the effects of YP in cartilage. Human cartilage explants were co-cultured with primary human synoviocytes and treated with IL-1β (Figure 4) and HAP (Figure 5) to simulate inflammatory and mineralizing conditions. Increased gene expression of COX-2, IL-6 and MMP3 in the co-culture cartilage explants treated with IL-1β, clearly indicated an induction of inflammatory reactions and ECM degradation at cartilage tissue level, which were consistently diminished in cartilage pre-treated with YP (Figure 4).

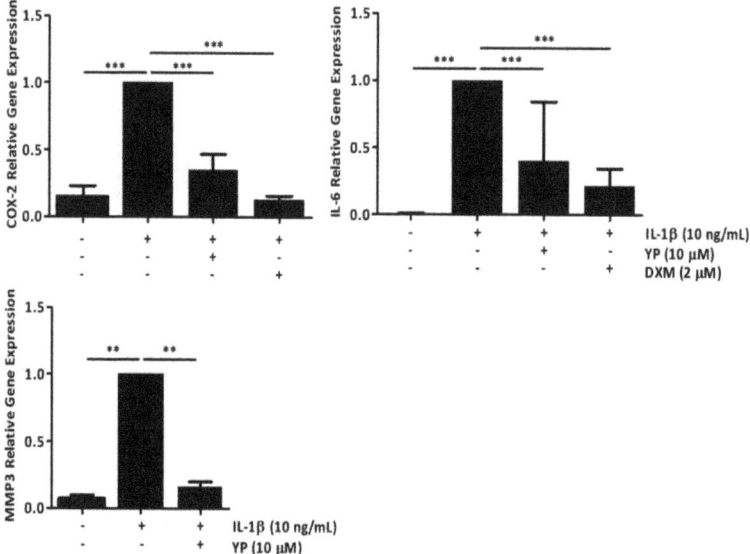

Figure 4. YP downregulates pro-inflammatory and ECM degradation markers associated with OA in the explant-based co-culture OA model under inflammatory stimulation with IL-1β. Cartilage explants co-cultured with human primary synoviocytes were pre-treated with 10 μM YP for 24 h, followed by 24 h of 10 ng/mL IL-1β stimulation. Relative gene expression of COX-2, IL-6 and MMP3 in cartilage explants were determined by qPCR. DXM indicates treatments with 2 μM dexamethasone. Data are presented as means of at least three independent experiments. One-way ANOVA and multiple comparisons were achieved with the Dunnett's test. All graphs show mean ±SD. Statistical significance was defined as $p \leq 0.005$ (**) and $p \leq 0.0005$ (***).

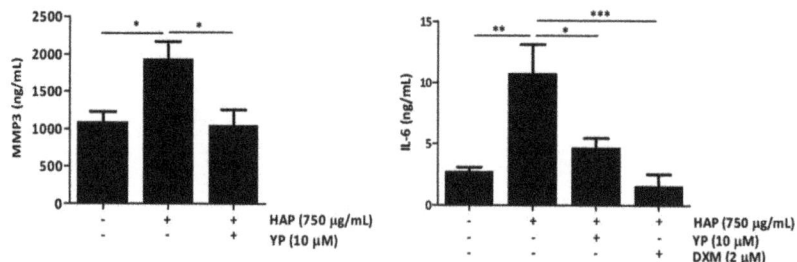

Figure 5. YP decreases the production of ECM degradation and pro-inflammatory markers in the explant-based co-culture OA model under mineralizing conditions. Cartilage explants co-cultured with human primary synoviocytes were pre-treated with 10 μM YP 24 h, followed by 72 h of 750 μg/mL HAP stimulation. Levels of MMP3 and IL-6 accumulation in the co-culture media were determined by ELISA. DXM indicates treatments with 2 μM dexamethasone. Data are presented as means of at least three independent experiments. One-way ANOVA and multiple comparisons were achieved with the Dunnett's test. All graphs show mean ±SD. Statistical significance was defined as $p \leq 0.05$ (*), $p \leq 0.005$ (**) and $p \leq 0.0005$ (***).

Additionally, increased levels of MMP3 and IL-6 in the cell culture media of co-culture cartilage explants treated with HAP demonstrated the interplay between mineralization and inflammation with consequent increased levels of inflammatory and ECM degrading markers, which were decreased with the YP pre-treatment (Figure 5).

Overall, considering the effects of YP at cartilage tissue level, evaluated using the cartilage explants and the explant-based co-culture models, the results suggest that YP exerts a cartilage protective effect, by reducing inflammatory reactions and preventing chondrocyte differentiation towards extracellular matrix mineralization and degradation.

2.4. YP Downregulates NF-kB Expression and Inhibits IkBα Phosphorylation in Primary Chondrocyte Cells

Since YP was able to downregulate several pro-inflammatory mediators known to be directly regulated by the nuclear factor-κB (NF-kB) signaling pathway, we investigated whether the anti-inflammatory action of YP was due to its effect on NF-kB transcription and phosphorylation of its inhibitor IkBα.

In human primary articular chondrocytes, pre-treated with YP for 24 h followed by IL-1β stimulation, NF-kB expression was significantly downregulated at all-time points tested (Figure 6a). To determine the effect of YP in IkBα phosphorylation (pIkBα), known to precede NF-kB nuclear translocation, an initial experiment was performed to determine the optimal time point of pIkBα under IL-1β stimulation. Western blot analysis of chondrocyte protein extracts indicated increased levels of pIkBα from 30 min to 60 min of IL-1β treatment (Figure S6). Based on that, detection of pIkBα in chondrocytes pre-treated with YP for 24 h followed by 30 min IL-1β stimulation suggests a reduction of pIkBα in the YP treated chondrocytes relatively to the untreated and IL-1β stimulated cells (Figure 6b). Specific ELISA assays measuring pIkBα and total IkBα at 30 min shown that YP treatment reduces the ratio of pIkBα/total IkBα (Figure 6c), strongly indicating an effect of YP on IkBα phosphorylation.

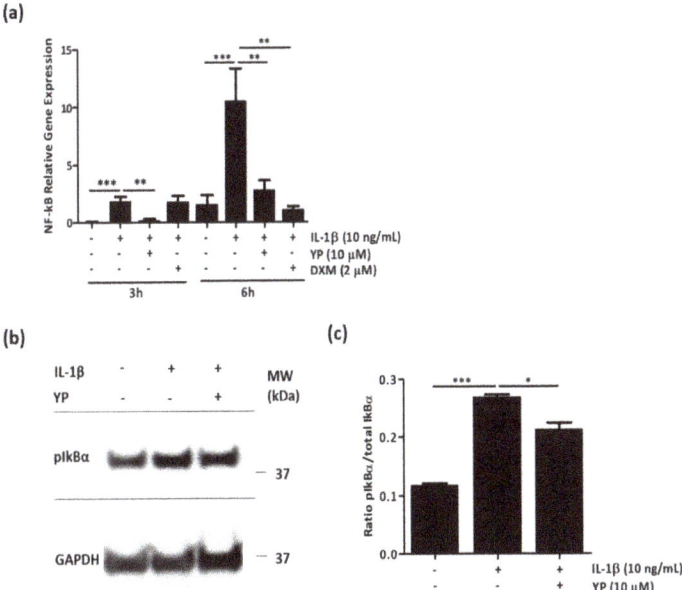

Figure 6. YP downregulates NF-kB expression and inhibits IkBα phosphorylation in IL-1β-stimulated primary articular chondrocytes. (**a**) Relative gene expression of NF-kB was determined by qPCR at 3 h and 6 h post 10 ng/mL IL-1β stimulation. Data is presented as mean of three independent experiments. (**b**) Total protein extracts of chondrocytes cultured in untreated conditions, stimulated with 10 ng/mL IL-1β for 30 min, and pre-treated with YP (μM) followed by 30 min of 10 ng/mL IL-1β treatment,

were analyzed by Western blot to detect pIkBα. Position of relevant molecular mass marker (kDa) is indicated on the right side and GAPDH was used as loading control. (c) The pIkBα ratio (pIkBα/total IkBα) was determined in total protein extracts of chondrocytes cultured in control conditions (Ctr); 30 min of IL-1β (10 ng/mL) treatment; and pre-treated with YP for 24 h followed by 30 min of IL-1β stimulation (YP), by measuring the content of total and pIkBα with the specific InstantOne ELISA assay kit. Data is presented as mean of two out of four representative experiments. All graphs show mean ±SD. One-way ANOVA and multiple comparisons were achieved with the Dunnett's test. Statistical significance was defined as $p \leq 0.05$ (*), $p \leq 0.005$ (**) and $p \leq 0.0005$ (***).

These results demonstrate an anti-inflammatory effect of YP in articular chondrocytes, by downregulation of NF-kB expression, and inhibition of its activation through modulation of IkBα phosphorylation, and consequent downregulation of several NF-kB-related target genes.

3. Discussion

In this study we demonstrated that YP, a meroterpenoid isolated from the brown alga *C. usneoides* [26], is able to decrease inflammation, cell differentiation and extracellular matrix (ECM) degradation in different osteoarthritis in vitro/ex vivo OA model systems. By using a pipeline with increasing complexity, from 2D monolayer cultures of THP-1 macrophages, primary chondrocytes and synoviocytes, to ex vivo culture of human cartilage explants and a newly developed OA explant-based co-culture model, YP consistently promoted a protective effect under pro-inflammatory and mineralizing stimuli. These results bring new evidences on the health benefits of YP as a protective OA agent by attenuating cartilage degrading processes under known OA promoting stimuli, with consequent cartilage maintenance promoting effects, with potential therapeutic application.

In OA, cartilage loss and synovial membrane inflammation are two major factors responsible for disease progression and associated outcomes. Complex and interconnected molecular events of cartilage homeostasis disruption associated to inflammation known to fuel cartilage degradation, are recognized as crucial for disease development and important targets for therapeutic approaches [32]. Cartilage degradation is associated with chondrocytes differentiation leading to apoptosis and deposition of a mineralized extracellular matrix, which in turn contributes to loss of ECM integrity and inflammation [33]. In fact, although the pathways involved in the crosstalk between inflammation and cartilage degradation are still not completely clarified, mineralizing and inflammatory events occur in a close related manner during OA progression [30]. BCP and calcium pyrophosphate (CPP) crystals, consistently associate with the early stage of OA and have a pathogenic role in the development and rapid progression to end-stage OA [11,12]. BCPs have been found in the synovial fluid and membrane, and cartilage from OA patients [34], and associated with the activation of macrophages, synovial fibroblasts and articular cells, resulting in increased cell proliferation and production of pro-inflammatory cytokines and MMPs [35,36]. In concordance, our results show an inflammatory response to hydroxyapatite stimulation in all tested OA models, similar to those obtained with the classical inflammatory cytokine IL-1β, and to previously reported effects in OA cell models [30,37]. Of particular relevance, at cartilage level, treatment with hydroxyapatite induced overexpression of Col10 and Runx2, indicative of triggered chondrocyte differentiation towards hypertrophy and calcification. In addition, up-regulation of COX-2 and IL-6, widely known to be associated with joint inflammation, and MMP3, a major responsible for ECM degradation, clearly demonstrate the detrimental potential of calcification in OA. This is in line with recent data showing that BCP upregulate IL-6 in in vivo murine OA models, which in turn induced the expression of genes involved in calcification, promoting BCP formation and potentiating a vicious cycle [38]. Increased levels of BCP and IL-6 were also associated with cartilage degradation through the induction of matrix-degrading enzymes activity in chondrocytes [38]. In another study, calcium-phosphate complexes were shown to induce MMP3 and MMP13, which in turn, promoted the release of calcium and phosphate through degradation of the ECM calcified cartilage, in a positive loop [39]. Additionally, the effect of IL-1β on cartilage is known to reflect not only the catabolic effect of aggrecanases and MMPs upregulation, but also the downregulation of chondrogenic extracellular matrix synthesis [40,41]. In concordance, our results showed that IL-1β induced an overexpression of MMP3. Overall, our results clearly demonstrated the potentialities of the developed ex vivo explant-based co-culture OA model to study the interplay between cartilage degradation and inflammation, reflecting early molecular events leading to subsequent phenotypic cartilage alterations, of critical value in drug development for potential anti-osteoarthritic compounds such as YP.

YP has previously shown to have anti-inflammatory properties associated with the inhibition of TNFα in LPS-activated human macrophages [26]. In the present study, we demonstrated that YP was able to counteract inflammation, cell differentiation and ECM degradation, induced not only by IL-1β but also by hydroxyapatite, in all OA models, including primary articular cells, cartilage explants and ex vivo explant-based co-culture systems. These effects were demonstrated at multiple levels. Through downregulation of master players involved in pro-inflammatory reactions, such as NF-kB, COX-2 and IL-6, and the ECM catabolic marker MMP3, YP is directly contributing to preserve cartilage homeostasis, by avoiding ECM disruption and cartilage collapse. Similarly, the capacity to downregulate crucial genes involved in chondrocyte differentiation such as Col10 and Runx2, suggests YP as an inhibitor of chondrocytes hypertrophic differentiation. The resulting decrease of apoptosis and ECM mineralization, indirectly contributes to a consequent decrease of pro-inflammatory reactions, ultimately preserving cartilage homeostasis. Although our studies were not directed to evaluate the effect of YP as a structural cartilage-modifying drug, its capacity to inhibit early molecular events leading to joint deterioration, suggests YP as a potential disease modifying OA drug, worth to be further investigated.

Additionally, this YP protective role might represent a promising alternative to the anti-inflammatory drugs commercially available to manage symptomatology associated with OA and chronic autoimmune and inflammatory diseases, mostly based on NSAIDs target to inactivate COX enzymes (COX-1 and COX-2) [42], or biologics targeting crucial pro-inflammatory cytokines such as TNFα and IL-1β [43,44]. Although some effectiveness has been shown in slowing inflammatory reactions, the growing list of adverse side effects and the high percentage of patients presenting no response to these treatments, clearly demonstrate the urgent need for safer and more effective anti-inflammatory drugs. In this field, natural derived products, such as YP, have been considered as promising and valid alternatives. Some examples are the tetracyclic triterpenoid glycoside Ginsenoside Rb1 (G-Rb1) and curcumin, which have shown both in vitro and in vivo the capacity of targeting the production of several pro-inflammatory species and promoting the synthesis of anti-inflammatory mediators, with cartilage protective effects [45–48].

Considering the pivotal role of NF-kB as a major regulator of inflammation, many strategies have been developed to block NF-kB signaling in a variety of inflammatory disease settings [49]. Although in the context of OA these strategies are still in their infancy, the crucial role of NF-kB signaling mediating inflammatory responses, but also the hypertrophic conversion of articular cartilage chondrocytes, leading to ECM damage and cartilage destruction, is of paramount importance in the disease context [50,51]. Our results demonstrate that YP is able to downregulate NF-kB expression and decrease IkBα phosphorylation in chondrocytes, strongly suggesting that YP cartilage protective properties are associated, at least in part, with the inhibition of NF-kB nuclear translocation and consequent decreased activation of catabolic pathways, including expression of cytokines and chemokines, inflammatory mediators, matrix degrading enzymes, and regulators of chondrocytes differentiation. In agreement, YP treatments consistently decreased levels of COX-2 and IL-6, MMP3, Col10 and Runx2 in cartilage tissue, clearly demonstrating the potential of YP in ameliorating cartilage homeostasis and integrity, a good rationale for the exploitation of YP in the treatment of OA.

4. Materials and Methods

4.1. Isolation of Amentadione (YP)

The meroditerpenoid amentadione (YP) was isolated from the brown alga *Cystoseira usneoides* collected off the coast of Tarifa (Spain) as previously described [26]. Briefly, the frozen alga was extracted with methanol and after evaporation of the solution under reduced pressure, the aqueous residue was extracted with diethyl ether. The resulting extract was subjected to column chromatography (CC) on silica gel (70–230 mesh) (Merck KGaA, Darmstadt, Germany) eluting with a mixture of *n*-hexane/diethyl ether (50:50, *v/v*), then diethyl ether, mixtures of chloroform/methanol (90:10 and 80:20, *v/v*), and finally methanol. The fraction that eluted with chloroform/methanol (90:10, *v/v*) was further separated by CC on silica gel using as eluents mixtures of *n*-hexane/ethyl acetate (50:50 to 30:70, *v/v*), then ethyl acetate, and finally methanol. The compound YP was obtained by reversed phase HPLC separation of selected subfractions using as eluent methanol/water (70:30, *v/v*). HPLC separations were performed on a LaChrom-Hitachi apparatus (Merck), equipped with Kromasil 100-5C18 columns (250 × 10 mm, 5 µm or 250 × 4.6 mm, 5 µm) (Hichrom, Reading, UK), using an RI-71 differential refractometer or L-7400 UV detector (Merck). The pure compound YP was identified as amentadione [52] by NMR and HRMS analysis (Figure S1) and the negative optical rotation. NMR spectra were recorded on an Agilent 500 spectrometer (Agilent Technologies, Santa Clara, CA, USA), HRMS spectra were obtained on a Waters SYNAPT G2 spectrometer (Waters, Milford, MA, USA), and optical rotation was measured on a JASCO P-2000 polarimeter (JASCO, Tokyo, Japan).

4.2. Cell Culture

Primary human chondrocytes and synoviocytes were commercially acquired (chondrocytes, Lonza, Visp, Switzerland; synoviocytes, ECACC, Sigma-Aldrich, St. Louis, MO, USA) and obtained from human tissue explants using well-defined methodology [53,54]. Both cell types were cultured in Advanced Dulbecco's Modified Eagle's Medium (Adv DMEM) (Invitrogen, Carlsbad, CA, USA) supplemented with 10% (*v/v*) of heat-inactivated Fetal Bovine Serum (FBS, Sigma-Aldrich), 1 mM of L-glutamine (L-Gln, Invitrogen) and 1% (*v/v*) of penicillin-streptomycin (PS, Invitrogen). THP-1 cell line was kindly given by Dr. Santos (CBME, University of Algarve, Faro) and was cultured according to ATCC instructions in RPMI Growth Medium (RPMI 1640 with L-glutamine (Lonza)) containing 10% heat-inactivated FBS (invitrogen) and 1% PS. Differentiation into THP-1 macrophage (THP-1 MOM) cells was achieved by culturing THP-1 cells in 25 ng/mL phorbol 12-myristate 13-acetate (PMA) (Sigma) in complete RPMI for 48 h. All cell cultures were maintained at 37 °C in a humidified atmosphere containing 5% CO_2, and experiments were performed on confluent cells.

4.3. Inflammatory Assays in Monolayer Cells

THP-1 MOM (1×10^6 cells/mL) were cultured in 500 µL of complete RPMI supplemented with different amentadione (YP) concentrations (2.5, 5 and 10 µM) in dose-dependence experiments and with 10 µM YP in subsequent experiments, or with 2 µM dexamethasone (DXM), during 24 h. After, 100 ng/mL of lipopolysaccharides (LPS) or synthetic hydroxyapatite nano-crystals (HAP) (Sigma) (750 µg/mL) were added to the culture media for another 24 h or 72 h, respectively. Confluent chondrocytes and synoviocytes were cultured in 1 mL of Adv DMEM supplemented with 10 µM of YP or 2 µM of DXM during 24 h, and further treated with: 10 ng/mL of interleukin-1β (IL-1β) for 3 and 6 h, or for 30 min in the assay for pIKBα content analysis; 750 µg/mL HAP for 6h. Control cells were cultured with respective media without any treatment. At determined time points, cell culture media were collected for ELISA analysis and cells harvested for RNA extraction.

4.4. Cell Proliferation

THP-1 MOM cells seeded in 96-well plates at 2×10^5 cells/well, and confluent chondrocytes and synoviocytes, were cultured in their respective growth media and supplemented with different concentrations of YP and HAP. Cell viability was determined at appropriate time points using the CellTiter 96 cell proliferation assay (Promega, Madison, WI, USA), following manufacturer's instructions.

4.5. Cartilage Collection and Tissue Explants Preparation

Knee articular cartilage was obtained from osteoarticular cuts performed on the femoral and tibial sides, from eight patients (4 male and 4 female, aged 71.5 ± 5.9 years) who had undergone arthroplasty surgeries at Hospital Particular do Algarve (Faro, Portugal). This study was approved by the ethics committee of the hospital, and written informed consent was obtained from all the participants. All principles of the Declaration of Helsinki of 1975, as revised in 2000, were followed. Macroscopically normal full-depth cartilage slices were removed in sterile conditions using a scalpel, collected in complete Adv DMEM media, and incubated for 24 h, at 37 °C, in a humidified atmosphere containing 5% CO_2, for tissue equilibration before preparation of tissue explants. After equilibration, 2 mm diameter and 1.71 ± 0.70 mm thickness cartilage explants, were obtained using a 2 mm biopsy punch (Integra-Miltex). Samples of the initial cartilage explant tissues were fixed in 4% PFA for histological evaluation.

4.6. Cartilage Explants Assays

Cartilage explants (8–10 per well), were plated in a 12 well plate and cultured at 37 °C, in a humidified atmosphere containing 5% CO_2, in 1 mL of complete Adv DMEM media supplemented with 10 µM of YP or 2 µM DXM for 24 h, and then treated with HAP (750 µg/mL), for further 72 h. As controls, explants were cultured without treatment. At the end of each experiment, cartilage explants were collected, washed twice with PBS, immediately processed for RNA extraction as described below, and the cell culture media collected for ELISA assays.

4.7. Co-Culture Assays

Cartilage explants (10 per well), were plated in a 12 well plate and co-cultured with synoviocytes in a transwell system (6.5 mm insert diameter, 3.0 µm polyester membrane, Corning Incorporated Life Sciences), in 1.8 mL of complete Adv DMEM, at 37 °C, in a humidified atmosphere containing 5% CO_2.

To evaluate the effect of YP, co-cultures were supplemented with 10 µM of YP or 2 µM DXM for 24 h, followed by treatment with IL-1β (10 ng/mL) during 24 h, or HAP (750 µg/mL) during 72 h. Cartilage explants were collected as described above for RNA extraction, and cell media collected for ELISA analysis.

4.8. RNA Extraction, cDNA Amplification and Quantitative Real-Time PCR (qPCR)

Cartilage tissue was immediately snap-frozen and manually grounded to powder in liquid nitrogen. Cells and tissue lysis was performed in a proportion of 1 mL of 4 M guanidine thiocyanate solution per 10^7 cells or 100 mg cartilage tissue, thoroughly mixed and passed 10 times through a 22G needle. Total RNA was further extracted as described by Chomczynski and Sacchi [55]. Briefly, homogenates were sequentially mixed with 2 M sodium citrate pH 4, phenol pH 4.2 and chloroform/isoamyl alcohol. After centrifugation, total RNA present in the aqueous phase was precipitated with isopropanol, redissolved in 4 M guanidine thiocyanate solution, reprecipitated in isopropanol, washed with 75% ethanol and resuspended in Sigma water. RNA concentration was determined by spectrophotometry at 260 nm (Nanodrop 1000, Thermo Scientific, Waltham, MA, USA). RNA was then treated with RQ1 RNase-free DNase (Promega, Madison, WI, USA) and reverse-transcribed using the qScipt cDNA SuperMix (Quanta bio, Beverly, MA, USA) according to manufacturer's recommendations. Quantitative real-time PCR reactions were performed using the CFX connect, Real time System (Bio-Rad, Richmond, CA, USA), SoFast Eva Green Supermix (Bio-Rad, Richmond, CA, USA), 300 nM of forward and reverse gene-specific primers for genes of interest (Table S2), and a 1:5 cDNA dilution. The following PCR conditions were used: initial denaturation/enzyme activation step at 95 °C for

13 min, 50 cycles of amplification (one cycle is 15 s at 95 °C and 30 s at 68 °C). Fluorescence was measured at the end of each extension cycle in the FAM-490 channel. Levels of gene expression were calculated using the comparative $\Delta\Delta Ct$ method, and normalized using gene expression levels of glyceraldehyde-3-phosphate dehydrogenase (GAPDH), with the iQ5 software (BioRad).

4.9. ELISA Assays

The cell culture media were used for the quantification of TNFα (Peprotech), IL-6 (Peprotech) and MMP3 (Life Technologies) following the manufacture's protocols.

4.10. Histological Evaluation

Paraffin-embedded cartilage tissue sections were processed at the Histopathology Department of Centro Hospitalar e Universitário do Algarve (CHUA, Faro) and used for histological assessment. Cartilage grading of initial tissue samples was conducted based on modified criteria originally established by Mankin et al., and the specimens were analyzed for abnormalities in structure, cellularity and matrix staining, based on hematoxylin-eosin (HE, Bio-Optica, Milano, Italy), safranin-O (SO)/Fast Green (Sigma-Aldrich, Steinheim, Germany) and toluidine blue (Merck, Darmstadt, Germany) stainings [56,57]. Four tissue sections from each sample were analyzed.

4.11. Protein Extraction and Quantification

Total protein from chondrocyte inflammatory assays and YP treatments was obtained by extraction with RIPA buffer (50 mM Tris HCl pH 8, 150 mM NaCl, 1% NP-40, 0.5% sodium deoxycholate, 0.1% SDS) for 1 h, at 4 °C, with agitation, followed by a centrifugation at 16× g for 15 min at 4 °C. Protein concentration was assessed using Micro BCA kit (Thermo Scientific), according to the manufacturer's instructions.

4.12. Electrophoresis and Western Blot

Aliquots of 20 µg of total protein extracts were size separated in a 4–12% (w/v) gradient polyacrylamide precast gel containing 0.1% (w/v) SDS (NuPage, Invitrogen, Carlsbad, CA, USA) and transferred onto a nitrocellulose membrane (Biorad, Richmond, CA, USA). Detection of pIKBα and GAPDH was performed through overnight (O/N) incubation with the pIKBα pSer32 ABfinity Rabbit Monoclonal antibody (2.5 µg/µL, Thermo Fisher, Waltham, MA, USA) and anti-GAPDH polyclonal antibody (1:500, Santa Cruz Biotechnology). Detection was achieved using Goat anti-rabbit IgG horseradish peroxidase-conjugated secondary antibody and Western Lightning Plus-ECL (PerkinElmer Inc., Waltham, MA, USA). Image acquisition was obtained using an IQ LAS 4000 mini biomolecular imager.

4.13. Determination of Total and Phosphorylated IkBα

Total IkBα and phosphorylated IkBα (pIkBα) were determined in chondrocyte cell lysates, using the InstantOne ELISA assay kit (Invitrogen) according to the manufacturer's protocol.

4.14. Statistical Analysis

Each independent experiment (n) was performed with different primary cell culture batches and cartilage from distinct patients. Replicates within an individual experiment were performed using the same batch of cells and cartilage from a single patient. Data are presented as mean ± standard deviation (SD). Multiple t tests were used for comparison between two groups. For more than two groups significance was determined using one-way analysis of variance (ANOVA) with comparison between groups by Dunnett test. Statistical significance was defined as $p \leq 0.05$ (*), $p \leq 0.005$ (**) and $p \leq 0.0005$ (***).

Supplementary Materials: The following are available online at http://www.mdpi.com/1660-3397/18/12/624/s1, Figure S1: Chemical structure, NMR and HRMS data of amentadione (YP); Figure S2: YP reduces the inflammatory response of THP-1 macrophages (THP-1 MOM) stimulated with LPS and hydroxyapatite (HAP); Figure S3: Viability of THP-1 macrophage cells (THP-1 MOM) exposed to different concentrations of amentadione (YP) for 24 h and exposed to different concentrations of HAP for 72 h; Figure S4: Viability of primary human chondrocytes and synoviocytes exposed to different amentadione (YP) concentrations for 24 h; Figure S5: Viability of primary human chondrocytes and synoviocytes exposed to different hydroxyapatite (HAP) concentrations for 72 h; Figure S6: Indication on the time point with increased pIkBα after IL-1β stimulation. Table S1: Modified Mankin score used for histological evaluation of human cartilage explants; Table S2: Gene-specific primers used for gene expression analysis by qPCR.

Author Contributions: Conceptualization, N.A., C.S.B.V. and D.C.S.; methodology, N.A. C.S.B.V., J.M., A.R., M.M.C., J.P.S. and H.C., investigation, N.A., C.S.B.V. and D.C.S.; resources, J.M. and E.Z.; writing—original draft preparation, N.A., C.S.B.V. and D.C.S.; writing—review and editing, C.S.B.V., J.M., F.J.B., C.V., E.Z. and D.C.S.; supervision, N.A., C.S.B.V. and D.C.S.; project administration, C.S.B.V. and D.C.S.; funding acquisition, C.S.B.V. and D.C.S. All authors have read and agreed to the published version of the manuscript.

Funding: This research was funded by the Portuguese national funds from FCT—Foundation for Science and Technology through the transitional provision DL57/2016/CP1361/CT0006 and project UIDB/04326/2020. N Araújo is the recipient of the Portuguese Science and Technology Foundation (FCT) fellowship SFRH/BD/111824/2015.

Acknowledgments: We would like to acknowledge José L. Enriquez and Alexandra Teixeira from the Centro Hospitalar e Universitário do Algarve (CHUAlgarve), Department of Histopathology, Faro, Portugal, for their collaboration in cartilage tissue paraffin embedding and sectioning.

Conflicts of Interest: Dina C. Simes and Carla Viegas are cofounders of GenoGla Diagnostics. The authors declare that there are no conflicts of interest regarding the publication of this paper.

References

1. Lawrence, R.C.; Felson, D.T.; Helmick, C.G.; Arnold, L.M.; Choi, H.; Deyo, R.A.; Gabriel, S.; Hirsch, R.; Hochberg, M.C.; Hunder, G.G.; et al. Estimates of the prevalence of arthritis and other rheumatic conditions in the United States. *Part II Arthritis Rheum.* **2008**, *58*, 26–35. [CrossRef] [PubMed]
2. Moe, R.H.; Uhlig, T.; Kjeken, I.; Hagen, K.B.; Kvien, T.K.; Grotle, M. Multidisciplinary and multifaceted outpatient management of patients with osteoarthritis: Protocol for a randomised, controlled trial. *BMC Musculoskelet. Disord.* **2010**, *11*, 253. [CrossRef] [PubMed]
3. Woolf, A.D.; Pfleger, B. Burden of major musculoskeletal conditions. *Bull. World Health Organ.* **2010**, *81*, 646–656.
4. Wallace, I.J.; Worthington, S.; Felson, D.T.; Jurmain, R.D.; Wren, K.T.; Maijanen, H.; Woods, R.J.; Lieberman, D.E. Knee osteoarthritis levels have recently doubled. *Proc. Natl. Acad. Sci. USA* **2017**, *114*, 9332–9336. [CrossRef] [PubMed]
5. Blanco, F.J. Osteoarthritis: Something is moving. *Reumatol. Clin.* **2014**, *10*, 4–5. [CrossRef]
6. Robinson, W.H.; Lepus, C.M.; Wang, Q.; Raghu, H.; Mao, R.; Lindstrom, T.M.; Sokolove, J. Low-grade inflammation as a key mediator of the pathogenesis of osteoarthritis. *Nat. Rev. Rheumatol.* **2016**, *12*, 580–592. [CrossRef]
7. Sokolove, J.; Lepus, C.M. Role of inflammation in the pathogenesis of osteoarthritis: Latest findings and interpretations. *Ther. Adv. Musculoskeletal Dis.* **2013**, *5*, 77–94. [CrossRef]
8. Sutton, S.; Clutterbuck, A.; Harris, P.; Gent, T.; Freeman, S.; Foster, N.; Barrett-Jolley, R.; Mobasher, A. The contribution of the synovium, synovial derived inflammatory cytokines and neuropeptides to the pathogenesis of osteoarthritis. *Vet. J.* **2009**, *179*, 10–24. [CrossRef]
9. Abramson, S.B.; Attur, M.; Amin, A.R.; Clancy, R. Nitric oxide and inflammatory mediators in the perpetuation of osteoarthritis. *Curr. Rheumatol. Rep.* **2001**, *3*, 535–541. [CrossRef]
10. Rose, B.J.; Kooyman, D.L. A Tale of Two Joints: The Role of Matrix Metalloproteases in Cartilage Biology. *Dis. Mark.* **2016**, *2016*, 4895050. [CrossRef]
11. Frallonardo, P.; Ramonda, R.; Peruzzo, L.; Scanu, A.; Galozzi, P.; Tauro, L.; Punzi, L.; Oliviero, F. Basic calcium phosphate and pyrophosphate crystals in early and late osteoarthritis: Relationship with clinical indices and inflammation. *Clin. Rheumatol.* **2018**, *37*, 2847–2853. [CrossRef] [PubMed]
12. Conway, R.; McCarthy, G.M. Calcium-Containing Crystals and Osteoarthritis: An Unhealthy Alliance. *Curr. Rheumatol. Rep.* **2018**, *20*, 13. [CrossRef]

13. Carlson, A.K.; McCutchen, C.N.; June, R.K. Mechanobiological implications of articular cartilage crystals Calcium. *Curr. Opin. Rheumatol.* **2017**, *29*, 157–162. [CrossRef] [PubMed]
14. Hochberg, M.C.; Altman, R.D.; April, K.T.; Benkhalti, M.; Guyatt, G.; McGowan, J.; Towheed, T.; Welch, V.; Wells, G.; Tugwell, P. American College of Rheumatology 2012 recommendations for the use of nonpharmacologic and pharmacologic therapies in osteoarthritis of the hand, hip, and knee. *Arthrit. Care Res.* **2012**, *64*, 465–474. [CrossRef]
15. Mobasheri, A. The future of osteoarthritis therapeutics: Targeted pharmacological therapy. *Curr. Rheumatol. Rep.* **2013**, *15*, 364. [CrossRef] [PubMed]
16. Samvelyan, H.J.; Hughes, D.; Stevens, C.; Staines, K.A. Models of osteoarthritis: Relevance and new insights [published online ahead of print, 2020 Feb 15]. *Calcif. Tissue Int.* **2020**. [CrossRef]
17. Schlichting, N.; Dehne, T.; Mans, K.; Endres, M.; Stuhlmüller, B.; Sittinger, M.; Kaps, C.; Ringe, J. Suitability of porcine chondrocyte micromass culture to model osteoarthritis in vitro. *Mol. Pharm.* **2014**, *11*, 2092–2105. [CrossRef] [PubMed]
18. Suroowan, S.; Mahomoodally, F. Herbal products for common auto-inflammatory disorders-novel approaches. *Comb. Chem. High Throughput Screen.* **2018**, *21*, 161–174. [CrossRef]
19. Henrotin, Y.; Mobasheri, A. Natural products for promoting joint health and managing osteoarthritis. *Curr. Rheumatol. Rep.* **2018**, *20*, 72. [CrossRef]
20. Castrogiovanni, P.; Trovato, F.M.; Loreto, C.; Nsir, H.; Szychlinska, M.A.; Musumeci, G. Nutraceutical supplements in the management and prevention of osteoarthritis. *Int. J. Mol. Sci.* **2016**, *17*, 2042. [CrossRef]
21. Liu, X.; Machado, G.C.; Eyles, J.P.; Ravi, V.; Hunter, D.J. Dietary supplements for treating osteoarthritis: A systematic review and meta-analysis. *Br. J. Sports Med.* **2018**, *52*, 167–175. [CrossRef]
22. Stoppoloni, D.; Politi, L.; Leopizzi, M.; Gaetani, S.; Guazzo, R.; Basciani, S.; Moreschini, O.; De Santi, M.; Scandurra, R.; Scotto d'Abusco, A. Effect of glucosamine and its peptidyl-derivative on the production of extracellular matrix components by human primary chondrocytes. *Osteoarth. Cart.* **2015**, *23*, 103–113. [CrossRef]
23. Paul, A.T.; Gohil, V.M.; Bhutani, K.K. Modulating TNF-alpha signaling with natural products. *Drug Discov. Today* **2006**, *11*, 725–732. [CrossRef] [PubMed]
24. Wang, G.; Tang, W.; Bidigare, R.R. Terpenoids as therapeutic drugs and pharmaceutical agents. Natural Products. In *Natural Products: Drug Discovery and Therapeutic Medicine*; Zhang, L., Demain, A.L., Eds.; Humana Press: Totowa, NJ, USA, 2017; pp. 197–227. [CrossRef]
25. De los Reyes, C.; Zbakh, H.; Motilva, V.; Zubía, E. Antioxidant and anti-inflammatory meroterpenoids from the brown alga *Cystoseira usneoides*. *J. Nat. Prod.* **2013**, *76*, 621–629. [CrossRef] [PubMed]
26. De los Reyes, C.; Ortega, M.J.; Zbakh, H.; Motilva, V.; Zubía, E. *Cystoseira usneoides*: A brown alga rich in antioxidant and anti-inflammatory meroditerpenoids. *J. Nat. Prod.* **2016**, *79*, 395–405. [CrossRef]
27. Zbakh, H.; Talero, E.; Avila, J.; Alcaide, A.; de los Reyes, C.; Zubía, E.; Motilva, V. The algal meroterpene 11-hydroxy-1'-O-methylamentadione ameloriates dextran sulfate sodium-induced colitis in mice. *Mar. Drugs* **2016**, *14*, 149. [CrossRef] [PubMed]
28. Zbakh, H.; Zubía, E.; Reyes, C.; Calderón-Montaño, J.M.; López-Lázaro, M.; Motilva, V. Meroterpenoids from the brown alga *Cystoseira usneoides* as potential anti-inflammatory and lung anticancer agents. *Mar. Drugs* **2020**, *18*, 207. [CrossRef]
29. Viegas, C.S.B.; Costa, R.M.; Santos, L.; Videira, P.A.; Silva, Z.; Araújo, N.; Macedo, A.L.; Matos, A.P.; Cees Vermeer, C.; Simes, D.C. Gla-rich protein function as an anti-inflammatory agent in monocytes/macrophages: Implications for calcification-related chronic inflammatory diseases. *PLoS ONE* **2017**, *12*, e0177829. [CrossRef]
30. Cavaco, S.; Viegas, C.S.B.; Rafael, M.S.; Ramos, A.; Magalhães, J.; Blanco, F.J.; Vermeer, C.; Simes, D.C. Gla-rich protein is involved in the cross-talk between calcification and inflammation in osteoarthritis. *Cell. Mol. Life Sci.* **2016**, *73*, 1051–1065. [CrossRef]
31. Pritzker, K.P.; Gay, S.; Jimenez, S.A.; Ostergaard, K.; Pelletier, J.P.; Revell, P.A.; Salter, D.; van den Berg, W.V. Osteoarthritis cartilage histopathology: Grading and staging. *Osteoarth. Cartil.* **2006**, *14*, 13–29. [CrossRef]
32. Houard, X.; Goldring, M.B.; Berenbaum, F. Homeostatic mechanisms in articular cartilage and role of inflammation in osteoarthritis. *Curr. Rheumatol. Rep.* **2013**, *15*, 375. [CrossRef] [PubMed]
33. Van der Kraan, P.M.; van den Berg, W.B. Chondrocyte hypertrophy and osteoarthritis: Role in initiation and progression of cartilage degeneration? *Osteoarth. Cartil.* **2012**, *20*, 223–232. [CrossRef] [PubMed]

34. Hernandez-Santana, A.; Yavorskyy, A.; Loughran, S.T.; McCarthy, G.M.; McMahon, G.P. New approaches in the detection of calcium-containing microcrystals in synovial fluid. *Bioanalysis* **2011**, *3*, 1085–1091. [CrossRef] [PubMed]
35. Corr, E.M.; Cunningham, C.C.; Helbert, L.; McCarthy, G.M.; Dunne, A. Osteoarthritis-associated basic calcium phosphate crystals activate membrane proximal kinases in human innate immune cells. *Arthritis Res. Ther.* **2017**, *19*, 23. [CrossRef] [PubMed]
36. Ea, H.K.; Nguyen, C.; Bazin, D.; Bianchi, A.; Guicheux, J.; Reboul, P.; Daudon, M.; Lioté, F. Articular cartilage calcification in osteoarthritis: Insights into crystal-induced stress. *Arthritis. Rheum.* **2011**, *63*, 10–18. [CrossRef]
37. Nadra, I.; Mason, J.C.; Philippidis, P.; Florey, O.; Smythe, C.D.; McCarthy, G.M.; Landis, R.C.; Haskardet, D.O. Proinflammatory activation of macrophages by basic calcium phosphate crystals via proteinkinase C and MAP kinase pathways: A vicious cycle of inflammation and arterial calcification? *Circ. Res.* **2005**, *96*, 1248–1256. [CrossRef]
38. Nasi, S.; So, A.; Combes, C.; Daudon, M.; Busso, N. Interleukin-6 and chondrocyte mineralisation act in tandem to promote experimental osteoarthritis. *Ann. Rheum. Dis.* **2016**, *75*, 1372–1379. [CrossRef]
39. Jung, Y.K.; Han, M.S.; Park, H.R.; Lee, E.J.; Jang, J.A.; Kim, G.-W.; Lee, S.Y.; Moon, D.; Han, S. Calcium-phosphate complex increased during subchondral bone remodelling affects early stage osteoarthritis. *Sci. Rep.* **2018**, *8*, 487. [CrossRef]
40. Wojdasiewicz, P.; Poniatowski, Ł.A.; Szukiewicz, D. The role of inflammatory and anti-inflammatory cytokines in the pathogenesis of osteoarthritis. *Mediators Inflamm.* **2014**, *2014*, 19. [CrossRef]
41. Ismail, H.M.; Yamamoto, K.; Vincent, T.L.; Nagase, H.; Troeberg, L.; Saklatvala, J. Interleukin-1 Acts via the JNK-2 Signaling Pathway to Induce Aggrecan Degradation by Human Chondrocytes. *Arthritis Rheumatol.* **2015**, *67*, 826–836. [CrossRef]
42. Zweers, M.C.; de Boer, T.N.; van Roon, J.; Bijlsma, J.W.; Lafeber, F.P.; Mastbergen, S.C. Celecoxib: Considerations regarding its potential disease-modifying properties in osteoarthritis. *Arthritis Res. Ther.* **2011**, *13*, 239. [CrossRef] [PubMed]
43. Aitken, D.; Laslett, L.L.; Pan, F.; Haugen, I.K.; Otahal, P.; Bellamy, N.; Bird, P.; Jones, G.A. Randomised double-blind placebo-controlled crossover trial of HUMira (adalimumab) for erosive hand Osteoarthritis-the HUMOR trial. *Osteoarth. Cart.* **2018**, *26*, 880–887. [CrossRef] [PubMed]
44. Rider, P.; Carmi, Y.; Cohen, I. Biologics for targeting inflammatory cytokines, clinical uses, and limitations. *Int. J. Cell Biol.* **2016**, *2016*, 11. [CrossRef] [PubMed]
45. Cheng, W.; Wu, D.; Zuo, Q.; Wang, Z.; Fan, W. Ginsenoside Rb1 prevents interleukin-1 beta induced inflammation and apoptosis in human articular chondrocytes. *Int. Orthop.* **2013**, *37*, 2065–2070. [CrossRef] [PubMed]
46. Aravinthan, A.; Hossain, M.A.; Kim, B.; Kang, C.W.; Kim, N.S.; Hwang, K.C.; Kim, J.H. Ginsenoside Rb1 inhibits monoiodoacetate-induced osteoarthritis in postmenopausal rats through prevention of cartilage degradation. *J. Ginseng Res.* **2020**, 1226–8453. [CrossRef]
47. Jurenka, J.S. Anti-Inflammatory Properties of curcumin, a major constituent of Curcuma Longa: A Review of Preclinical and Clinical Research. *Altern. Med. Rev.* **2009**, *14*, 141–153.
48. Zhang, Z.; Leong, D.J.; Xu, L.; He, Z.; Wang, A.; Navati, M.; Kim, S.J.; Hirsh, D.M.; Hardin, J.A.; Cobelli, N.J.; et al. Curcumin slows osteoarthritis progression and relieves osteoarthritis-associated pain symptoms in a post-traumatic osteoarthritis mouse model. *Arthritis Res. Ther.* **2016**, *18*, 28. [CrossRef] [PubMed]
49. Marcu, K.B.; Otero, M.; Olivotto, E.; Borzi, R.M.; Goldring, M.B. NF-kappaB signaling: Multiple angles to target OA. *Curr. Drug Targets* **2010**, *11*, 599–613. [CrossRef]
50. Olivotto, E.; Otero, M.; Marcu, K.B.; Goldring, M.B. Pathophysiology of osteoarthritis: Canonical NF-κB/IKKβ-dependent and kinase-independent effects of IKKα in cartilage degradation and chondrocyte differentiation. *RMD Open.* **2015**, *1*, e000061. [CrossRef] [PubMed]
51. Choi, M.C.; Jo, J.; Park, J.; Kang, H.K.; Park, Y. NF-κB Signaling pathways in osteoarthritic cartilage destruction. *Cells* **2019**, *8*, 734. [CrossRef]
52. Amico, V.; Oriente, G.; Neri, P.; Piatelli, M.; Ruberto, G. Tetraprenyltoluquinols from the brown alga *Cystoseira stricta*. *Phytochemistry* **1987**, *26*, 1715–1718. [CrossRef]

53. Burguera, E.F.; Vela, A.A.; Magalhães, J.; Meijide-Faílde, R.; Blanco, F.J. Effect of hydrogen sulfide sources on inflammation and catabolic markers on interleukin 1b-stimulated human articular chondrocytes. *Osteoarth. Cartil.* **2014**, *22*, 1026–1035. [CrossRef]
54. Cillero, P.B.; Martin, M.; Arenas, J.; Lopez-Armada, M.J.; Blanco, F.J. Effect of nitric oxide on mitochondrial activity of human synovial cells. *BMC Musculoskelet. Disord.* **2011**, *12*, 42. [CrossRef]
55. Single-step method of RNA isolation by acid guanidinium thiocyanate phenol chloroform extraction. *Anal. Biochem.* **1987**, *162*, 156–159. [CrossRef]
56. Rosenberg, L. Chemical basis for the histological use of safranin O in the study of articular cartilage. *J. Bone Joint Surg. Am.* **1971**, *53*, 69–82. [CrossRef] [PubMed]
57. López-Senra, E.; Casal-Beiroa, P.; López-Álvarez, M.; Serra, J.; González, P.; Valcarcel, J.; Vázquez, J.A.; Burguera, E.F.; Blanco, F.J.; Magalhães, J. Impact of prevalence ratios of chondroitin sulfate (CS)- 4 and -6-isomers derived from marine sources in cell proliferation and chondrogenic differentiation processes. *Mar. Drugs* **2020**, *18*, 94. [CrossRef] [PubMed]

Publisher's Note: MDPI stays neutral with regard to jurisdictional claims in published maps and institutional affiliations.

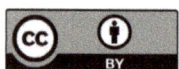

© 2020 by the authors. Licensee MDPI, Basel, Switzerland. This article is an open access article distributed under the terms and conditions of the Creative Commons Attribution (CC BY) license (http://creativecommons.org/licenses/by/4.0/).

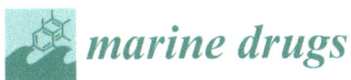

Article

Anti-Fouling Effects of Saponin-Containing Crude Extracts from Tropical Indo-Pacific Sea Cucumbers

Elham Kamyab [1,*], Norman Goebeler [1,2], Matthias Y. Kellermann [1], Sven Rohde [1], Miriam Reverter [1], Maren Striebel [1] and Peter J. Schupp [1,3,*]

1. Institute for Chemistry and Biology of the Marine Environment (ICBM), Carl-von-Ossietzky University Oldenburg, Schleusenstrasse 1, 26382 Wilhelmshaven, Germany; norman.gobeler@helsinki.fi (N.G.); matthias.kellermann@uol.de (M.Y.K.); sven.rohde@uol.de (S.R.); miriam.reverter@uol.de (M.R.); maren.striebel@uol.de (M.S.)
2. Tvärminne Zoological Station, University of Helsinki, J.A. Palmènin tie 260, 10900 Hanko, Finland
3. Helmholtz Institute for Functional Marine Biodiversity at the University of Oldenburg (HIFMB), Ammerländer Heerstrasse 231, D-26129 Oldenburg, Germany
* Correspondence: elham.kamyab@uol.de (E.K.); peter.schupp@uni-oldenburg.de (P.J.S.); Tel.: +49(0)-4421-944-218 (E.K.); +49-4421-944-100 (P.J.S.)

Received: 6 March 2020; Accepted: 28 March 2020; Published: 31 March 2020

Abstract: Sea cucumbers are bottom dwelling invertebrates, which are mostly found on subtropical and tropical sea grass beds, sandy reef flats, or reef slopes. Although constantly exposed to fouling communities in these habitats, many species are surprisingly free of invertebrate epibionts and microfouling algae such as diatoms. In our study, we investigated the anti-fouling (AF) activities of different crude extracts of tropical Indo-Pacific sea cucumber species against the fouling diatom *Cylindrotheca closterium*. Nine sea cucumber species from three genera (i.e., *Holothuria*, *Bohadschia*, *Actinopyga*) were selected and extracted to assess their AF activities. To verify whether the sea cucumber characteristic triterpene glycosides were responsible for the observed potent AF activities, we tested purified fractions enriched in saponins isolated from *Bohadschia argus*, representing one of the most active anti-fouling extracts. Saponins were quantified by vanillin-sulfuric acid colorimetric assays and identified by LC-MS and LC-MS/MS analyses. We were able to demonstrate that AF activities in sea cucumber extracts were species-specific, and growth inhibition as well as attachment of the diatom to surfaces is dependent on the saponin concentration (i.e., *Actinopyga* contained the highest quantities), as well as on the molecular composition and structure of the present saponins (i.e., *Bivittoside D* derivative was the most bioactive compound). In conclusion, the here performed AF assay represents a promising and fast method for selecting the most promising bioactive organism as well as for identifying novel compounds with potent AF activities for the discovery of potentially novel pharmacologically active natural products.

Keywords: holothurian; diatom; anti-fouling compounds; marine natural products; saponins; triterpene glycosides; mass spectrometry

---

1. Introduction

Biofouling is the colonization process of micro- (i.e., protozoa, bacteria, fungi and diatoms) or macro-organisms (i.e., algae and invertebrates) on either living (known as epibiosis) or artificial substrates [1,2]. Mckenzie and Grigolava (1996) described that epibiosis decreased host fitness, their survival rate, and species abundance, as well as affects their community composition [3]. Fouling on living surfaces of marine invertebrates can increase their friction as well as their body weight, and thus reduces speed, elasticity, and flexibility of the fouled organism, which in turn may lead to reduced viability and death [4,5]. Shading by fouling organisms can also impact negatively on the growth rate of the fouled organisms due to a reduced photosynthetic rate of macroalgae [6]. Biofouling processes are however not only relevant from an ecological perspective, but they have also important economic implications [4]. Marine biofouling shortens the lifespan and increases the maintenance costs of underwater constructions like ship hulls and aquaculture cages [7,8]. It also increases the weight and the friction of a ship, which in turn decreases the maximum cruising speed as well as increases fuel consumption [7,9]. In order to counteract the biofilm production on these structures, various synthetic anti-fouling (AF) paints that contain toxicants such as mercury (mercuric oxide (HgO), mercuric arsenate (AsO_4Hg_3)), arsenic (arsenic trioxide (As_2O_3)), copper (cuprous arsenite (AsO_3Cu_3)), as well as organotins (mainly tributyltin (TBT) based compounds) and rosin-based paint, have been applied in the past [7,9]. However, there are numerous studies showing that all the latter paints are hazardous for the environment and negatively affect the growth rate and reproduction of both fouling and non-fouling marine organisms [7,8,10–12]. As a result of such studies, production and application of TBT-based AF paints was internationally banned in the 1990s [7,13], and substituted with copper-based and booster biocides. However, recent research showed that these compounds still display toxic effects on marine organisms. The use of natural products as biological-based AF biocides in coating has been suggested as a new sustainable alternative, since they generally show biocompatibility, biodegradability, and thus their toxicity effects (if any) will not accumulate and generate long-lasting perturbations in the environment [14–18]. Engineering of an effective biological-based AF coating may not only protect the marine environment, but could also have substantial economic benefits by increasing the lifespan of underwater structures and by reducing the fuel consumption rate in the shipping industry (i.e., 60$ billion per annum). Furthermore, reduced fuel consumption also decreases carbon dioxide and sulfur dioxide emissions to the atmosphere [19–21] and therefore mitigate the effects of world-wide shipping to climate change.

In order to avoid the negative effects from unwanted epibioses, organisms can either accept and tolerate the presence of the fouling organisms (i.e., by developing a symbiosis) or avoid them, by either changing their habitat or developing chemical defenses [3,22–24]. AF defenses of marine organisms include mucus secretion (e.g., in sea star *Marthasterias glacialis*; [25]), shedding, microroughness, burrowing, scraping, and cleaning their body wall as well as chemical defense [4,26–28]. Chemical anti-fouling compounds can have various modes of action. They can be toxic to epibionts [29–31], inhibit settlement of larvae from fouling organisms [5,32,33] or prevent development of bacterial biofilms by disrupting bacterial communication via inhibition of the bacterial acylated homoserine lactone (AHL) signaling pathways [34]. Until 2017, almost 200 different AF compounds were described from marine invertebrates such as echinoderms, sponges, gorgonians and soft corals [35]. These AF compounds belong to various groups of terpenoids (i.e., triterpenes, sesquiterpenes and diterpenes), alkaloids, steroids, triterpene glycosides (saponins), polyacetylenes, butenolides, peptides and phenol derivatives [30,35,36]. More recently, the AF activities of compounds isolated from sea cucumbers such as *Holothuria atra* [37,38], *H. nobilis* [38], *H. edulis* [39], *H. glaberrima* [40], *H. tubulosa* and *H. polii* [41] were reported, as these sea cucumbers keep their body surfaces conspicuously free of fouling organisms [3]. Echinoderms, and especially sea cucumbers, are known to produce a wide variety of triterpene glycosides or saponins [42]. Saponins are composed of a hydrophilic glycone and a hydrophobic aglycone (i.e., sapogenin; Figure 1) that, depending on the holothuroids (*cf.* Figure 2), are located in the Cuverian Tubules (CT), in its body wall and its viscera [43]. Because of the membranolytic activities of saponin, a wide range of bioactivities such as anti-bacterial, anti-fungal, anti-viral, anti-inflammatory, ichthyotoxic, as well as anti-fouling properties have been reported [42,44,45].

The colonization process of fouling organisms starts after the first contact of the respective surface to sea water [4]. After "biochemical conditioning," which is initiated by adsorption of macromolecules to the surface, a bacterial biofilm develops. This is followed by the colonization of unicellular eukaryotes and algae such as diatoms [4]. One such algae is the meroplanktonic diatom *Cylindrotheca closterium*, that showed rapid growth particularly on surfaces [46,47]. This diatom species is also known to produce different types of hydrophilic and carbohydrate-rich extracellular polymeric substances (EPS) that often represent the major component of the extracellular aggregative matrix [46]. EPS plays a crucial role in the biofilm formation, and the microbial and physicochemical defenses of the diatom [48,49], their motility [50], cell to cell and cell to substratum adhesion [51], as well as in the settlement success and post larval growth of other organisms [52–54]. Thus, *C. closterium* has been used as a model organism in the past for early stage fouling studies [50,52,55].

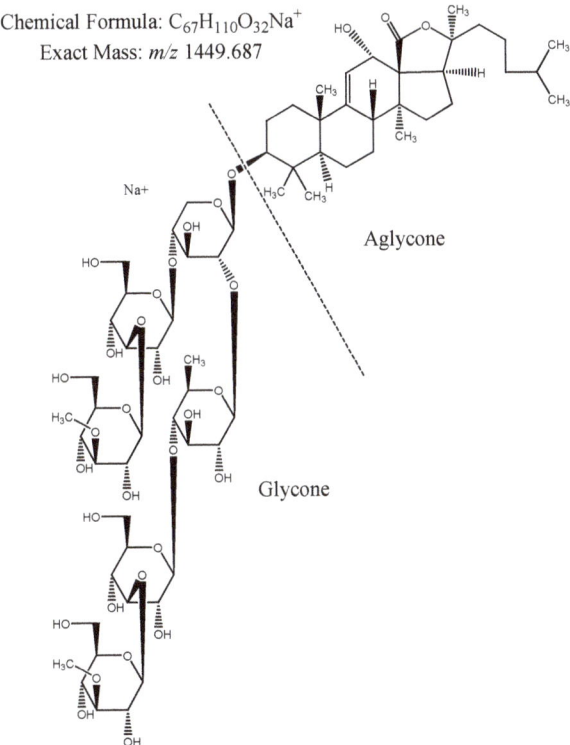

Figure 1. Structure of the saponin molecule "bivittoside D", m/z 1449.687 [M + Na]$^+$ [56], consisting of the glycone and aglycone moieties (produced with ChemDraw, version 16.0.1.4 (77)).

The aim of this study is to determine AF activities of different crude extracts of tropical Indo-Pacific sea cucumber species against the fouling diatom species *C. closterium*. To identify phylogenetic differences in AF activities of sea cucumber species, we choose nine species from three different genera (i.e., *Holothuria, Bohadschia, Actinopyga*). Also, we tested purified fractions enriched in saponins as well as pure saponin compounds to verify whether these sea cucumber characteristic compounds were involved in the observed AF activities of sea cucumbers.

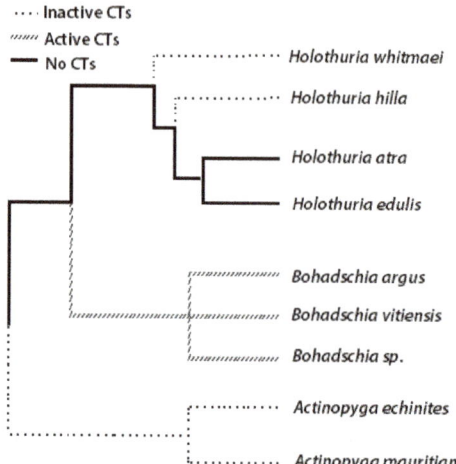

Figure 2. Phylogeny tree of the here studied sea cucumbers (CT = cuvierian tubule; adapted from [57–60]).

2. Results

2.1. Anti-Fouling Effects of the Crude Extracts

Antifouling activity of the sea cucumber crude extracts was assessed by measuring biomass and attachment of the diatom *C. closterium*. To assess suspended algal biomass, chlorophyll a *(Chl a)* was extracted from the water samples, while *Chl a* content of diatoms attached to the substrate was used to evaluate diatom attachment. *Chl a* measurements are well established as a proxies for monitoring water quality, assessing phytoplankton biomass, and estimating primary production [61–63], while fluorometric measurements of *Chl a* concentrations are an efficient proxy to monitor the total biomass of diatoms in the water column and on the substrate. To determine the anti-fouling effects of the holothurian's crude extracts, a logarithmic response ratio (LRR; see Section 4.1.5) of measured *Chl a* concentrations was calculated. Negative LRR reveals an anti-fouling effect of the extract with less *Chl a* in the treated compared to the control samples, while a positive LRR indicates a higher *Chl a* concentration and thus an increase in algal growth in the treatments compared to the control samples.

Measurements of *Chl a* concentration of the suspended cells in the water and the attached cells at the flasks surface showed that the sea cucumbers crude extracts had a concentration-dependent effect on growth and settlement of *C. closterium* (Figure S1A–F). The LRR supports this finding (Figure 3A,B), showing the highest negative effect ($p < 0.05$) on diatom growth in the water column at the highest extract concentrations (150 µg mL^{-1}, Figure 3A), except for extracts from *H. whitmaei* and *H. hilla* where no negative effects could be observed ($p = 0.371$ and $p = 0.65$, respectively; Table S1). *Actinopyga* spp. and *Bohadschia* extracts (except *B. vitiensis*) exhibited negative LRR at 15 µg mL^{-1} concentration, indicating significant anti-fouling effects. Extracts of the genera *Holothuria* (except *H. atra*) had no inhibitory effects at the same concentration. At the lowest concentration (1.5 µg mL^{-1}; Figure 3A), all the crude extracts showed a positive LRR, except *B. argus* and *A. echinites* extracts, which had significant inhibitory activity toward the tested diatom in the water column.

Similar to the LRR in the water column, the highest crude extract concentrations (150 µg mL^{-1}) inhibited diatom settlement (Figure 3B). The treatment containing 15 µg mL^{-1} of extract of the genus *Holothuria* stimulated diatom settlement, whereas *Bohadschia* (except *B. vitiensis*) and *Actinopyga* extracts suppressed it. At the lowest concentration (1.5 µg mL^{-1}) all crude extracts (except *B. vittiensis*) showed a significant inhibition on diatom settlement (Table S1).

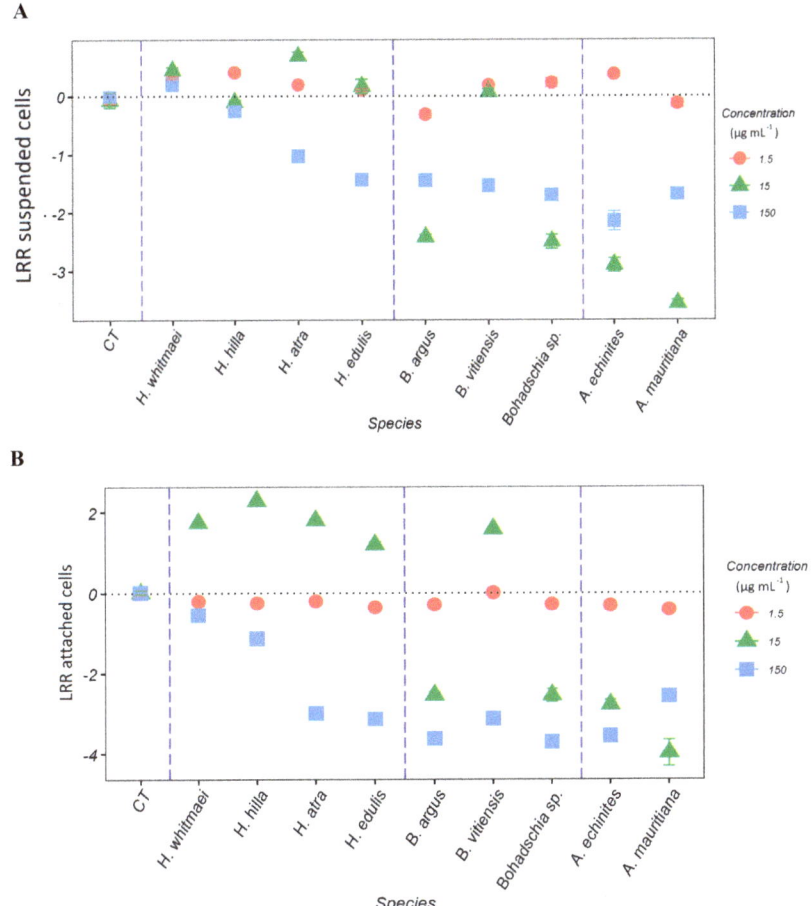

Figure 3. Logarithmic response ratio (LRR) of *C. closterium* after exposure to three different concentrations (150, 15 and 1.5 µg mL^{-1}) of nine sea cucumber extracts in total (genera *Holothuria*, *Bohadschia* and *Actinopyga*) for (**A**) suspended cells in the water and (**B**) attached to the surface of the incubation flask. Significant differences compared to the control (CT = control) are shown in Table S1.

2.2. Saponin Profile of the Crude Extracts

2.2.1. Saponin Composition

Identification of the most prominent saponins in the crude extracts of the nine sea cucumber species (peak areas > 10,000 mu) yielded 102 different saponin-like molecules (Table S2). However, several of the saponins showed the same exact molecular mass, but different retention times, indicating unknown isomers of potentially known saponin compounds (Table S3).

A hierarchical cluster analysis was performed to explore the similarity of saponin compositions between the different holothurian species. Except for *H. edulis*, we observed that all sea cucumber species cluster with species from the same genus (using the Kelley-Gardner-Sutcliffe (KGS) penalty function for identifying significant clusters, Figure 4). Note, that all species from the genus *Bohadschia* formed a clear separated cluster compared to *Actinopyga* and *Holothuria*.

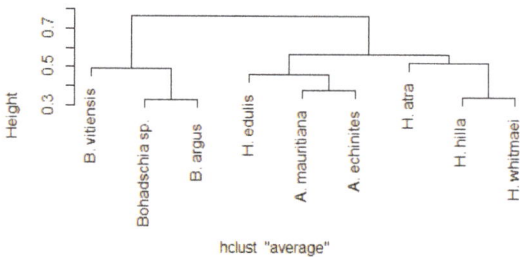

Figure 4. Cluster dendrogram of sea cucumber species based on their studied saponin and sapogenin compositions ("average" distance type, log-transformed data, R version 1.2.5019).

More detailed analysis of the various saponin compounds revealed that compound M1104T11.1 (abbreviation indicates molecular mass (M) and retention time (T)) was present in all nine sea cucumber species, M1118T8.9 in eight and M600T9.3 and M1374T9 in seven species (*cf.* Table S3). Composition and relative intensities of both saponins and sapogenins, which are visualized for each sea cucumber species (Figure 5A,B), showed that *Bohadschia* species contained the highest number of known saponins, as well as the highest intensities, whereas signal intensities of sapogenins were especially high in the genus *Holothuria*. Interestingly, the three investigated *Bohadschia* species, which were among the most active in inhibiting *C. closterium* growth (Figure 5A), were the only ones containing M1426T10.3 (*m/z* 1426.698; $C_{67}H_{110}O_{32}$), M1410T11.3 (*m/z* 1410.703; $C_{67}H_{110}O_{31}$), and M1424T9.8 (*m/z* 1424.6823; $C_{67}H_{108}O_{32}$), which represent analogous molecular formulas to the known saponins *bivittoside D-like*, *bivittoside C-like*, and *marmoratoside A-like*, respectively (Figures S2–S4).

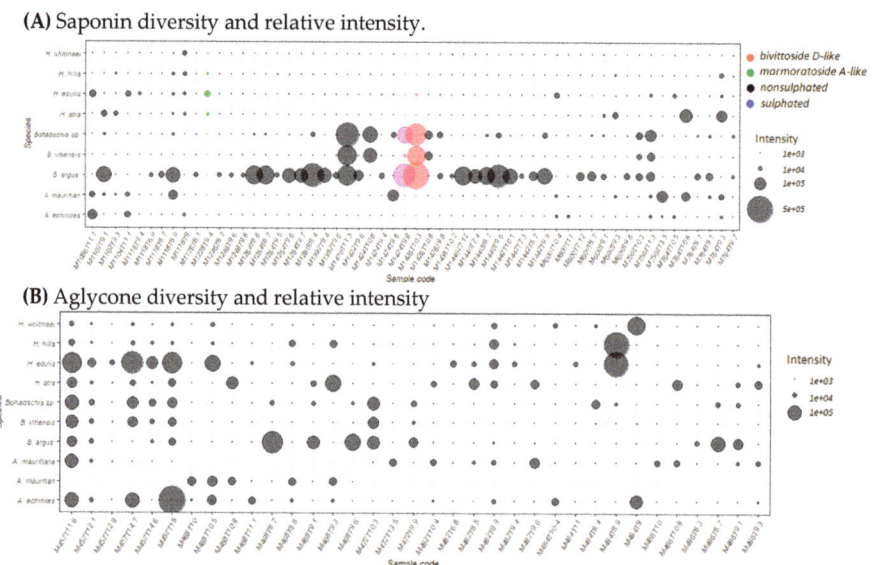

Figure 5. Major saponin compounds detected in the studied sea cucumbers (peak area $\geq 10^4$). (**A**) saponin diversity and relative intensity and (**B**) sapogenin (aglycon) diversity and relative intensity. Sample codes represent exact mass (M in Da), and retention time (T in min). Different colors represent the presence of sulphate groups (in blue), non-sulphate groups (in black) and pure compounds (in purple and red). Bubble size correlates with differences in relative peak areas of the respective molecules.

2.2.2. Total Saponin Concentration

The total triterpene glycoside concentration of the crude extracts was assessed using the vanillin-sulfuric acid colorimetric assay (Figure 6). *H. atra* (0.456 mg mL^{-1} ± 0.08) and *H. whitmaei* (0.496 mg mL^{-1} ± 0.08) had the lowest saponin concentration, whereas *A. echinites* (2.106 mg mL^{-1} ± 0.16), *A. mauritiana* (1.880 mg mL^{-1} ± 0.15), *B. vitiensis* (1.181 mg mL^{-1} ± 0.01), and *B. argus* (1.130 mg mL^{-1} ± 0.01) contained the highest concentrations of saponins. Saponin concentration in the genus *Actinopyga* was significantly higher than within *Holothuria* and *Bohadschia* (Kruskal-Wallis test; $p < 0.05$).

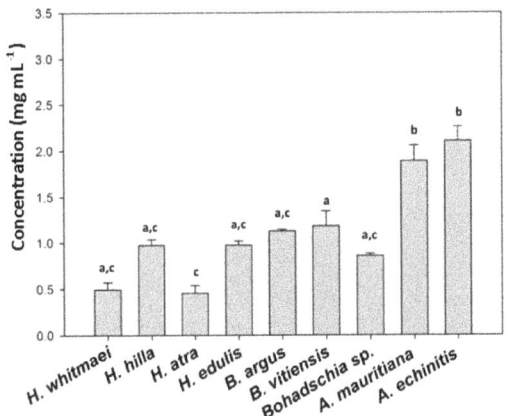

Figure 6. Absolute saponin concentration of the tested crude extracts. (**a–c**) indicate significant differences between different sea cucumber crude extracts. Kruskal–Wallis, Dunn's method as a multiple comparison test. Significance level at $p < 0.05$ was applied.

2.3. Anti-Fouling Effects of Purified Saponin Fractions and Pure Compounds

2.3.1. AF Assay with an Emphasis on Saponins

Based on the LRR of *Chl a* calculated for 1.5 µg mL^{-1} of different fractions, the Kruskal-Wallis test revealed that fraction 3 and 4 had a significant negative effect on the growth of *C. closterium* ($p < 0.05$). The first two fractions, on the other hand, had a significant positive effect on the growth of the diatom species (Figure 7A,B).

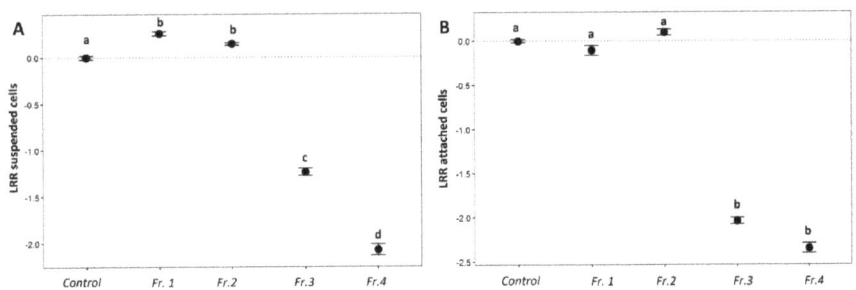

Figure 7. Logarithmic response ratio (LRR) of *C. closterium* following exposure to *B. argus* extract fractions in suspended cells in the water (**A**) and attached to the substrate (**B**). Fr.1 and Fr.2: impure, Fr. 3: semi-pure, Fr. 4: pure singular saponin species (*bivittoside D-like*). a–d represent result of Kruskal-Wallis test; $p < 0.05$.

2.3.2. Saponin Profile of the Fractions

The most abundant saponin compounds in *B. argus* (i.e., $C_{67}H_{110}O_{32}$, *bivittoside D-like* and $C_{67}H_{108}O_{32}$, *marmoratoside A-like*; Figure S5, Table S4) were isolated to examine whether saponins are responsible for the observed anti-fouling activities. As shown in Figure S6, the mixed fraction 3, containing the saponin species M1426T10.3 (*bivittoside D-like*), M1454T10.7 (*stichoposide D-like*) and 1424T10.4 (*marmoratoside A-like*), as well as the relatively pure fraction 4 with mainly saponin M1426T10.3 (*bivittoside D-like*) strongly inhibited growth as well as attachment of the diatom. Fraction 1 and 2, on the other hand, contained a mixture of saponins (except *bivittoside D-like*), which did not affect the growth and attachment of *C. closterium*. Currently, the main three saponin species from fraction 3 are further purified and their molecular structure is being elucidated via NMR spectroscopy.

3. Discussion

Many marine benthic organisms (e.g., sponges, mussels, starfishes, sea urchins, algae) are known to harbor anti-fouling metabolites that protect them from deleterious fouling organisms (e.g., [33,64–67]). Sea cucumbers do not have visible defensive mechanisms, however their surfaces are free of fouling organisms [40]. Several molecules with various biological activities (e.g., anti-bacterial, anti-fungal, ichtyotoxic) are reported from sea cucumbers, including their anti-fouling properties [38,68]. The AF potential was found to be species specific, and saponins were identified as the main bioactive molecules responsible for these activities [69].

This study demonstrated that the AF properties of the crude extracts of nine sea cucumber species were related to the presence of particular chemical compounds. Our results showed a clear dose-effect for the genus *Actinopyga* and *Bohadschia*, with minimal growth and settlement inhibition at the lowest concentration. Only two of the four tested *Holothuria* species (*H. atra* and *H. edulis*) inhibited algal growth and settlement at the highest concentration, whereas their lower doses (15 and 1.5 µg mL^{-1}) actually induced diatom growth, which is following the hormetic effects described by Stebbing ([70,71]; Figure 3). Similar patterns have been reported for crude extracts of *Holothuria leucospilota* against the diatoms *Nitzschia closterium* and *Navicola subinflata*, where lower concentrations (i.e., < 400 µg mL^{-1}) of *H. leucospilota* crude extract induced diatom settlement, and at higher concentrations (i.e., > 400 µg mL^{-1}) inhibited their growth [69].

Previous studies have shown that steroidal and triterpene glycosides in sponges, gorgonians, sea stars, sea urchins, and sea cucumbers are responsible for the observed anti-fouling activities [15,36,38,41,65,72,73]. Saponins have often been described from holothurians including their various biological activities [74]. For example, studies on *Holothuria glaberrima* [40], *H. atra* and *Holothuria nobilis* [38] showed that saponins were responsible for the observed anti-fouling activities. Also, Selvin and Lipton (2004), and Ozupeck and Cavas (2017) found that the saponin-enriched fraction of different sea cucumbers (i.e., *Holothuria scabra, Holothuria polii* and *Holothuria tubulosa*) had pronounced anti-fouling properties [41,75]. In this study, we demonstrated that the composition of saponins is more similar within species of the same genus. For example, the saponin compositions of the genus *Bohadschia* was rather different from the genus *Holothuria* and *Actinopyga* (Figure 4). These observations were in line with the strong AF effects of *B. argus* and *Bohadschia sp.* crude extracts (Figure 3). As apparent from our AF assays, not only *Bohadschia*, but also the genus *Actinopyga* showed much stronger activities compared to *H. atra* and *H. edulis* (Figure 3), which may be explained by significantly higher concentrations of total saponins (*cf.* Figure 6).

Looking at the saponin profile of the studied genera, we observed similar patterns as described by Kalinin and his colleagues (2015), that non-sulphated saponins with molecular weights of *m/z* 1426.698, and *m/z* 1410.703 were found in the highest intensity in the genus *Bohadschia* [76–78]. All these saponins contain six monosaccharide units in their glycone parts, and were present nearly 1–5-fold higher than the tetraosides (*m/z* 1118.551 and *m/z* 1102.556), which were present in the other sea cucumber species. Whereas, sulphated saponins (e.g., molecular weights of *m/z* 1206.510 and *m/z* 868.389), putatively annotated as *echinoside A* and *echinoside B* respectively, were observed only in the two genera of *Actinopyga* and *Holothuria*. This is in accordance with the results from Kitagawa and colleagues (1981; 1989), and Grauso and colleagues (2019), who reported *echinoside A* and *B* from *Holothuria* (i.e., *H. atra*; [79]), and *Actinopyga* species [80]. *Actinopyga* and *Holothuria* extracts also contained mixtures of biosides including *bivittoside A* like compounds ($C_{41}H_{66}O_{12}$; *m/z* 750.455), tetraosides such as the saponin *desholothurin A* ($C_{54}H_{86}O_{24}$; *m/z* 1118.551) and *pervicoside B* ($C_{54}H_{86}O_{22}$; *m/z* 1086.561). Our data indicated that the AF activity may correlate with the amount and/or type of sugar units in their glycone part (in genus *Bohadschia*). A similar result has been observed by Van Dyck and colleagues (2010), who analyzed the saponin profile of *Holothuria forskali* in undisturbed and under predator stress conditions [43]. In the undisturbed state, the body wall of *H. forskali* produced mainly tetraosides (i.e., *holothurinoside C* (*m/z* 1102) and *desholothurin A* (*m/z* 1118)), while under stressed conditions *holothurinoside C* was converted to the hexaosides *holothurinoside F* (*m/z* 1410) and *holothurinoside H* (*m/z* 1440) and *desholothurin A* was converted to the hexaosides *holothurinoside G* (*m/z* 1426). However, Van Dyck and colleagues (2010) also pointed out that *m/z* 1426 is produced under both environmental states in the tested sea cucumber, suggesting that *m/z* 1426 is a "background prevention signal," and other molecules might play more important roles under stressful conditions [81]. Also, Kalinin and colleagues (2015) described a molecule with the same molecular mass, but different side chain (*m/z* 1426) as a characteristic saponin of *Bohadschia*, which was identified as "*bivittoside D*." A remarkable similarity observed between *H. forskali* and genus *Bohadschia* is the presence of chemically defended CTs (*cf.* Figure 1), each containing different saponin mixtures [43,82].

The mechanism of action of many extracted and isolated molecules with anti-fouling effects are usually unclear because of multiple possible interactions involved [83]. As mentioned earlier, saponins are amphiphilic molecules with hydrophilic and hydrophobic properties. The amount of monosaccharides attached on the C-3 position (Figure 2) of the steroid affects the hydrophilicity of the saponin molecule, which can affect the permeability of the cell membranes by inducing curvature and forming pores in the membrane [84]. Therefore, high integration values of hexaosidic saponins, containing lanosterol as the major sterol within the genus *Bohadschia* [85], may explain their strong AF activities [81].

It can be concluded that the AF activity is species-specific in sea cucumbers and related to not only total saponin concentration (e.g., in *Actinopyga*), but also saponin composition (such as shown in *B. argus*). AF activities of the studied crude extracts showed that *B. argus* contained compounds affecting fouling by the diatom *C. closterium*. Consequently, purified fractions and pure compounds of *B. argus* (Figure 7) confirmed that particular saponin compounds (here *m/z* 1426.698) had strong inhibitory effects on growth and settlement of the diatom *C. closterium*. Furthermore, the here performed anti-fouling assays can be a promising and fast method for identifying compounds with anti-fouling activity and for pre-selecting bioactive extracts and/or compound from various organism to discover ecologically and potentially pharmaceutically active natural products.

4. Materials and Methods

In this study we investigated nine holothurian species from the family Holothuriidae that were collected from Guam in 2016. These nine species were members of three different genera, *Holothuria* (*H. whitmaei*, *H. hilla*, *H. atra*, *H. edulis*), *Bohadschia* (*B. argus*, *B. vittiensis*, *Bohadschia* sp.) and *Actinopyga* (*A. echinites*, *A. mauritiana*; Figure 2).

4.1. Experimental Setup

4.1.1. Cylindrotheca Closterium Culture

The AF assays were conducted using the diatom species *C. closterium* as the test organism. The diatom cultures were kept in climate chamber with constant temperature of 18 °C with a light and dark cycle of 12 h and a light intensity of 90 µmol m^{-2} s^{-1}. The initial stock culture (strain number CCAP-1017/8) was obtained from Culture Collection of Algae and Protozoa (CCAP), and was prepared in 250 mL polystyrene culture flasks, filled with sterile artificial seawater enriched with F/2 nutrients, which has shown to be an optimal nutrient supply for this algal species [86,87].

4.1.2. Preparation of Sea Cucumber Crude Extracts

Extractions of sea cucumbers were performed by freeze dried material. For each extraction a 1:10 ratio (w/v) of freeze-dried sea cucumber tissue (in g) and organic solvent mixture (in mL) was used. In brief, the ground tissue samples were extracted twice with a 1:1 mixture (v/v) of methanol (MeOH) and ethyl acetate (EtOAc) and a third and final time with 100% MeOH. Samples were shaken for at least 3 h during each subsequent extraction. After filtering through filter paper (Diameter: 150 mm, Grade: 3 hw, Sartorius GmbH, 37979, Goettingen, Germany), extracts were dried by rotary evaporation (Rotavapor RII, BUCHI, Flawil, Switzerland) and finally transferred and dried using a centrifugal vacuum concentrator (Speedvac, Christ RVC 2–25 Co plus; Freeze dryer: Christ Alpha 2–4 LD plus). The dried crude extracts were weighted and stored at −20 °C until further usage.

4.1.3. Anti-Fouling Assay: Experimental Design

The effect of the sea cucumber crude extracts on the growth and settlement behavior of *C. closterium* was tested by monitoring the biomass of the diatom after 24 and 72 h incubation, based on chlorophyll a (*Chl a*) concentration of suspended cells in the water as well as attached cells on the flask surface. The AF assays were performed in 40 mL culture flasks (TC Flask T25, SARSTEDT AG & Co. KG, 51588, Nümbrecht, Germany). All crude extracts were dissolved in MeOH and added in triplicates to empty the cell culture flasks in order to obtain three different final concentrations of the crude extracts (150, 15 and 1.5 µg mL^{-1}, Figure 8). After the MeOH evaporated, 10% of the diatom stock (i.e., 1.5 mL of algae inoculated in 15 mL F/2 medium; OD$_{442}$ = 0.46 ± 0.01) was inoculated to the culture flask pre-filled with 18 mL of sterile artificial seawater. For three days, the flasks were stored horizontally in a growth chamber under the above-mentioned culturing conditions (Section 4.1.1) to perform the diatom surface attachment experiment. Treatments with only MeOH and no sea cucumber crude extract served as control experiment.

The potential AF effects of particular saponin species were assessed using fractions isolated from *B. argus*. The assay with the purified saponin fraction and pure saponin compounds were conducted with only the lowest concentrations of 1.5 µg mL^{-1}.

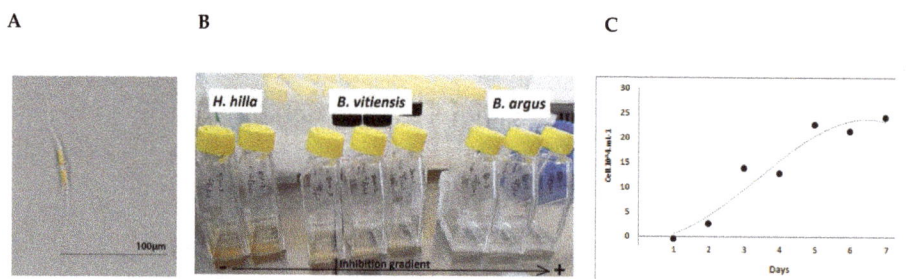

Figure 8. (A–C). The test organism *C. closterium* under the microscope (**A**), culture flasks demonstrating high growth rates (left, not-inhibited), medium growth rates (middle) and low growth rates (inhibited) of *C. closterium* (**B**), growth curve of *C. closterium* in 7 days in the stock solution (**C**).

4.1.4. Diatom Growth and Settlement Analyses

Chlorophyll a measurements: To assess diatom biomass, *Chl a* was extracted from the water samples after 24 and 72 h of inoculation. Furthermore, to study the attachment behavior of the diatom, the *Chl a* content of *C. closterium* attached to the substrate was extracted after 72 h (end of the experiment), except for the highest concentration. Since we observed that algae biomass was dramatically reduced in most of the extracts exposed to the highest extract concentration (150 µg mL^{-1}), Chl a concentrations in both, suspended in water and attached to substrate, were measured only after 24 h of inoculation. Experimental procedure included filtering water samples through a combusted and acid-washed glass microfiber filter (GF/C, Whatman, GE Healthcare life sciences, Pittsburg, PA 15264-3065, USA) and storing at −80 °C until extraction. For extraction, ethanol (90%) was added to the samples, vortexed, and then placed in an ultrasonic bath filled with ice for 30 min. Before measuring pigment concentrations, all samples were stored for 24 h at 4 °C. Measurements were conducted with a microplate reader (BioTek, SYNERGY H1, Winooski, VT, USA) to determine the Chl a concentration using a fluorescence excitation (Ex) wavelength of 395 nm and emission (Em) wavelength of 680 nm. Chl a concentrations were obtained by converting fluorescence data to concentrations using a Chl a standard from *Anacystis nidulans* algae (Product Number C 6144, Sigma-Aldrich, St. Louis, MO, USA).

4.1.5. Anti-Fouling Effects: Data and Statistical Analyses

Statistical analyses were performed with R (version 1.1.423, R Foundation for Statistical Computing, Vienna, Austria), and SPSS (Version 26, IBM, NY 10504, USA). We assessed the effect of different sea cucumber extracts and concentrations on diatom settlement, as well as cell density of the diatom *C. closterium*. After testing for normality and homoscedastity, Kruskal-Wallis test was conducted for each extract concentration, followed by Kruskal–Wallis post hoc test. The same method was applied for the purified fractions and pure compounds (Section 4.3). Differences were considered significant at a 95% confidence level. The logarithmic response ration (LRR; Equation (1)) was calculated as the ratio of Chl a concentration affected by crude extracts to the controls. LRR > 0 illustrates higher Chl a concentration and thus a positive effect in extract treatments, while LRR < 0 identifies decreased Chl a concentrations, and thus a negative effect compared to control samples.

$$LRR = Ln\left(\frac{treatment}{control}\right) \qquad (1)$$

4.2. Saponins as Potential Bioactive Compounds Affecting the Fouling Organism C. closterium

4.2.1. Dereplication of Saponins

To analyze the content of the most abundant saponin species within the different sea cucumber crude extracts (dissolved in MeOH), an aliquot was analyzed using ultra performance liquid chromatography-high resolution mass spectrometry (UPLC-HRMS; Tables S2 and S3). Chromatographic separation was achieved on a Waters Acquity BEH C_{18} column (1.7 µm, 2.1 mm × 50 mm) with an ACQUITY ultra performance liquid chromatography (UPLC) H-Class System (Waters Co., Milford, MA, USA) coupled to a Synapt G2-Si HDMS high-resolution Q-ToF-MS (Waters Co., Manchester, UK) equipped with a LockSpray dual electrospray ion source operated in positive (POS) ionization modes. The Q-ToF-MS was calibrated in resolution mode over a mass-to-charge (m/z) ranging from 50 to 2000 Dalton by using a 0.5 mmol L^{-1} sodium formate solution. For each run leucine enkephalin was used as the lock mass, generating a reference ion for POS mode ([m/z 556.277 M + H]$^+$) to ensure a mass tolerance for all LC-MS or LC-MS/MS experiments of less than one ppm. Mass spectral data were collected using the MS^e data acquisition function to simultaneously obtain information on the intact molecule (no collision energy applied) as well as their fragmentation data (collision energy ramp reaching from 15 to 75 eV). Analytes were eluted at a flow rate of 0.6 mL min^{-1} using a linear gradient of milliQ water (H_2O, 100%, eluent A) to acetonitrile (ACN, 100%, eluent B) both with 0.1% formic acid. The initial condition was 100% A held for 0.5 min, followed by a linear gradient to 100% B in 19 min. The column was then washed with 100% B for 9.5 min and subsequently returned and held for 2.9 min to the initial conditions (100% eluent A) to equilibrate the column for the following run. The column temperature was set to 40 °C.

Data treatment: To identify different saponin compounds in the holothurian extracts we compared the molecular masses of known saponins to the here-analyzed mass data (MS[1]) and by confirmation the saponin nature (Figure 1) by identifying their diagnostic key fragments. Therefore, we used different diagnostic key fragments corresponding to oligosaccharides residues [88], and the sapogenin molecule (aglycone) part (Table 1). Unknown saponin molecules (with different molecular formulas than previously reported) were not considered in this analysis. Given that we identified several saponins with the same exact mass (probably isomers), we retained the following information for compound identification: (1) retention time (RT), (2) molecular weight and (3) the integrated area of the respective peak (Table S3).

Table 1. Key diagnostic fragments of saponins detected via the MS/MS analysis of the studied sea cucumbers.

Diagnostic Ions	Reported Exact Mass (m/z)	Molecular Formula	Organism	References
Sapogenin	472.3552	$C_{30}H_{48}O_4$	*B. vitiensis*	[89]
Sapogenin 1	482.3032	$C_{30}H_{42}O_5$	Octacoral (*Anthomastus bathyproctus*)	[90]
Sapogenin 3	457.3318	$C_{29}H_{45}O_4$	Gorgonian (*Eunicella cavolini*)	[91]
Caudinoside A	468.3239	$C_{30}H_{44}O_4$	*Paracaudina ransonetii*	[92]
Stichopogenin A4	486.3345	$C_{30}H_{46}O_5$	*Stichopus japonicus*	[93]
16 Keto holothurinogenin	484.3189	$C_{30}H_{44}O_5$	*A. mauritiana*	[94,95]
MeGlc-Glc-Qui + Na+	507.164	$C_{19}H_{32}O_{14}Na^+$	*H. lesson, H. forskali*	[96,97]

4.2.2. Saponin Compounds Composition: Data and Statistical Analyses

The integrated areas have been log transformed to reduce the skewness. Principal component analysis (PCA) was used to evaluate the differences between saponin compositions of the studied sea cucumbers. In order to identify the saponin similarity among different sea cucumber species, a hierarchical cluster analysis (function *hclust*, using packages ape for R) was used. After choosing the best cluster method using cophenetic correlation distances (pearson correlation), the penalty function of Kelley Gardner Sutcliffe (*KGS*; package maptree in R) was used to trim the dendrogram. Compounds with integration values higher than 10,000 were then selected to further study the saponin composition of each of the sea cucumber species.

4.2.3. Total Saponin Concentration within the Examined Sea Cucumber Species

Since only known saponins could be identified by the LC-MS/MS data, we also quantified total saponin concentration of different sea cucumbers using a spectrophotometric method with vanillin-sulfuric acid, which was adapted after Hiai and colleagues [98]. Based on their method, sulfuric acid oxidizes saponins and transformes glycone chains to furfural. The free hydroxyl group at the C-3 position of the agylcone part reacts with vanillin and produces a distinctive yellow-brown color [41]. According to this methodology, we prepared 8% vanillin solution (w/v) dissolved in ethanol (analytical grade), and sulfuric acid 72% (v/v) dissolved in distilled water. Crude extracts as well as double distilled water (used as blanks), were mixed with vanillin (8%; AppliChem GmbH, Germany) and sulfuric acid (72%) in a 1:1:10 (v/v/v) proportion in an ice bath. Next, we incubated the obtained solution at 60 °C in a water bath for 10 min. To stop the reaction, samples were cooled down on ice. A standard curve was measured, using a concentration gradient of Quillaja bark saponin (AppliChem GmbH, 64291, Darmstadt, Germany), diluted in distilled water. Finally, the absorbance was measured at 540 nm using a microplate reader.

4.3. Anti-Fouling Effects of Purified Saponin Fractions

We further fractionated the crude extract of *B. argus*, since it had exhibited one of the highest AF activity among the tested organic extracts. The aim was the identification of one or multiple saponin compounds responsible for the anti-fouling activity observed in the crude extract.

4.4. Sample Fractionation and Purification

Liquid/liquid partitioning: The crude extracts of *B. argus* were first partitioned using (1) EtOAc:H_2O (1:1) followed by partitioning of the H_2O fraction with (2) n-BuOH:H_2O (1:1).

Solid Phase Extraction (SPE) chromatography: The BuOH fraction which contained the saponins was further fractionated by SPE chromatography [99]. Therefore, the SPE column (SUPELCLEAN LC_{18}, 60 mL/10 g; Supleco Park, USA) was desalted/washed with 60 mL MeOH and preconditioned with 120 mL distilled water. Then, the concentrated BuOH fraction was added to the column and washed with five elution gradients: (1) Elution with H_2O (Fraction A, 120 mL), (2) MeOH:H_2O (Fraction B, 50:50, 180 mL), (3) ACN: H_2O (Fraction C, 70:30, 180 mL), (4) ACN 100% (Fraction D, 180 mL) and (5) CH_2Cl_2: MeOH (fraction E, 90:10, 180 mL; Figure 9).

Preparative HPLC: Preliminary biological and chemical screening of each SPE fraction showed that fractions B (MeOH:H_2O 50:50) and C (CH_3CN:H_2O 70:30) contained not only diverse and high amounts of saponins, they also had high activities against the fungi *Rhodotorula glutinis* and *Candida albicans* (unpublished data). Therefore, these fractions were selected for further purification by semi-preparative HPLC (Agilent Technologies, 1260 Infinity) with a PDA detector (Agilent, G4212-60008, CA, USA). Chromatographic separation was achieved using a C_{18} column (Pursuit XRs 5 µm, 250 mm × 10 mm, Agilent, CA, USA) with a pre-column (2.7 µm, 2.1 mm × 5 mm, Agilent, CA, USA) and applying a linear gradient: initial 50% A/50% B, 0–4 min 50% A/50% B; 4–36 min 38% A/62% B; 36–39 min 100% B, and a column reconditioning phase for 39–59 min 100% B, and 8 min to 50% A/50% B. (flow rate 1.5 mL min^{-1}; eluent **A:** 95% H_2O and 0.1% of formic acid 98% (Roth); eluent **B:** ACN and 0.1% formic acid). Several fractions were collected by peak picking at specific retention times. In order to determine the saponin composition of the obtained fractions and pure compounds, the fractions and compounds were dissolved in HPLC-grade MeOH, filtered through a 0.2 µm syringe filter, and injected into the HPLC-DAD-MS system, as previously described in Section 4.2.1. The peak integration of saponins in the final fractions has been assessed (Table S4), and these fractions have been used for AF assay.

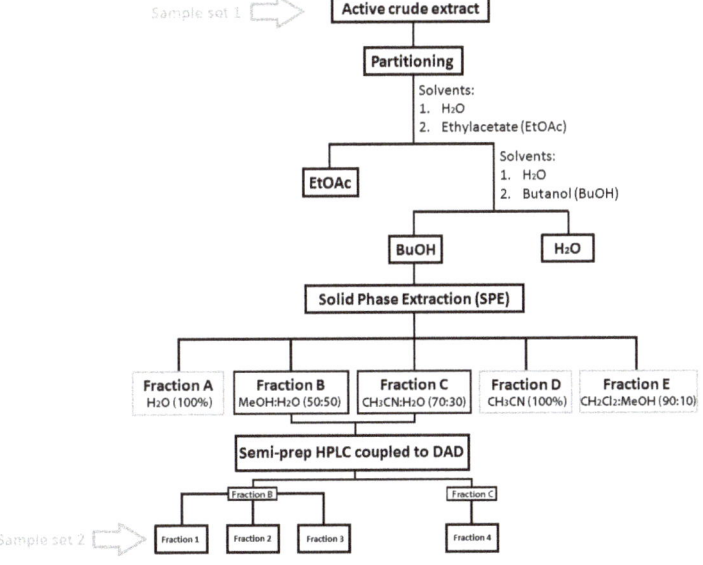

Figure 9. Flow chart showing the applied procedure for isolating the bioactive saponin compounds (Cutignano et al., 2015; Ebada et al., 2008 [99,100]). Sample set 1 and 2 refers to the samples that were tested for anti-fouling (AF) activity in this study.

Supplementary Materials: Figure S1A–F: *Chl a* concentrations in the suspended cells in the water after incubation of *C. closterium* with different concentrations of sea cucumbers extracts (A = 150 µg mL^{-1}; C = 15 µg mL^{-1}; E = 1.5 µg mL^{-1}) and of *C. closterium* attached to the flask surface (B = 150 µg mL^{-1}; D = 15 µg mL^{-1}; F = 1.5 µg mL^{-1}). Dashed lines separate different genera of sea cucumbers (*Holothuria, Bohadschia, Actinopyga*). CT = Control. (a–e) indicate significance levels according to post hoc test. Figure S2: LC/MS spectra of the crude extracts of genus *Holothuria* (Y-axis relative intensity in % of maximum peak, x-axis retention time in minutes). Figure S3: LC/MS spectra of the crude extracts of genus *Bohadschia* (Y-axis relative intensity in % of maximum peak, x-axis retention time in minutes). Figure S4: LC/MS spectra of the crude extracts of genus *Actinopyga* (Y-axis relative intensity in % of maximum peak, x-axis retention time in minutes). Figure S5: LC/MS spectra of fractions isolated from *B. argus* (see Table S4; Y-axis relative intensity in % of maximum peak, x-axis retention time in minutes). Figure S6: Identified saponins species presented in different fractions isolated from *B. argus*. The red color referred to the presence of a semi-purified saponin species (bivittoside D-like at *m/z* 1426.698). Size of bubbles represented the peak area of the molecules obtained from LC/MS analysis. Table S1. Significant differences (reported as *p-values*) of sea cucumber crude extracts compared to control experiments using the Kruskal–Wallis test. Table S2: Saponins reported, and found in studied species. Table S3: Exact mass (*m/z*), molecular formula, retention time (RT), and intensity signal (IntSig) of saponins, and sapogenins (aglycone parts) presented in the three sea cucumber genera *Holothuria, Bohadschia* and *Actinopyga*. Table S4: Exact mass (*m/z*), molecular formula, retention time (RT in minutes) and intensity signal of saponins presented in isolated fractions of *B. argus*.

Author Contributions: E.K., M.Y.K., M.S., S.R., and P.J.S. conceived and designed the experiments; E.K., N.G., M.Y.K. performed the experiments; E.K., N.G., M.S., M.Y.K., M.R., S.R. analyzed the data; E.K., M.Y.K., M.R., M.S., P.J.S. wrote the paper; E.K., N.G., M.Y.K., S.R., M.R., M.S., P.J.S. reviewed and edited the paper. All authors have read and agreed to the published version of the manuscript.

Funding: The authors acknowledge funding by the Federal Ministry of Education and Research (BMBF) via the Germany-Indonesia Anti-infective Cooperation (GINAICO) grant number 16GW0106 and Deutsche Forschungsgemeinschaft (DFG) funding INST 1841147.1FUGG for the high-resolution mass spectrometer Waters Synapt G2-Si.

Acknowledgments: We would like to thank Sabine Flöder and Christian Spindler for their support in phytoplankton cultivation and media preparation, also Pedro Martinez Arbizu for his advices in developing the R codes. The authors acknowledge funding by the BMBF via the GINAICO grant (16GW0106) and DFG funding (INST 1841147.1FUGG). We also thank anonymous reviewers for valuable comments, and their time which helped to improve the manuscript.

Conflicts of Interest: The authors declare no conflict of interest.

References

1. Briand, J.F. Marine antifouling laboratory bioassays: An overview of their diversity. *Biofouling* **2009**, *25*, 297–311. [CrossRef] [PubMed]
2. Railkin, A. *Marine biofouling: Colonization processes and defenses*; CSC Press: Boca Raton, FL, USA, 2004.
3. McKenzie, J.D.; Grigolava, I.V. The echinoderm surface and its role in preventing microfouling. *Biofouling* **1996**, *10*, 261–272. [CrossRef] [PubMed]
4. Wahl, M. Marine epibiosis.I. fouling and antifouling: Some basice aspects. *Mar. Ecol. Prog. Ser.* **1989**, *58*, 175–189. [CrossRef]
5. Davis, A.R.; Targett, N.M.; McConnell, O.J.; Young, C.M. *Epibiosis of Marine Algae and Benthic Invertebrates: Natural Products Chemistry and Other Mechanisms Inhibiting Settlement and Overgrowth*; Scheuer, P.J., Ed.; Bioorganic; Springer: Berlin/Heidelberg, Germany, 1989; Vol. 3.
6. Rohde, S.; Hiebenthal, C.; Wahl, M.; Karez, R.; Bischof, K. Decreased depth distribution of *Fucus vesiculosus* (Phaeophyceae) in the Western Baltic: Effects of light deficiency and epibionts on growth and photosynthesis. *Eur. J. Phycol.* **2008**, *43*, 143–150. [CrossRef]
7. Yebra, D.M.; Kiil, S.; Dam-Johansen, K. Antifouling technology—Past, present and future steps towards efficient and environmentally friendly antifouling coatings. *Prog. Org. Coatings* **2004**, *50*, 75–104. [CrossRef]
8. Amara, I.; Miled, W.; Slama, R.B.; Ladhari, N. Antifouling processes and toxicity effects of antifouling paints on marine environment. A review. *Environ. Toxicol. Pharmacol.* **2018**, *57*, 115–130. [CrossRef]
9. Puentes, C.; Carreño, K.; Santos-Acevedo, M.; Gómez-León, J.; García, M.; Pérez, M.; Stupak, M.; Blustein, G. Anti-fouling paints based on extracts of marine organisms from the colombian varibbean. *Sh. Sci. Technol.* **2014**, *8*, 75–90.
10. Alzieu, C.; Sanjuan, J.; Michel, P.; Borel, M.; Dreno, J.P. Monitoring and assessement of butyltins in Atlantic coastal waters. *Mar. Pollut. Bull.* **1989**, *20*, 22–26. [CrossRef]

11. Ellis, D.V. New dangerous chemicals in the environment: Lessons from TBT. *Mar. Pollut. Bull.* **1991**, *22*, 8–10. [CrossRef]
12. Tsukamoto, S.; Kato, H.; Hirota, H.; Fusetani, N. Antifouling terpenes and steroids against barnacle larvae from marine sponges. *Biofouling* **1997**, *11*, 283–291. [CrossRef]
13. Champ, M.A. The status of the treaty to ban TBT in marine antifouling paints and alternatives. In Proceedings of the 24th UJNR (US/Japan) Marine Facilities Panel Meeting, Honolulu, HI, USA, 7–8 November 2001; pp. 1–7.
14. Singh, P.; Cameotra, S.S. Potential applications of microbial surfactants in biomedical sciences. *Trends Biotechnol.* **2004**, *22*, 142–146. [CrossRef] [PubMed]
15. Qi, S.H.; Zhang, S.; Yang, L.H.; Qian, P.Y. Antifouling and antibacterial compounds from the gorgonians *Subergorgia suberosa* and *Scripearia gracillis*. *Nat. Prod. Res.* **2008**, *22*, 154–166. [CrossRef] [PubMed]
16. Armstrong, E.; Boyd, K.G.; Pisacane, A.; Peppiatt, C.J.; Burgess, J.G. Marine microbial natural products in antifouling coatings. *Biofouling* **2000**, *16*, 215–224. [CrossRef]
17. Dusane, D.H.; Pawar, V.S.; Nancharaiah, Y.V.; Venugopalan, V.P.; Kumar, A.R.; Zinjarde, S.S. Anti-biofilm potential of a glycolipid surfactant produced by a tropical marine strain of *Serratia marcescens*. *Biofouling* **2011**, *27*, 645–654. [CrossRef] [PubMed]
18. Tello, E.; Castellanos, L.; Arevalo-Ferro, C.; Rodríguez, J.; Jiménez, C.; Duque, C. Absolute stereochemistry of antifouling cembranoid epimers at C-8 from the Caribbean octocoral *Pseudoplexaura flagellosa*. Revised structures of plexaurolones. *Tetrahedron* **2011**, *67*, 9112–9121. [CrossRef]
19. Salta, M.; Wharton, J.A.; Stoodley, P.; Dennington, S.P.; Goodes, L.R.; Werwinski, S.; Mart, U.; Wood, R.J.K.; Stokes, K.R. Designing biomimetic antifouling surfaces. *Philos. Trans. R. Soc. A Math. Phys. Eng. Sci.* **2010**, *368*, 4729–4754. [CrossRef]
20. Jadhav, S.; Shah, R.; Bhave, M.; Palombo, E.A. Inhibitory activity of yarrow essential oil on Listeria planktonic cells and biofilms. *Food Control* **2013**, *29*, 125–130. [CrossRef]
21. Majik, M.; Parvatkar, P. Next Generation Biofilm Inhibitors for *Pseudomonas aeruginosa*: Synthesis and Rational Design Approaches. *Curr. Top. Med. Chem.* **2014**, *14*, 81–109. [CrossRef]
22. Okino, T.; Yoshimura, E.; Hirota, H.; Fusetani, N. New antifouling kalihipyrans from the marine sponge *Acanthella cavernosa*. *J. Nat. Prod.* **1996**, *59*, 1081–1083. [CrossRef]
23. Bryan, P.J.; Mcclintock, J.B.; Hopkins, T.S. Structural and chemical defenses of echinoderms from the northern Gulf of Mexico. *Exp. Mar. Biol. Ecol.* **1997**, *210*, 173–186. [CrossRef]
24. Wright, A.D.; McCluskey, A.; Robertson, M.J.; MacGregor, K.A.; Gordon, C.P.; Guenther, J. Anti-malarial, anti-algal, anti-tubercular, anti-bacterial, anti-photosynthetic, and anti-fouling activity of diterpene and diterpene isonitriles from the tropical marine sponge *Cymbastela hooperi*. *Org. Biomol. Chem.* **2011**, *9*, 400–407. [CrossRef] [PubMed]
25. Canicattí, C.; D'Ancona, G. Biological protective substances in Marthasterias glacialis (Asteroidea) epidermal secretion. *J. Zool.* **1990**, *222*, 445–454. [CrossRef]
26. Pawlik, J.R. Marine Invertebrate Chemical Defenses. *Chem. Rev.* **1993**, *93*, 1911–1922. [CrossRef]
27. Key, M.M.; Jeffries, W.B.; Voris, H.K. Epizoic bryozoans, sea snakes, and other nektonic substrates. *Bull. Mar. Sci.* **1995**, *56*, 462–474.
28. Krupp, D.A. An immunochemical study of the mucus from the solitary coral *Fungia scutaria* (Scleractinia, Fungiidae). *Bull. Mar. Sci.* **1985**, *36*, 163–176.
29. Wahl, M.; Kröger, K.; Lenz, M. Non-toxic protection against epibiosis. *Biofouling* **1998**, *12*, 205–226. [CrossRef]
30. Fusetani, N. Biofouling and antifouling. *Nat. Prod. Rep.* **2004**, *21*, 94–104. [CrossRef]
31. Qian, P.Y.; Xu, Y.; Fusetani, N. Natural products as antifouling compounds: Recent progress and future perspectives. *Biofouling* **2010**, *26*, 223–234. [CrossRef]
32. Faulkner, D.J. Marine Natural Products. *Nat. Prod. Chem. Biol.* **1994**, *11*, 355–394. [CrossRef]
33. Ortlepp, S.; Sjögren, M.; Dahlström, M.; Weber, H.; Ebel, R.; Edrada, R.A.; Thoms, C.; Schupp, P.; Bohlin, L.; Proksch, P. Antifouling activity of bromotyrosine-derived sponge metabolites and synthetic analogues. *Mar. Biotechnol.* **2007**, *9*, 776–785. [CrossRef] [PubMed]
34. Kjelleberg, S.; Steinberg, P.; Givskov, M.; Gram, L.; Manefield, M.; De Nys, R. Do marine natural products interfere with prokaryotic AHL regulatory systems? *Aquat. Microb. Ecol.* **1997**, *13*, 85–93. [CrossRef]
35. Qi, S.H.; Ma, X. Antifouling compounds from marine invertebrates. *Mar. Drugs* **2017**, *15*, 263.

36. De Marino, S.; Iorizzi, M.; Zollo, F.; Amsler, C.D.; Greer, S.P.; McClintock, J.B. Three new asterosaponins from the starfish *Goniopecten demonstrans*. *European J. Org. Chem.* **2000**, *2000*, 4093–4098. [CrossRef]
37. Dobretsov, S.; Al-Mammari, I.M.; Soussi, B. Bioactive Compounds from Omani Sea Cucumbers. *Agric. Mar. Sci.* **2009**, *14*, 49–53. [CrossRef]
38. Soliman, Y.A.; Ibrahim, A.M.; Tadros, H.R.Z.; Abou-Taleb, E.A.; Moustafa, A.H.; Hamed, M.A. Antifouling and antibacterial activities of marine bioactive compounds extracted from some Red Sea sea cucumber. *Int. J. Contemp. Appl. Sci.* **2016**, *3*, 83–103.
39. Dobretsov, S.; Teplitski, M.; Paul, V. Mini-review: Quorum sensing in the marine environment and its relationship to biofouling. *Biofouling* **2009**, *25*, 413–427. [CrossRef]
40. Acevedo, M.S.; Puentes, C.; Carreño, K.; León, J.G.; Stupak, M.; García, M.; Pérez, M.; Blustein, G. Antifouling paints based on marine natural products from Colombian Caribbean. *Int. Biodeterior. Biodegrad.* **2013**, *83*, 97–104. [CrossRef]
41. Ozupek, N.M.; Cavas, L. Triterpene glycosides associated antifouling activity from *Holothuria tubulosa* and *Holothuria polii*. *Reg. Stud. Mar. Sci.* **2017**, *13*, 32–41. [CrossRef]
42. Kamyab, E.; Kellermann, M.Y.; Kunzmann, A.; Schupp, P.J. Chemical Biodiversity and Bioactivities of Saponins in Echinodermata with an Emphasis on Sea Cucumbers (Holothuroidea). In *YOUMARES 9-The Oceans: Our Research, Our Future*; Jungblut, S., Liebich, V., Bode-Dalby, M., Eds.; Springer: Cham, Switzerland, 2020; pp. 121–157.
43. Van Dyck, S.; Flammang, P.; Meriaux, C.; Bonnel, D.; Salzet, M.; Fournier, I.; Wisztorski, M. Localization of secondary metabolites in marine invertebrates: Contribution of MALDI MSI for the study of saponins in Cuvierian tubules of *H. forskali*. *PLoS ONE* **2010**, *5*, e13923. [CrossRef]
44. Popov, A.M. A comparative study of the hemolytic and cytotoxic activities of triterpenoids isolated from ginseng and sea cucumbers. *Biol. Bull.* **2002**, *29*, 120–128. [CrossRef]
45. Van Dyck, S.; Gerbaux, P.; Flammang, P. Qualitative and quantitative saponin contents in five sea cucumbers from the Indian ocean. *Mar. Drugs* **2010**, *8*, 173–189. [CrossRef] [PubMed]
46. Kingston, M.B. Growth and motility of the diatom *Cylindrotheca closterium*: Implications for commercial applications. *J. North Carolina Acad. Sci.* **2009**, *125*, 138–142.
47. Tanaka, N. The cell division rates of ten species of attaching diatoms in natural seawater. *Bull. Japanese Soc. Sci. Fish.* **1984**, *50*, 969–972. [CrossRef]
48. Aslam, S.N.; Strauss, J.; Thomas, D.N.; Mock, T.; Underwood, G.J.C. Identifying metabolic pathways for production of extracellular polymeric substances by the diatom *Fragilariopsis cylindrus* inhabiting sea ice. *ISME J.* **2018**, *12*, 1237–1251. [CrossRef]
49. Decho, A.W. Microbial exopolymer secretions in ocean environments: Their role(s) in food webs and marine processes. *Ocean. Mar. Biol. Annu. Rev.* **1990**, *28*, 73–153.
50. Stal, L.J.; Défarge, C. Structure and dynamics of exopolymers in an intertidal diatom biofilm. *Geomicrobiol. J.* **2005**, *22*, 341–352. [CrossRef]
51. Wimpenny, J.; Manz, W.; Szewzyk, U. Heterogeneity in biofilms. *FEMS Microbiol. Rev.* **2000**, *24*, 661–671. [CrossRef]
52. Apoya-Horton, M.D.; Yin, L.; Underwood, G.J.C.; Gretz, M.R. Movement modalities and responses to environmental changes of the mudflat diatom *Cylindrotheca closterium* (Bacillariophyceae). *J. Phycol.* **2006**, *42*, 379–390. [CrossRef]
53. Roberts, R.D.; Kawamura, T.; Handley, C.M. Factors affecting settlement of abalone (*Haliotis Iris*) larvae on benthic diatom films. *J. Shellfish Res.* **2007**, *26*, 323–334. [CrossRef]
54. Gallardo, W.G.; Buen, S.M.A. Evaluation of mucus, Navicula, and mixed diatoms as larval settlement inducers for the tropical abalone Haliotis asinina. *Aquaculture* **2003**, *221*, 357–364. [CrossRef]
55. Hellio, C.; Berge, J.P.; Beaupoil, C.; Le Gal, Y.; Bourgougnon, N. Screening of marine algal extracts for anti-settlement activities against microalgae and macroalgae. *Biofouling* **2002**, *18*, 205–215. [CrossRef]
56. Kitagawa, I.; Kobayashi, M.; Hori, M.; Kyogoku, Y. Structures of four new triterpenoidal oligoglycosides, Bivittoside A, B, C, and D, from the sea cucumber *Bohadschia bivittata* MITSUKURI. *Chem. Pharm. Bull* **1981**, *29*, 282–285. [CrossRef]
57. Kerr, A.M.; Kim, J. Phylogeny of Holothuroidea (Echinodermata) inferred from morphology. *Zool. J. Linn. Soc.* **2001**, *133*, 63–81. [CrossRef]

58. Kamarudin, K.R.; Ridzwan, H.; Usup, G. Phylogeny of sea cucumber (Echinodermata: Holothuroidea) as inferred from 16s mitochondrial rRNA gene sequences. *Sains Malaysiana* **2010**, *39*, 209–218.
59. Wen, J.; Hu, C.; Zhang, L.; Fan, S. Genetic identification of global commercial sea cucumber species on the basis of mitochondrial DNA sequences. *Food Control* **2011**, *21*, 72–77. [CrossRef]
60. Miller, A.K.; Kerr, A.M.; Paulay, G.; Reich, M.; Wilson, N.G.; Carvajal, J.I.; Rouse, G.W. Molecular phylogeny of extant Holothuroidea (Echinodermata). *Mol. Phylogenet. Evol.* **2017**, *111*, 110–131. [CrossRef]
61. Antoine, D.; Andre, J.; Morel, A. Oceanic primary production 2. Estimation at global scale from satellite (coastal zone color scanner) chlorophyll. *Global Biogeochem. Cycles* **1996**, *10*, 57–69. [CrossRef]
62. Thrane, J.E.; Kyle, M.; Striebel, M.; Haande, S.; Grung, M.; Rohrlack, T.; Andersen, T. Spectrophotometric analysis of pigments: A critical assessment of a high-throughput method for analysis of algal pigment mixtures by spectral deconvolution. *PLoS ONE* **2015**, *10*. [CrossRef]
63. Gerhard, M.; Koussoroplis, A.M.; Hillebrand, H.; Striebel, M. Phytoplankton community responses to temperature fluctuations under different nutrient concentrations and stoichiometry. *Ecology* **2019**, *100*, e02834. [CrossRef]
64. Iorizzi, M.; Bryan, P.; McClintock, J.; Minale, L.; Palagiano, E.; Maurelli, S.; Riccio, R.; Zollo, F. Chemical and biological investigation of the polar constituents of the starfish *Luidia clathrata*, collected in the gulf of mexico. *J. Nat. Prod.* **1995**, *58*, 653–671. [CrossRef] [PubMed]
65. Kubanek, J.; Whalen, K.E.; Engel, S.; Kelly, S.R.; Henkel, T.P.; Fenical, W.; Pawlik, J.R. Multiple defensive roles for triterpene glycosides from two Caribbean sponges. *Oecologia* **2002**, *131*, 125–136. [CrossRef] [PubMed]
66. Bers, A.V.; D'Souza, F.; Klijnstra, J.W.; Willemsen, P.R.; Wahl, M. Chemical defence in mussels: Antifouling effect of crude extracts of the periostracum of the blue mussel *Mytilus edulis*. *Biofouling* **2006**, *22*, 251–259. [CrossRef] [PubMed]
67. Schwartz, N.; Dobretsov, S.; Rohde, S.; Schupp, P.J. Comparison of antifouling properties of native and invasive Sargassum (Fucales, Phaeophyceae) species. *Eur. J. Phycol.* **2017**, *52*, 116–131. [CrossRef]
68. Hellio, C.; De La Broise, D.; Dufossé, L.; Le Gal, Y.; Bourgougnon, N. Inhibition of marine bacteria by extracts of macroalgae: Potential use for environmentally friendly antifouling paints. *Mar. Environ. Res.* **2001**, *52*, 231–247. [CrossRef]
69. Gonsalves, C.O.L. Effect of holothurian and zoanthid extracts on growth of some bacterial and diatom species. *Indian J. Mar. Sci.* **1997**, *26*, 377–379.
70. Stebbing, A.R.D. Hormesis-The stimulation of growth by low levels of inhibitors. *Sci. Total Environ.* **1982**, *22*, 213–234. [CrossRef]
71. Stebbing, A.R.D. A theory for growth hormesis. *Mutat. Res. Mol. Mech. Mutagen.* **1998**, *403*, 249–258. [CrossRef]
72. Riccio, R.; Iorizzi, M.; Minale, L.; Oshima, Y.; Yasumoto, T. Starfish saponins. Part 34. Novel steroidal glycoside sulphates from the starfish *Asterias amurensis*. *J. Chem. Soc. Perkin Trans. 1* **1988**, *6*, 1337–1347. [CrossRef]
73. Haug, T.; Kjuul, A.K.; Styrvold, O.B.; Sandsdalen, E.; Olsen, Ø.M.; Stensvag, K. Antibacterial activity in *Strongylocentrotus droebachiensis* (Echinoidea), *Cucumaria frondosa* (Holothuroidea), and *Asterias rubens* (Asteroidea). *J. Invertebr. Pathol.* **2002**, *81*, 94–102. [CrossRef]
74. Lorent, J.H.; Quetin-Leclercq, J.; Mingeot-Leclercq, M.P. The amphiphilic nature of saponins and their effects on artificial and biological membranes and potential consequences for red blood and cancer cells. *Org. Biomol. Chem.* **2014**, *12*, 8803–8822. [CrossRef]
75. Selvin, J.; Lipton, A.P. Antifouling activity of bioactive substances extracted from *Holothuria scabra*. *Hydrobiologia* **2004**, *513*, 251–253. [CrossRef]
76. Kalinin, V.I.; Avilov, S.A.; Silchenko, A.S.; Stonik, V.A. Triterpene glycosides of sea cucumbers (Holothuroidea, Echinodermata) as Taxonomic Markers. *Nat. Prod. Commun.* **2015**, *10*, 21–26. [CrossRef] [PubMed]
77. Caulier, G.; Van Dyck, S.; Gerbaux, P.; Eeckhaut, I.; Flammang, P. Review of saponin diversity in sea cucumbers belonging to the family Holothuriidae. *SPC Beche-de-mer Inf. Bull.* **2011**, *31*, 48–54.
78. Kitagawa, I.; Kobayashi, M.; Hori, M.; Kyogoku, Y. Marine Natural Producs. XVIII. Four lanostane-type triterpene oligoglycosides, bivittosides A,B,C, and D from the Okinawan sea cucumber *Bohadschia bivittata* (Mitsukuri). *Chem. Pharm. Bull.* **1989**, *37*, 61–67. [CrossRef]

79. Grauso, L.; Yegdaneh, A.; Sharifi, M.; Mangoni, A.; Zolfaghari, B.; Lanzotti, V. Molecular networking-based analysis of cytotoxic saponins from sea cucumber *Holothuria atra*. *Mar. Drugs* **2019**, *17*, 86. [CrossRef] [PubMed]
80. Kitagawa, I.; Inamoto, T.; Fuchida, M.; Okada, S.; Kobayashi, M.; Nishino, T.; Kyoboku, Y. Structures of Echinoside A and B, two antifungal oligoglycosides from the sea cucumber *Actinopyga echinites* (JAEGER). *Chem. Pharm. Bull.* **1980**, *28*, 1651–1653. [CrossRef]
81. Van Dyck, S.; Caulier, G.; Todesco, M.; Gerbaux, P.; Fournier, I.; Wisztorski, M.; Flammang, P. The triterpene glycosides of *Holothuria forskali*: Usefulness and efficiency as a chemical defense mechanism against predatory fish. *J. Exp. Biol.* **2011**, *214*, 1347–1356. [CrossRef]
82. Honey-Escandón, M.; Arreguín-Espinosa, R.; Solís-Marín, F.A.; Samyn, Y. Biological and taxonomic perspective of triterpenoid glycosides of sea cucumbers of the family Holothuriidae (Echinodermata, Holothuroidea). *Comp. Biochem. Physiol. Part-B Biochem. Mol. Biol.* **2015**, *180*, 16–39. [CrossRef]
83. Olsen, S.M. Controlled release of environmentally friendly antifouling agents from marine coatings. Kgs. Lyngby, Denmark: Technical University of Denmark. 2009. Available online: https://backend.orbit.dtu.dk/ws/portalfiles/portal/5008364/Stefan+M%C3%B8ller+Olsen.pdf (accessed on 20 October 2019).
84. Lorent, J.; Le Duff, C.S.; Quetin-Leclercq, J.; Mingeot-Leclercq, M.P. Induction of highly curved structures in relation to membrane permeabilization and budding by the triterpenoid saponins, α- And δ-hederin. *J. Biol. Chem.* **2013**, *288*, 14000–14017. [CrossRef]
85. Kobayashi, M.; Hori, M.; Kan, K.; Yasuzawa, T.; Matsu, M.; Suzuki, S.; Kitagawa, I. Marine Natural Products. XXVII Distribution of Lanostane-type triterpene oligoglycosides in ten kind of Okinawan sea cucumbers. *Chem. Pharm. Bull.* **1991**, *39*, 2282–2287. [CrossRef]
86. Guillard, R.R.L. Culture of Phytoplankton for Feeding Marine Invertebrates. In *Culture of Marine Invertebrate Animals: Proceedings-1st Conference on Culture of Marine Invertebrate Animals Greenport*; Smith, W.L., Chanley, M.H., Eds.; Springer: Boston, MA, USA, 1975; pp. 29–60. ISBN 978-1-4615-8714-9.
87. Affan, A.; Heo, S.J.; Jeon, Y.J.; Lee, J.B. Optimal growth conditions and antioxidative activities of *Cylindrotheca closterium* (bacillariophyceae). *J. Phycol.* **2009**, *45*, 1405–1415. [CrossRef] [PubMed]
88. Bahrami, Y.; Zhang, W.; Franco, C. Discovery of novel saponins from the viscera of the sea cucumber *Holothuria lessoni*. *Mar. Drugs* **2014**, *12*, 2633–2667. [CrossRef] [PubMed]
89. Clastres, A.; Ahond, A.; Poupat, C.; Potier, P.; Intes, A. Marine invertebrates from New-Caledonian Lagoon. I. Structural study of a new sapogenin isolated from a sea-cucumber: *Bohadschia vitiensis* Semper. *Experientia* **1978**, *34*, 973–974. [CrossRef]
90. Mellado, G.G.; Zubía, E.; Ortega, M.J.; López-González, P.J. Steroids from the antarctic octocoral *Anthomastus bathyproctus*. *J. Nat. Prod.* **2005**, *68*, 1111–1115. [CrossRef]
91. Ioannou, E.; Abdel-Razik, A.F.; Alexi, X.; Vagias, C.; Alexis, M.N.; Roussis, V. 9,11-Secosterols with antiproliferative activity from the gorgonian *Eunicella cavolini*. *Bioorganic Med. Chem.* **2009**, *17*, 4537–4541. [CrossRef]
92. Kalinin, V.I.; Malyutin, A.N.; Stonik, V.A. Caudinoside A—A novel triterpene glycoside from the holothurian *Paracaudina ransonetii*. CA 105: 169209x. *Khim. Prir. Soedin* **1986**, 378–379.
93. Elyakov, G.B.; Kuznetsova, T.A.; Dzizenko, A.K.; Elkin, Y.N. A chemical investigation of the trepang (*Stichopus Japonicus* Selenka): The structure of triterpenoid aglycones obtained from trepang glycosides. *Tetrahedron Lett.* **1969**, *10*, 1151–1154. [CrossRef]
94. Bhatnagar, S.; Dudouet, B.; Ahond, A.; Poupat, C.; Thoison, O.; Clastres, A.; Laurent, D.; Potier, P. Invertebres marins du lagon Neocaledonien IV. Saponines et sapogenines d'une holothurie, *Actinopyga flammea*. *Bull. Soc. Chim. Fr.* **1985**, 124–129.
95. Radhika, P.; Anjaneyulu, V.; Subba Rao, P.V.; Makarieva, T.N.; Kalinovsky, A.I. Chemical examination of the echinoderms of Indian Ocean: The triterpene glycosides of the sea cucumbers: *Holothuria nobilis*, *Bohadschia aff. tenuissima* and *Actinopyga mauritana* from Lakshadweep, Andaman and Nicobar Islands. *Indian J. Chem.-Sect. B Org. Med. Chem.* **2002**, *41*, 1276–1282.
96. Bahrami, Y.; Zhang, W.; Chataway, T.; Franco, C. Structural elucidation of novel saponins in the sea cucumber *Holothuria lessoni*. *Mar. Drugs* **2014**, *12*, 4439–4473. [CrossRef]
97. Van Dyck, S.; Gerbaux, P.; Flammang, P. Elucidation of molecular diversity and body distribution of saponins in the sea cucumber *Holothuria forskali* (Echinodermata) by mass spectrometry. *Comp. Biochem. Physiol.-B* **2009**, *152*, 124–134. [CrossRef] [PubMed]

98. Hiai, S.; Oura, H.; T, N. Color Reaction of Some Sapogenins. *Planta Med.* **1976**, *29*, 116–122. [CrossRef] [PubMed]
99. Cutignano, A.; Nuzzo, G.; Ianora, A.; Luongo, E.; Romano, G.; Gallo, C.; Sansone, C.; Aprea, S.; Mancini, F.; D'Oro, U.; et al. Development and application of a novel SPE-method for bioassay-guided fractionation of marine extracts. *Mar. Drugs* **2015**, *13*, 5736–5749. [CrossRef] [PubMed]
100. Ebada, S.; Edrada, R.A.; Lin, W.; Proksch, P. Methods for isolation, purification and structural elucidation of bioactive secondary metabolites from marine invertebrates. *Nature Protocols* **2008**, *3*, 1820–1831. [CrossRef] [PubMed]

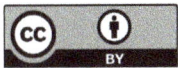

© 2020 by the authors. Licensee MDPI, Basel, Switzerland. This article is an open access article distributed under the terms and conditions of the Creative Commons Attribution (CC BY) license (http://creativecommons.org/licenses/by/4.0/).

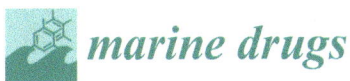

Article

New Benthic Cyanobacteria from Guadeloupe Mangroves as Producers of Antimicrobials

Sébastien Duperron [1,2,*], Mehdi A. Beniddir [3], Sylvain Durand [1], Arlette Longeon [1], Charlotte Duval [1], Olivier Gros [4], Cécile Bernard [1] and Marie-Lise Bourguet-Kondracki [1,*]

1. Molécules de Communication et Adaptation des Microorganismes, UMR 7245 CNRS, Muséum National d'Histoire Naturelle, 57 rue Cuvier (CP54), 75005 Paris, France; sylvain.durand@orange.fr (S.D.); arlette.longeon@mnhn.fr (A.L.); charlotte.duval@mnhn.fr (C.D.); cecile.bernard@mnhn.fr (C.B.)
2. Institut Universitaire de France, 75005 Paris, France
3. Équipe "Pharmacognosie-Chimie des Substances Naturelles" BioCIS, CNRS, Université Paris-Saclay 5 rue Jean-Baptiste Clément, 92290 Châtenay-Malabry, France; mehdi.beniddir@u-psud.fr
4. UMR 7205 ISYEB et Université des Antilles, Pointe à Pitre, 97157 Guadeloupe, France; olivier.gros@univ-antilles.fr
* Correspondence: sebastien.duperron@mnhn.fr (S.D.); marie-lise.bourguet@mnhn.fr (M.-L.B.-K)

Received: 27 November 2019; Accepted: 19 December 2019; Published: 23 December 2019

Abstract: Benthic cyanobacteria strains from Guadeloupe have been investigated for the first time by combining phylogenetic, chemical and biological studies in order to better understand the taxonomic and chemical diversity as well as the biological activities of these cyanobacteria through the effect of their specialized metabolites. Therefore, in addition to the construction of the phylogenetic tree, indicating the presence of 12 potentially new species, an LC-MS/MS data analysis workflow was applied to provide an overview on chemical diversity of 20 cyanobacterial extracts, which was linked to antimicrobial activities evaluation against human pathogenic and ichtyopathogenic environmental strains.

Keywords: benthic cyanobacteria; tropical mangrove; Guadeloupe; phylogenetic diversity; chemical diversity; molecular networking; antimicrobial activity

1. Introduction

Cyanobacteria are among the important primary producers in various coastal ecosystems including mangroves. Besides their occurrence in the bacterioplankton, various cyanobacteria occur in biofilms on the sediment surface, on rocks, and on biological surfaces as part of the periphyton [1,2]. Biofilm-forming cyanobacteria contribute to locale trophic networks through carbon fixation, and depending on species also to nitrogen fixation, accumulation of calcium, magnesium, and phosphorous [3]. The benthic species, especially in tropical zones, may form dense biofilms on various types of substrates and may have major ecological roles [2] but are still poorly known, compared to pelagic species. Although cyanobacteria are of particular interest as ecologically-relevant microorganisms, they are also regarded as producers of a broad diversity of bioactive secondary metabolites including cyanotoxins and various antimicrobial compounds which influence their interactions with other organisms [1,4,5]. Some of these compounds are of pharmacological interest, as illustrated by the use of Brentuxymab vedotin, based on dolastatin 10 from *Symploca*, in the treatment of Hodgkin's lymphoma [1,6].

Currently, the 1700 described cyanobacterial species [7] are probably only a small subset of the group's true diversity. The tropical regions and the benthic compartment are particularly ill-explored compared to the potential diversity their harbor [2]. Chemical investigations have focused on an even smaller subset of this diversity, with over 50% of characterized metabolites reported from the order Oscillatoriales, and 35% in the sole genus *Lyngbya* [5].

In this study, we investigated both the phylogenetic and chemical diversity of cultivable cyanobacteria isolated from coastal habitats in Guadeloupe (French West Indies). Marine benthic cyanobacteria from Guadeloupe have indeed received very little attention despite the fact that they can form biofilms that may cover large areas of sediment and plant surfaces. Three filamentous morphotypes were, for example, recently characterized, but were not maintained in culture collections [8]. In the present study, 20 bacterial strains were isolated from various biofilms in Guadeloupe collected from the benthic sediment surface or from the surface of immersed mangrove tree branches and roots in the Manche-à-Eau mangrove lagoon, the Marina Bas-du-Fort harbor, and the Canal Des Rotours, a 6-km long canal connecting the city of Morne-à-l'eau to the coastal mangrove. Strains were characterized by means of 16S rRNA comparative gene sequence analysis, and their metabolites were analyzed using LC-MS/MS. A molecular network was built to establish chemical entities families, which were compared among strains [9]. Finally, the antibacterial activities were evaluated against six human and four marine pathogen reference strains. This study provides a first glimpse of the taxonomic and chemical diversity of the benthic cyanobacteria occurring in Guadeloupe coastal mangroves.

2. Results

A total of 20 cyanobacterial strains were successfully isolated, and grown from green biofilms collected from distinct locations in Guadeloupe, namely the Manche-à-Eau lagoon close to red mangrove trees (two stations ST1 and ST2 and five strains), the Marina Bas-du-Fort (one station ST4, one strain), and the Canal Des Rotours (three stations ST5, ST6, and ST7 and 14 strains, Figure 1 and Table 1). Biofilms were found either covering the sediment surface, attached to immersed roots of mangrove trees, or attached to sunken deadwood.

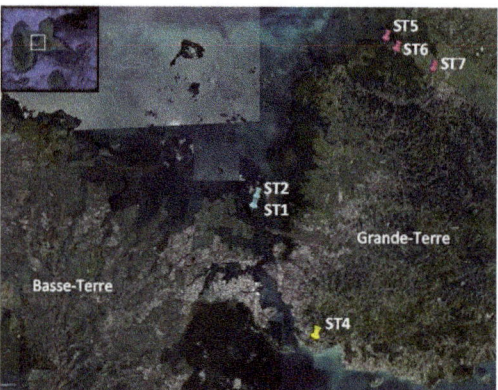

Figure 1. Google map showing the collection sites (ST: stations) located in Grande-Terre (ST4, ST5, ST6, and ST7) and in Basse-Terre (ST1 and ST2), the two main islands constituting Guadeloupe.

2.1. Phylogenetic and 16S rRNA Dissimilarity-Based Identification of Strains

The 16S rRNA-encoding gene sequences from the 20 strains clustered within the three cyanobacterial orders Oscillatoriales, Synechococcales and Nostocales (ten, eight, and two strains, respectively, Figure 2). Strains were affiliated to hypothetical species and genera based on widely accepted 16S rRNA similarity cutoff values for species and genus delimitation [7,10], respectively, and monophyly with members of these species and genera. A large-scale comparison of 6787 genomes from 22 prokaryotic phyla established that a 99% 16S rRNA similarity cutoff value should be retained to delimit species [10]; and reference taxonomic works on Cyanobacteria recommend a 95% cutoff of cyanobacterial genera delimitation [7].

Five of the ten Oscillatoriales strains clustered with sequences from uncultured *Oscillatoria* and a strain assigned to *Kamptonema formosum* (formely *Oscillatoria formosa*). Using the aforementioned criteria, these strains are congeneric, and can be assigned to three new hypothetical species represented by strain PMC 1075.18, strains PMC 1068.18 and 1076.18, and strains PMC 1050.18 and 1051.18, respectively (Table 1 and Table S1). Strains PMC 1056.18 and 1057.18 (0.8% dissimilarity) from Manche-à-Eau represent one hypothetical new species that displays 4% dissimilarity with the closest described genus, *Arthrospira*, and thus probably belong to this genus. Strains PMC 1071.18 (7.8% dissimilarity with *Symploca* sp. NAC 12/21/08-3), and PMC 1072.18 (5.1% dissimilarity with *Ramsaria avicennae* and *Coleofasciculus chthonoplastes*) represent two new species, each belonging to a new genus based on the 95% similarity threshold. Strain PMC 1092.19 displayed 2.2% dissimilarity with *Lyngbya* sp. ALCB114379 and thus likely represents a new species within this genus. Within the Synechococcales, five strains (PMC 1073.18, 1074.18, 1078.18, 1079.18, and 1080.18, all from Canal des Rotours) clustered with genus *Jaaginema* and represent a single new hypothetical species. Strain PMC 1066.18 was closely related (0.5% sequence dissimilarity) to a sequence from an uncultured *Nodosilinea* sp. CENA 322, isolated from leaves of the mangrove tree *Avicennia schaueriana* in Brazil [11]. Sequence from strain PMC 1064.18 was highly similar (0.5% dissimilarity) to sequences from two unpublished strains of *Limnothrix*. Strain PMC 1052.18 displayed at least 7.4% dissimilarity to all other sequences in databases, and represents a new species within a new undescribed genus. Finally, strains PMC 1069.18 and 1070.18 from Canal des Rotours were the only two Nostocales, clustering together and representing a single new hypothetical species belonging to the genus *Scytonema*.

2.2. MS/MS Analysis and Annotation of Cyanobacterial Specialized Metabolites

In an attempt to map the chemical diversity of the 20 cyanobacterial extracts, their LC-MS/MS data were preprocessed using MZmine 2 [12] and the obtained 2468 mass features were organized into a molecular network consisting of 156 clusters (two or more connected nodes of a graph, Figure 3). In order to visualize the distribution of the cyanobacterial metabolites across the 20 extracts, the whole molecular network was mapped at the genus identification level using a typical color tag (Figure 3). An examination of the network reveals that certain clusters are constrained to specific genera. This observation highlighted the distribution of closely related yet different chemical structures in each genus (See supporting information for further details). Moreover, MS/MS data constituting the entire molecular network were searched against the GNPS spectral libraries [13] and yielded only 9 hits (triangle shapes on the network), including a nucleotide, diketopiperazines and phosphocholines (https://gnps.ucsd.edu/ProteoSAFe/result.jsp?task=9581427a15b7422d8bd2b3b4b086189e&view=view_all_annotations_DB). To further expand the annotation coverage, we applied DEREPLICATOR, a recently developed dereplication algorithm that enables high-throughput peptide natural products (PNPs) identification from their tandem mass spectra [14–17]. Interestingly, this tool allows to putatively identify an unknown PNP from its known variants (for example, with a substitution, a modification or an adduct) through the so-called variable dereplication process (as opposed to the strict dereplication when a PNP is described in the database). This dereplication process allowed the annotation of 54 peptide spectrum matches (PSMs) (red ellipses on the network, Figure 3) analogues closely related to known ones (Table S2). Even though, no perfect match was generated through DEREPLICATOR algorithm, marine peptide natural products were proposed and therefore support the relevance of this tool for the exploration of peptide diversity. Furthermore, on the basis of the taxonomic annotation, some clusters were restricted to a single genus indicating the chemical uniqueness of the features within the whole map and, potential structural originality (Figure S1) [18].

Table 1. Cyanobacterial strains isolated from Guadeloupe habitats (see map on Figure 1). Strain ID corresponds to the reference number in the Paris Museum Collection (PMC) of cyanobacteria from which strains are available upon request. Affiliation is according to the 16SrRNA-based phylogenetic analysis displayed on Figure 2 and to the distance matrix in Table S1.

Strain ID	Order	Affiliation	Sampling Site	Coordinates	Isolation Source	Best BLAST Hit and % 16S rRNA Sequence Similarity
PMC 1050.18	Oscillatoriales	*Oscillatoria* n. sp. 3	Manche-à-Eau, ST1	16°16′32″ N/61°33′18″ W	Dense filamentous brown mat	*Oscillatoria/Kamptonema formosum* BDU 92022 (KU958133)/99%
PMC 1051.18	Oscillatoriales	*Oscillatoria* n. sp. 3			Dense filamentous brown mat	*Oscillatoria/Kamptonema formosum* BDU 92022 (KU958133)/99%
PMC 1052.18	Synechococcales	Gen. Nov. 3, n. sp. 1			Benthic mat with Cyanobacteria and *Beggiatoa*-like morphotypes	*Synechocystis* sp. (KU951820)/92%
PMC 1056.18	Oscillatoriales	*Arthrospira*, n. sp. 1	Manche-à-Eau, ST2	16°16′49″ N/61°33′13″ W	Benthic blue-green mat	Uncultured bacterium clone TV002_28 (JX521753)/98%
PMC 1057.18	Oscillatoriales	*Arthrospira*, n. sp. 1			Periphytic biofilm covering immersed roots of *Rhizophora mangle*	Uncultured bacterium clone TV002_28 (JX521753)/97%
PMC 1064.18	Synechococcales	*Limnothrix* n. sp. 1	Marina Bas du Fort, ST4	16°13′13″ N/61°31′24″ W	Dense green benthic biofilm containing Oscillatoriales, *Spirulina* and *Beggiatoa*-like morphotypes	*Limnothrix* sp. TK01 (LC383431)/99%
PMC 1066.18	Synechococcales	*Nodosilinea* n. sp. 1	Canal des Rotours, ST5	16°21′8.4″ N/61°29′20″ W	Dense periphytic biofilm covering immersed roots of *Rhizophora mangle*	*Nodosilinea* sp. CENA322 (KT731143)/99%
PMC 1068.18	Oscillatoriales	*Oscillatoria* n. sp. 2			Dense periphytic biofilm covering immersed roots of *Rhizophora mangle*	*Oscillatoria/Kamptonema formosum* BDU 92022 (KU958133)/98%
PMC 1069.18	Nostocales	*Scytonema* n. sp. 1			Dense periphytic biofilm covering immersed roots of *Rhizophora mangle*	*Scytonema* cf. *mirabile* ER0515.01 (MG970546)/96%
PMC 1070.18	Nostocales	*Scytonema* n. sp. 1			Dense periphytic biofilm covering immersed roots of *Rhizophora mangle*	*Scytonema* cf. *mirabile* ER0515.01 (MG970546)/96%
PMC 1071.18	Oscillatoriales	Gen. Nov. 1, n. sp. 1			Dense periphytic biofilm covering immersed roots of *Rhizophora mangle*	*Symploca* sp. NAC 12/21/08-3 (JQ388601)/92%
PMC 1072.18	Oscillatoriales	Gen. Nov. 2, n. sp. 1			Dense periphytic biofilm covering immersed roots of *Rhizophora mangle*	Uncultured bacterium clone DM1-166 (KC329581)/94%
PMC 1073.18	Synechococcales	*Jaaginema* n. sp. 1	Canal des Rotours, ST 6	16°20′50″ N/61°29′03″ W	Dense periphytic blue-green biofilm covering immersed roots of *Rhizophora nigra*	*Jaaginema* sp. PsrJGgm14 (KM438189)/98%
PMC 1074.18	Synechococcales	*Jaaginema* n. sp. 1			Dense periphytic blue-green biofilm covering immersed roots of *Rhizophora nigra*	*Jaaginema* sp. PsrJGgm14 (KM438189)/91%
PMC 1075.18	Oscillatoriales	*Oscillatoria* n. sp. 1			Dense periphytic blue-green biofilm covering immersed roots of *Rhizophora nigra*	*Oscillatoria/Kamptonema formosum* BDU 92022 (KU958133)/94%
PMC 1076.18	Oscillatoriales	*Oscillatoria* n. sp. 2	Canal des Rotours, ST7	16°20′19″ N/61°27′55″ W	Dense periphytic biofilm covering immersed branch fragment	*Oscillatoria/Kamptonema formosum* BDU 92022 (KU958133)/99%
PMC 1078.18	Synechococcales	*Jaaginema* n. sp. 1			Dense periphytic biofilm covering immersed branch fragment	*Jaaginema* sp. PsrJGgm14 (KM438189)/98%
PMC 1079.18	Synechococcales	*Jaaginema* n. sp. 1			Dense periphytic biofilm covering immersed branch fragment	*Jaaginema* sp. PsrJGgm14 (KM438189)/98%
PMC 1080.18	Synechococcales	*Jaaginema* n. sp. 1			Dense periphytic biofilm covering immersed branch fragment	*Jaaginema* sp. PsrJGgm14 (KM438189)/97%
PMC 1092.19	Oscillatoriales	*Lyngbya*, n. sp. 1			Dense periphytic biofilm covering immersed branch fragment	*Lyngbya* sp. ALCB114379 (KY824052)/98%

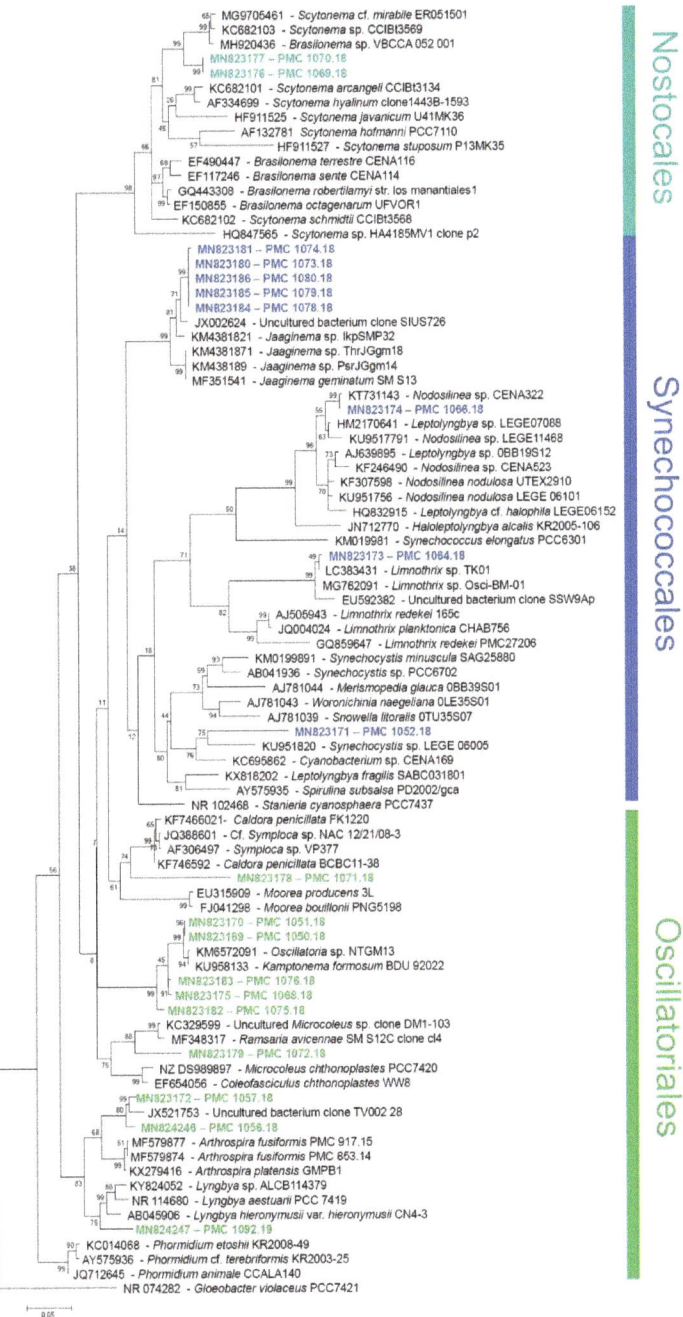

Figure 2. Phylogenetic tree based on the maximum-likelihood analysis of the bacterial 16S rRNA-encoding gene. Sequences from this study are in bold and colored. Support values at nodes were obtained from 100 boostrap replicates. Scale bar represents estimated 5% sequence difference.

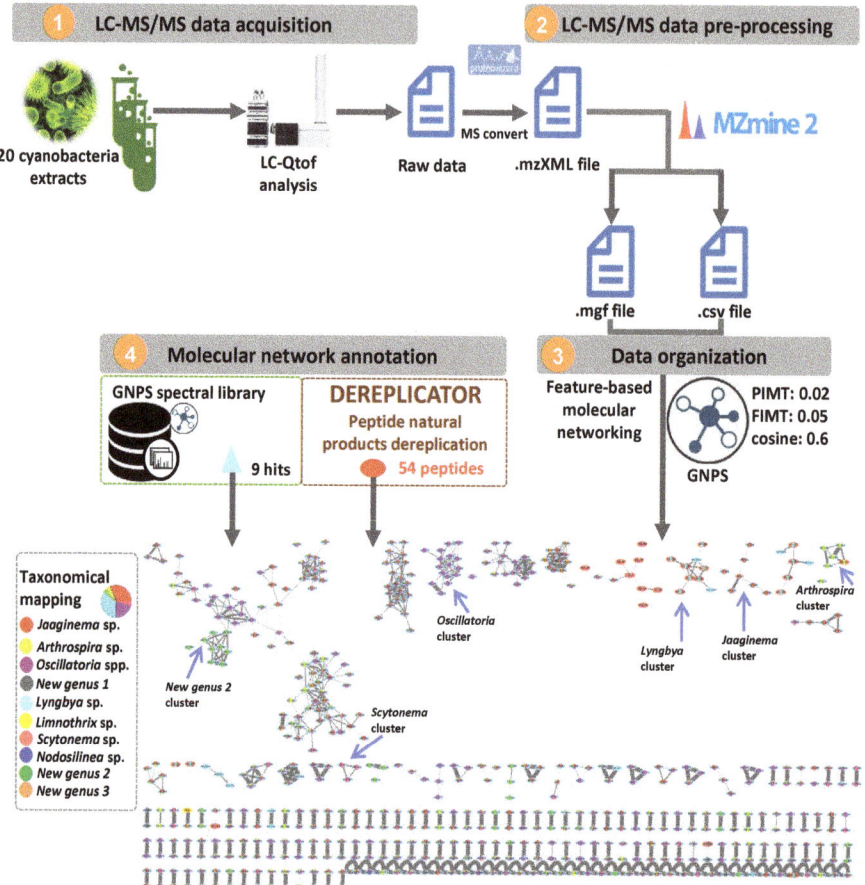

Figure 3. The molecular network obtained through the LC-MS/MS analysis of the 20 extracts of cyanobacterial strains collected in Guadeloupe. Peptides dereplicated via DEREPLICATOR are visualized in red ellipses. Nodes (round shape) are colored according to the mean precursor ion intensity per cyanobacterium genus (For further details See Figure S1).

2.3. Evaluation of the Antimicrobial Activity

The evaluation of the antimicrobial activity was performed against six human pathogenic bacteria (*Escherichia coli*, *Klebsiella pneumoniae*, *Pseudomonas aeruginosa*, *Enterococcus faecalis*, *Staphylococcus aureus*, and *Bacillus cereus*) and four marine environmental pathogenic bacteria (*Vibrio alginolyticus*, *Vibrio anguillarum*, *Pseudoalteromonas atlantica*, and *Pseudoalteromonas distincta*). All the cyanobacterial strains extracts were tested in triplicates at a concentration of 100 µg/mL. Only positive results (i.e., inhibition above 50%) are presented in Table 2.

Most of the cyanobacterial strains showed moderate activity against *P. atlantica* with a mean growth inhibition of 20% to 60%; three *Jaaginema* strains PM 1078.18, 1079.18 and 1080.18 as well as *Oscillatoria n. sp.* 2 PMC 1076.18 displayed highest growth inhibition properties.

Table 2. Summary of significant antibacterial activities among the 20 cyanobacterial strains expressed as percentage of growth inhibition against pathogenic human and marine environmental bacteria.

Strain ID	Gram-Negative Pathogenic Bacteria	
	Human *E. coli*	Environmental *P. atlantica*
Oscillatoria spp.		
PMC 1051.18	100 ± 4.17	n.a.
PMC 1076.18	n.a.	50.87 ± 1.37
Jaaginema sp.		
PMC 1078.18	n.a.	54.07 ± 8.50
PMC 1079.18	n.a.	60.95 ± 5.52
PMC 1080.18	n.a.	53.01 ± 4.42

n.a.: not active at the concentration of 100 µg/mL (i.e., inhibition below 50%); Chloramphenicol was used as positive control in both human *E. coli* and marine environmental *P. atlantica* pathogenic bacteria. Values presented as the mean ± SEM ($n = 3$).

Interestingly, *Oscillatoria/Kamptonema* strain PMC 1051.18 was the only strain to reveal significant activity against *E. coli* with 100 % growth inhibition at 100 µg/mL, while its conspecific strain PMC 1050.18 did not show significant activity.

3. Discussion and Conclusions

3.1. Mangroves of Guadeloupe are a Source of Novel Cyanobacteria

This study yielded 20 new cyanobacterial strains including ten Oscillatoriales, eight Synechococcales and two Nostocales [7]. Based on 16S rRNA phylogeny and similarity criteria, these possibly represent 12 new species within three new and seven already known genera (*Jaaginema*, *Scytonema*, *Oscillatoria*, *Nodosilinea*, *Lyngbya*, *Arthrospira*, and *Limnothrix*). Ascertaining the exact status of strains as new species or genera requires further characterization beyond simple 16S rRNA dissimilarity- and phylogeny-based criteria considered here. A polyphasic approach is required in order to offer a proper taxonomic description, that is beyond the scope of this paper [7,19]. However, this result based on the analysis of 16S rRNA-encoding genes alone, already emphasizes the high level of taxonomic novelty found in Guadeloupe coastal environments. Apart from a recent paper describing three cyanobacteria not closely related to strains described herein, namely *Oscillatoria* sp. clone gwada strain OG (displaying over 5 % 16S rRNA sequence dissimilarity with our *Oscillatoria/Kamptonema* sequences), 'Candidatus Planktothricoides niger' strain OB and 'Candidatus Planktothricoides rosea' strain OP, very little data is available regarding cyanobacterial taxonomic diversity in Guadeloupe [8]. Overall the level of novelty documented here reveals mostly untapped cyanobacterial diversity in Guadeloupe. Various authors have highlighted the potential of tropical ecosystems, in particular mangroves, as reservoirs of cyanobacterial diversity and bioactive molecules [11,20], and the predominance of orders Oscillatoriales and Synechococcales among recovered strains [21,22], so this novelty is not unexpected and warrants further investigations.

3.2. The Benthic Cyanobacterial Strains Reveal a High Level of Chemical Novelty

The presence of 54 peptides, variants of known previously identified peptides, was documented using the DEREPLICATOR algorithm. These latter include eleven peptides previously isolated from yanobacteria (Table 3 and Figure S2) but also twelve known peptides from marine Sponges, three from Chordata, five from Fungi (including two marine fungi), and ten from Bacteria, whose one marine bacterium (Table S2). These results suggest that some of the previously isolated peptides from marine organisms could have a symbiotic origin and could be in fact produced by cyanobacteria associated with these organisms.

Table 3. Eleven peptide natural products (PNPs) previously isolated from cyanobacteria (in the increasing order of P values) dereplicated by DEREPLICATOR.

Variant PNP	Producer	Detected in	Score	P-Value	Variant PNP Mass	Peptide Mass *
Viequeamide A	Marine Button Cyanobacterium (unidentified)	Oscillatoria sp., Scytonema sp., Arthrospira sp.	12	$2.8\ 10^{-17}$	803.50	892.55
Nostophycin	Nostoc 152	Lyngbya sp.	11	$2.1\ 10^{-15}$	888.48	943.55
Wewakamide A	Lyngbya semiplena Lyngbya majuscula	Oscillatoria sp., Scytonema sp., Arthrospira sp.	12	$4.4\ 10^{-15}$	994.65	891.59
Majusculamide C_Demethoxy	Lyngbya majuscula	Oscillatoria sp., Scytonema sp., Arthrospira sp.	11	$4.6\ 10^{-13}$	954.58	892.49
Wewakazole	Lyngbya majuscula	Lyngbya sp.	12	$6.7\ 10^{-12}$	1140.54	1058.54
Anacyclamide A10	Anabaena sp. 90	Lyngbya sp.	10	$9.6\ 10^{-11}$	1052.53	1009.49
Aerucyclamide C	Microcystis aeruginosa	Lyngbya sp.	7	$9.5\ 10^{-9}$	516.22	645.28
Microcystin LR	Microcystis bloom	Lyngbya sp.	7	$1.5\ 10^{-8}$	980.53	846.91
Pitipeptolide A	Lyngbya majuscula	Oscillatoria sp., Scytonema sp., Arthrospira sp.	7	$1.6\ 10^{-8}$	807.48	795.51
Microcystin RA	Microcystis	Lyngbya sp.	7	$1.7\ 10^{-8}$	952.50	825.38
Raocyclamide B	Oscillatoria raoi	Arthrospira sp.	6	$6.5\ 10^{-8}$	568.21	581.17

*: Peptide mass (in Da) found in our extracts and previously isolated from Cyanobacteria.

The comparison of ions observed in the chemical extracts of the 20 strains also revealed high heterogeneity in chemical composition despite that strains were grown under similar conditions (temperature, Z8 media, photoperiod). This indicates high levels of inter-strain variability.

The assessment of those cyanobacterial extracts using molecular networking and in silico annotation tool finally pointed out a high level of chemical novelty. Notably, this endeavor will allow prioritizing cyanobacterial strains for further chemical studies that will be pursued with full structure elucidation of each isolated compound through detailed NMR analyses.

3.3. Certain Cyanobacterial Strains Reveal Promising Antimicrobial Activities

All strains inhibited the growth of *P. atlantica* to a certain extent. The most active strains, namely PMC 1078.18, 1079.18, and 1080.18, displaying more than 50% of inhibitory activity, belong to a single hypothetical new species of the genus *Jaaginema* and were isolated from the Canal des Rotours. The two other conspecific strains PMC 1073.18 and 1074.18 did not display a significant inhibition, suggesting that this property is limited to certain strains within this species. More interestingly, a single strain of *Oscillatoria*/*Kamptonema*, namely PMC 1051.18, isolated in the Manche à Eau lagoon, showed a very high inhibition against the human pathogenic bacterium strain *E. coli* with 100% of inhibition at the concentration of 100 µg/mL. This promising activity stimulates a deeper chemical study of this strain in order to isolate and identify the molecule(s) responsible for the detected activity. The antimicrobial activity assay will also be enlarged with assays against resistant pathogenic bacterial strains. Surprisingly, its closest relative in the phylogenetic tree, strain PMC 1050.18 did not display such an activity, again suggesting a strain-specific level of activity.

Altogether these findings support that activities are limited to certain strains of a given cyanobacterial species. Inter-strain variability is most often attributed to the existence of certain genes or pathways that are found in some, but not all strains of a given species [23]. This could explain some of the chemical and activity differences observed herein between closely related strains. Alternatively, recent studies on cyanobacterial strains maintained in culture have revealed the existence of an overlooked associated cyanosphere, i.e., a cohort of other microorganisms (mostly bacteria) that is co-isolated and co-cultured with the cyanobacterium [24]. In this case, as observed in other organisms that co-exist with a microbiota, this cyanosphere certainly interacts and influences the cyanobacterial strains physiology, possibly being in obligate symbiosis, a consequence being the reported difficulty to obtain axenic cultures in Cyanobacteria [24]. These interactions might result in strain-specific differences in chemical composition and activities, either by modulating cyanobacterial gene expression, or because compounds and activities are in fact due to other members of the cyanosphere, and not the cyanobacterium itself. This may explain why different strains within a single species and cultured under similar conditions can display very different compounds and properties, and emphasizes the necessity to account for this heterogeneity by investigating various strains in parallel within each species.

In conclusion, easy-to-sample coastal areas in Guadeloupe harbor an untapped diversity of benthic cyanobacteria that probably represent novel lineages and display a diversity of potentially novel molecules, some of which have promising antimicrobial properties. The taxonomic affiliation of the strains has to be further investigated using polyphasic approaches (that include morphological, ultrastructural and molecular analyses). The different types of activities of the isolated peptides have also to be further explored. It certainly emphasizes the need to further investigate the different habitats in Guadeloupe, in particular mangroves, and more generally tropical coastal habitats, as environmental conditions have a major impact on cyanobacterial diversity [20]. To understand the significance of these Cyanobacteria in these ecosystems, and the possible roles of antibacterial compounds in nature, work is under way to address the actual abundance and functions of isolated strains in biofilms in natura using additional approaches including metagenomics, metabolomics and metatranscriptomics. This study paves the way for further promising investigations on benthic cyanobacteria from tropical mangroves.

4. Materials and Methods

4.1. Sampling and Strain Isolation

Green biofilms, presumed to contain abundant cyanobacteria, were sampled in July 2018 from distinct locations in Guadeloupe, namely two stations located in the Manche-à-Eau lagoon close to red mangrove trees (*Rhizophora mangle*, [25], five strains), the Marina Bas-du-Fort (one strain), and the Canal Des Rotours, a 6-km long canal build between 1826 and 1830 connecting the city of Morne-à-l'eau to the sea on three stations, representing a transition between the coastal mangrove (stations 5 and 6 with six and three strains, respectively) and freshwater (station 7 with five strains, Table 1). In accordance with Article 17, paragraph 2, of the Nagoya Protocol on Access and Benefit-sharing, a sampling permit was issued and published (https://absch.cbd.int/database/ABSCH-IRCC-FR-246959). Biofilms, either benthic or attached to submerged tree roots or branches (periphyton) were sampled by snorkeling. Back to the lab, biofilms were examined under a binocular and individual cyanobacterial morphotypes were transferred to plates containing solid Z8 medium [26] containing 0, 20, and 35 g/L salt (Instant Ocean, Aquarium Systems, France). Isolation in liquid Z8 medium was also attempted.

4.2. Strain Cultivation and Biomass Production

Back to the laboratory, surviving non-axenic strains were stabilized. Strains were registered in the Paris Museum Collection (PMC) under labels PMC 1050.18 to PMC 1092.19 (Table 1). They are maintained in liquid medium and are available upon request (https://www.mnhn.fr/fr/collections/ensembles-collections/ressources-biologiques-cellules-vivantes-cryoconservees/microalgues-cyanobacteries). Biomass was produced for two months in increasing volumes of liquid Z8 media (25 ± 1 °C; 15 µmol/m^2/s white light; 16 h light: 8 h dark) without salt (PMC1069.18, 1070.18, 1071.18, 1072.18, 1073.18, 1092.18) or with 20 g/L salt (other strains).

4.3. Strain Identification

DNA was extracted from cultures using the ZymoBIOMICS Fecal/Soil Kit (Zymo Research, Irvine, CA, USA) following manufacturer's instructions including a 3 min disruption of cells using ceramic beads. Concentrations were measured using Nanodrop and Qubit. Fragments of the 16S rRNA-encoding gene were amplified by PCR for 35 cycles using two primer sets commonly used to specifically amplify cyanobacterial genes. Annealing temperature of 58 °C was used for primer set 8F (5′-AGAGTTTGATCCTGGCTCAG 3′) and 920R (5′-TTGTAAGGTTCTTCGCGTTG-3′), and annealing at 55 °C was used for primer set 861F (5′-TAACGCGTTAAGTATCCC-3′) and 1380R (5′-TAACGACTTCGGGCGTGACC-3′) [27,28]. For each strain, sequence chromatograms (Genoscreen, Lille, France) were examined, assembled using Geneious (https://www.geneious.com/), and compared to the GENBANK database using BLAST. Sequences are deposited in GENBANK under accession numbers MN823169 to MN823186; MN824246 and MN824247.

A dataset was built consisting of sequences from the 20 isolated strains, their best BLAST hits, and representatives of major cyanobacterial lineages. Sequences from genus *Gloeobacter* were used as an outgroup. Sequences were aligned using the secondary structure-aware Infernal Aligner v. 1.0 tool available on the Ribosomal Database Project website [29]. Alignment was controlled to remove ambiguously-aligned zones. Phylogenetic tree was reconstructed using the software MEGA7 [30]. Relationships were inferred using a Maximum Likelihood approach using a General Time Reversible model (5 categories and invariants), and 1280 nucleotide positions. Support values at nodes were obtained from 100 boostrap replicates analyzed using the same method. A pairwise p-distance matrix (Table S1) was built to support preliminary genus and species delimitation.

4.4. Preparation of Cyanobacteria Chemical Extracts

An aliquot each culture was deposited in a 15 mL Falcon tube containing 10 mL of unsalted Z8 medium. After centrifugation at 4000 g and three successive washes with unsalted Z8 medium, the pellets were lyophilized under vacuum at −40 °C for 12 h. The dry extracts were weighed and then re-suspended in a MeOH/CH$_3$CN/H$_2$O mixture (40:40:20) for having a final concentration of 1 mg /100 µL of solvent mixture. After three successive sonications (6 min cycle: 1 min ON/30 s OFF) and centrifugations at 14,000 g for 5 min, the supernatants were evaporated and the dry extracts were prepared for having a final concentration of 1 mg/mL and were then filtered on a membrane of 13 mm in diameter and 0.2 µm in pores (VWR International). An aliquot of 30 µL was reserved for LC-MS^2 analysis. The remaining samples were evaporated and diluted in DMSO at a concentration of 10 µg/µL for antibacterial activities evaluation.

4.5. LC-MS^2 Analyzes of Extracts

The extracts were subjected to an Agilent 1260 HPLC (Agilent Technologies, Les Ulis, France) coupled to an Agilent 6530 Q-ToF-MS equipped with a Dual ESI source. The chromatographic separation was performed using an HPLC (C18 Sunfire® Waters 150 × 2.1 mm, 3.5 µm column, 250 µL/min gradient elution (A: CH$_3$CN, B: H$_2$O + 0.1% formic acid) from 5% to 100% A, over 20 min). The divert valve was set to waste for the first 3 min. In positive ion mode, purine C$_5$H$_4$N$_4$ [M + H]$^+$ ion (*m/z* 121.0509) and hexakis (1H, 1H, 3H-tetrafluoropropoxy) phosphazine C$_{18}$H$_{18}$F$_{24}$N$_3$O$_6$P$_3$ [M + H]$^+$ ion (*m/z* 922.0098) (HP 0921) were used as internal lock masses. Source parameters were set as follow: capillary voltage at 3500 V, gas temperature at 320 °C, drying gas flow at 10 L/min, nebulizer pressure at 40 psi. Fragmentor was set at 175 V. Acquisition was performed in auto MS^2 mode on the range *m/z* 100–1200 with an MS rate of 1 spectra/sec and an MS/MS scan rate of 3 spectra/sec. Isolation MS/MS width was 2 *m/z*. Fixed collision energies 45 eV was used. MS/MS events were performed on the three most intense precursor ions per cycle with a minimum intensity of 5000 counts. Full scans were acquired at a resolution of 11,000 [FWHM] (*m/z* 922).

4.5.1. MS/MS Data Pretreatment

The MS data were converted from RAW (Thermo) standard data format to mzXML format using the MSConvert software, part of the ProteoWizard package [31]. The converted files were treated using the MZmine software suite v. 2.38 [12].

The parameters were adjusted as following: the centroid mass detector was used for mass detection with the noise level set to 1.0E6 for MS level set to 1, and to 0 for MS level set to 2. The ADAP [32] chromatogram builder was used and set to a minimum group size of scans of 2, minimum group intensity threshold of 3.0E3, minimum highest intensity of 3.0E3 and m/z tolerance of 10.0 ppm. For chromatogram deconvolution, the algorithm used was the wavelets (ADAP). The intensity window S/N was used as S/N estimator with a signal to noise ratio set at 10, a minimum feature height at 1000, a coefficient area threshold at 10, a peak duration range from 0.02 to 1.0 min and the RT wavelet range from 0.02 to 0.6 min. Isotopes were detected using the isotopes peaks grouper with a m/z tolerance of 10.0 ppm, a RT tolerance of 0.3 min (absolute), the maximum charge set at 1 and the representative isotope used was the most intense. Peak alignment was performed using the RANSAC alignment method (m/z tolerance at 10 ppm), RT tolerance 0.3 min, RT tolerance after correction 0.5 min, RANSAC iterations 0, Minimum number of points: 80.0 %, Threshold value: 0.3, requiring the same charge state. The peak list was gap-filled with the same RT and m/z range gap filler (m/z tolerance at 10 ppm). Eventually the resulting aligned peaklist was filtered using the peak-list rows filter option in order to keep only features associated with MS^2 scans.

4.5.2. Molecular Networks Generation

In order to keep the retention time, the exact mass information and to allow for the separation of isomers, a feature-based molecular network (https://ccms-ucsd.github.io/GNPSDocumentation/featurebasedmolecularnetworking/) was created using the mgf file resulting from the MZmine pretreatment step detailed above. Spectral data was uploaded on the GNPS molecular networking platform. A network was then created where edges were filtered to have a cosine score above 0.7 and more than six matched peaks. Further edges between two nodes were kept in the network if and only if each of the nodes appeared in each other's respective top 10 most similar nodes. The spectra in the network were then searched against GNPS' spectral libraries. All matches kept between network spectra and library spectra were required to have a score above 0.7 and at least six matched peaks. The output was visualized using Cytoscape 3.6 software [33]. The GNPS job parameters and resulting data are available at the following address (https://gnps.ucsd.edu/ProteoSAFe/status.jsp?task=9581427a15b7422d8bd2b3b4b086189e). The DEREPLICATOR job resulting data is available at the following address (https://gnps.ucsd.edu/ProteoSAFe/status.jsp?task=0c058507ac774dd7b881c2ee36d57720).

4.6. Evaluation of the Antibacterial Activity of Cyanobacterial Strains

The antibacterial activities of the chemical extracts of the various cyanobacterial strains were tested against six human pathogenic bacteria (*Escherichia coli* ATCC 8739, *Klebsiella pneumoniae* ATCC 11296, *Pseudomonas aeruginosa* ATCC 13388, *Enterococcus faecalis* ATCC 29212, *Staphylococcus aureus* ATCC 6538 and *Bacillus cereus* ATCC 14579) and four marine pathogenic bacteria (*Vibrio alginolyticus* ATCC 17749, *Vibrio anguillarum* ATCC 19264, *Pseudoalteromonas atlantica* ATCC 19262 and *Pseudoalteromonas distincta* ATCC 700518). The selected pathogenic human and marine bacteria were cultured in LB (Luria Bertoni) medium at 37 °C or in MB (Marine Broth) at 25 °C, respectively. The different bacteria were isolated on LB or MB agar by incubation at 37 °C or 25 °C overnight. A pre-culture of 5 mL was prepared by inoculating a colony of each bacterial strain, and incubated at 37 °C or 25 °C and stirring overnight. The bacterial suspension was adjusted by dilution to obtain an optical density (OD) of 0.03 at 620 nm. The antibacterial assays were performed by a liquid method in 96-well microplates. Briefly, 100 µL of the bacterial suspension of different bacteria strains were distributed in each well. The extracts, diluted in DMSO, were tested in triplicate at a concentration of 100 µg/mL. The 96-well microplates were incubated overnight at 37 °C or 25 °C and shaked at 450 rpm. The OD of each well was measured at 620 nm using an absorbance reader plate (Multiscan, Thermofisher, Saint-Herblain, France). The percentage of growth inhibition was calculated using the formula: % inhibition = 100 − [(ODS − ODB)/(ODT − ODB) × 100] where T = bacterial suspension without test sample, B = culture medium without bacteria and S = bacterial suspension test sample. Standard antibiotics were used as positive controls (ampicillin against *E. faecalis*, *B. cereus*, *P. distincta*, *V. anguillarum*; chloramphenicol against *E. coli*, *P. aeruginosa*, *V. alginolyticus*, *P. atlantica*; gentamycin against *S. aureus*, *K. pneumoniae*).

Supplementary Materials: The following are available online at http://www.mdpi.com/1660-3397/18/1/16/s1, Table S1: Pairwise distance values among new cyanobacterial strains isolated during this study. Values below 0.05 (5% divergence, as congenerics) are in bold. Table S2. List of the 54 candidate structures, which are consistent with previously identified peptides using DEREPLICATOR algorithm. Figure S1. Global molecular network obtained from LC-MS/MS data of 20 cyanobacteria extracts (red ellipses are DEREPLICATOR peptide matches). Figure S2. A selection of clusters and self-loops annotated with putative cyanobacterial peptides and their origin.

Author Contributions: Conceptualization and supervision: S.D. (Sébastien Duperron) and M.-L.B.-K., Phylogenetic studies: C.D., S.D (Sylvain Durand) and S.D. (Sébastien Duperron), Chemical studies: S.D. (Sylvain Durand), A.L., and M.-L.B.-K., Molecular Network: M.A.B. and S.D. (Sylvain Durand). Antimicrobial assays: S.D. (Sylvain Durand), A.L. and M.-L.B.-K. All the authors contributed to the writing and editing the manuscript. All authors have read and agreed to the published version of the manuscript.

Funding: We obtained financial support from the CNRS MITI X-Life 2018-2019 program (CABMAN project) and the ATM CHEMCYANGROV from the 2019 MNHN grant "biodiversity of microorganisms".

Acknowledgments: We acknowledge the financial support of the CNRS and the MNHN.

Conflicts of Interest: The authors declare no conflict of interest.

References

1. Shah, S.A.A.; Akhter, N.; Auckloo, B.N.; Khan, I.; Lu, Y.; Wang, K.; Wu, B.; Guo, Y.-W. Structural diversity, biological properties and applications of natural products from Cyanobacteria. *Mar. Drugs* **2017**, *15*, 354. [CrossRef] [PubMed]
2. Alvarenga, D.O.; Rigonato, J.; Branco, L.H.Z.; Fiore, M.F. Cyanobacteria in mangrove ecosystems. *Biodivers. Conserv.* **2015**, *24*, 799–817. [CrossRef]
3. Lovelock, C.; Grinham, A.; Adame, F.; Penros, H. Elemental composition and productivity of cyanobacterial mats in an arid zone estuary in north Western Australia. *Wetl. Ecol. Manag.* **2010**, *18*, 37–47. [CrossRef]
4. Kleigrewe, K.; Almaliti, J.; Tian, I.Y.; Kinnel, R.B.; Korobeynikov, A.; Monroe, E.A.; Duggan, B.M.; Di Marzo, V.; Sherman, D.H.; Dorrestein, P.C.; et al. Combining Mass Spectrometric Metabolic Profiling with Genomic Analysis: A Powerful Approach for Discovering Natural Products from Cyanobacteria. *J. Nat. Prod.* **2015**, *78*, 1672–1682. [CrossRef] [PubMed]
5. Demay, J.; Bernard, C.; Reinhardt, A.; Marie, B. Natural Products from Cyanobacteria: Focus on Beneficial Activities. *Mar. Drugs* **2019**, *17*, 320. [CrossRef]
6. Mi, Y.; Zhang, J.; He, S.; Yan, X. New peptides isolated from marine cyanobacteria, an overview over the past decade. *Mar. Drugs* **2017**, *15*, 132. [CrossRef]
7. Komarek, J.; Kastovsky, J.; Mares, J.; Johansen, J.R. Taxonomic classification of cyanoprokaryotes (cyanobacterial genera) 2014, using a polyphasic approach. *Preslia* **2014**, *86*, 295–335.
8. Guidi-Rontani, C.; Jean, M.R.N.; Gonzalez-Rizzo, S.; Bolte-Kluge, S.; Gros, O. Description of new filamentous toxic Cyanobacteria (Oscillatoriales) colonizing the sulfidic periphyton mat in marine mangroves. *FEMS Microbiol. Lett.* **2014**, *359*, 173–181. [CrossRef]
9. Fox Ramos, A.E.; Evanno, L.; Poupon, E.; Champy, P.; Beniddir, M.A. Natural products targeting strategies involving molecular networking: Different manners, one goal. *Nat. Prod. Rep.* **2019**, *36*, 960–980. [CrossRef]
10. Kim, M.; Oh, H.S.; Park, S.C.; Chun, J. Towards a taxonomic coherence between average nucleotide identity and 16S rRNA gene sequence similarity for species demarcation of prokaryotes. *Int. J. Syst. Evol. Microbiol.* **2014**, *64*, 346–351. [CrossRef]
11. Alvarenga, D.O.; Rigonata, J.; Branco, L.E.; Mele, I.S.; Fiore, M.F. *Phyllonema aviceniicola* gen. nov., sp nov and *Foliisarcina bertiogensis* gen. nov., sp nov., epiphyllic cyanobacteria associated with *Avicennia schaueriana* leaves. *Int. J. Syst. Evol. Microbiol.* **2016**, *66*, 689–700. [CrossRef] [PubMed]

12. Pluskal, T.; Castillo, S.; Villar-Briones, A.; Orešič, M. MZmine 2: Modular framework for processing, visualizing, and analyzing mass spectrometry-based molecular profile data. *BMC Bioinform.* **2010**, *11*, 395. [CrossRef] [PubMed]
13. Wang, M.; Carver, J.J.; Phelan, V.V.; Sanchez, L.M.; Garg, N.; Peng, Y.; Nguyen, D.D.; Watrous, J.; Kapono, C.A.; Luzzatto-Knaan, T.; et al. Sharing and community curation of mass spectrometry data with Global Natural Products Social Molecular Networking. *Nat. Biotechnol.* **2016**, *34*, 828–837. [CrossRef] [PubMed]
14. Mohimani, H.; Gurevich, A.; Mikheenko, A.; Garg, N.; Nothias, L.-F.; Ninomiya, A.; Takada, K.; Dorrestein, P.C.; Pevzner, P.A. Dereplication of peptidic natural products through database search of mass spectra. *Nat. Chem. Biol.* **2016**, *13*, 30–33. [CrossRef] [PubMed]
15. Martin, H.C.; Ibá#xF1;ez, R.; Nothias, L.-F.; Boya, P.C.A.; Reinert, L.K.; Rollins-Smith, L.A.; Dorrestein, P.C.; Gutiérrez, M. Viscosin-like lipopeptides from frog skin bacteria inhibit *Aspergillus fumigatus* and *Batrachochytrium dendrobatidis* detected by imaging mass spectrometry and molecular networking. *Sci. Rep.* **2019**, *9*, 3019. [CrossRef]
16. Saurav, K.; Macho, M.; Kust, A.; Delawská, K.; Hájek, J.; Hrouzek, P. Antimicrobial activity and bioactive profiling of heterocytous cyanobacterial strains using MS/MS-based molecular networking. *Folia Microbiol.* **2019**, *64*, 645–654. [CrossRef]
17. Paulo, B.S.; Sigrist, R.; Angolini, C.F.F.; De Oliveira, L.G. New Cyclodepsipeptide Derivatives Revealed by Genome Mining and Molecular Networking. *Chem. Sel.* **2019**, *4*, 7785–7790. [CrossRef]
18. Olivon, F.; Allard, P.-M.; Koval, A.; Righi, D.; Genta-Jouve, G.; Neyts, J.; Apel, C.; Pannecouque, C.; Nothias, L.-F.; Cachet, X.; et al. Bioactive Natural Products Prioritization Using Massive Multi-informational Molecular Networks. *ACS Chem. Biol.* **2017**, *12*, 2644–2651. [CrossRef]
19. Cellamare, M.; Duval, C.; Drelin, Y.; Djediat, C.; Touibi, N.; Agogué, H.; Leboulanger, C.; Ader, M.; Bernard, C. Characterization of phototrophic microorganisms and description of new cyanobacteria isolated from the saline-alkaline crater-lake Dziani Dzaha (Mayotte, Indian Ocean). *FEMS Microbiol. Ecol.* **2018**, *94*, 108. [CrossRef]
20. Rigonato, J.; Alvarenga, D.O.; Andreote, F.; Dias, A.C.; Melo, I.S.; Kent, A.; Fiore, M.F. Cyanobacterial diversity in the phyllosphere of a mangrove forest. *FEMS Microbiol. Ecol.* **2012**, *80*, 312–322. [CrossRef]
21. Zubia, M.; Turquet, J.; Golubic, S. Benthic cyanobacterial diversity of Iles Eparses (Scattered Islands) in the Mozambique Channel. *Acta Oecol.* **2016**, *72*, 21–32. [CrossRef]
22. Zubia, M.; Vieira, C.; Palinska, K.A.; Roue, M.; Gaertner, J.C.; Zloch, I.; Grellier, M.; Golubic, S. Benthic cyanobacteria on coral reefs of Moorea Island (French Polynesia): Diversity response to habitat quality. *Hybrobiologia* **2019**, *843*, 61–78. [CrossRef]
23. Beck, C.; Knoop, H.; Steuer, R. Modules of co-occurrence in the cyanobacterial pan-genome reveal functional associations between groups of ortholog genes. *PLoS Genet.* **2018**, *14*, e1007239. [CrossRef] [PubMed]
24. Alvarenga, D.O.; Fiore, M.F.; Varani, A.M. A metagenomic approach to cyanobacterial genomics. *Front. Microbiol.* **2017**, *8*, 809. [CrossRef] [PubMed]
25. Gontharet, S.; Crémière, A.; Blanc-Valleron, M.M.; Sébilo, M.; Gros, O.; Laverman, A.M.; Dessailly, D. Sediment characteristics and microbial mats in a marine mangrove, Manche-à-eau lagoon (Guadeloupe). *J. Soils Sediments* **2017**, *17*, 1999–2010. [CrossRef]
26. Rippka, R. Isolation and purification of cyanobacteria. *Meth. Enzym.* **1988**, *167*, 3–27.
27. Lane, D.L. 16S/23S rRNA sequencing. In *Nucleic Acid Techniques in Bacterial Systematics*; Stackenbrandt, E., Goodfellow, M., Eds.; John Wiley and Sons: New York, NY, USA, 1991; pp. 115–175.
28. Gugger, M.; Lyra, C.; Henriksen, P.; Couté, A.; Humbert, J.-F.; Sivonen, K. Phylogenetic comparison of the cyanobacterial genera *Anabaena* and *Aphanizomenon*. *Int. J. Syst. Evol. Microbiol.* **2002**, *52*, 1867–1880.
29. Nawrocki, E.P.; Kolbe, D.L.; Eddy, S.R. Infernal 1.0: Inference of RNA alignments. *Bioinformatics* **2009**, *10*, 1335–1337. [CrossRef]
30. Kumar, S.; Stecher, G.; Tamura, K. MEGA7: Molecular Evolutionary Genetics Analysis version 7.0 for bigger datasets. *Mol. Biol. Evol.* **2016**, *33*, 1870–1874. [CrossRef]
31. Chambers, M.C.; Maclean, B.; Burke, R.; Amodei, D.; Ruderman, D.L.; Neumann, S.; Gatto, L.; Fischer, B.; Pratt, B.; Egertson, J.; et al. A cross-platform toolkit for mass spectrometry and proteomics. *Nat. Biotechnol.* **2012**, *30*, 918–920. [CrossRef]

32. Myers, O.D.; Sumner, S.J.; Li, S.; Barnes, S.; Du, X. One Step Forward for Reducing False Positive and False Negative Compound Identifications from Mass Spectrometry Metabolomics Data: New Algorithms for Constructing Extracted Ion Chromatograms and Detecting Chromatographic Peaks. *Anal. Chem.* **2017**, *89*, 8696–8703. [CrossRef]
33. Shannon, P.; Markiel, A.; Ozier, O.; Baliga, N.S.; Wang, J.T.; Ramage, D.; Amin, N.; Schwikowski, B.; Ideker, T. Cytoscape: A Software Environment for Integrated Models of Biomolecular Interaction Networks. *Genome Res.* **2003**, *13*, 2498–2504. [CrossRef]

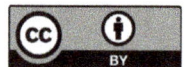

© 2019 by the authors. Licensee MDPI, Basel, Switzerland. This article is an open access article distributed under the terms and conditions of the Creative Commons Attribution (CC BY) license (http://creativecommons.org/licenses/by/4.0/).

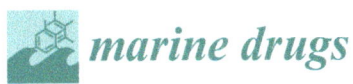

Article

Uncovering the Core Microbiome and Distribution of Palmerolide in *Synoicum adareanum* Across the Anvers Island Archipelago, Antarctica

Alison E. Murray [1,*], Nicole E. Avalon [2], Lucas Bishop [1], Karen W. Davenport [3], Erwan Delage [4], Armand E.K. Dichosa [3], Damien Eveillard [4], Mary L. Higham [1], Sofia Kokkaliari [2], Chien-Chi Lo [3], Christian S. Riesenfeld [1], Ryan M. Young [2], Patrick S.G. Chain [3,*] and Bill J. Baker [2,*]

1. Division of Earth and Ecosystem Science, Desert Research Institute, Reno, NV 89512, USA; bishoplucas95@gmail.com (L.B.); mary.higham@dri.edu (M.L.H.); csriesenfeld@gmail.com (C.S.R.)
2. Department of Chemistry, University of South Florida, Tampa, FL 33620, USA; neavalon@usf.edu (N.E.A.); skokkaliari@usf.edu (S.K.); ryan.young@nuigalway.ie (R.M.Y.)
3. Bioscience Division, Los Alamos National Laboratory, Los Alamos, NM 87545, USA; kwdavenport@lanl.gov (K.W.D.); armand@lanl.gov (A.E.K.D.); chienchi@lanl.gov (C.-C.L.)
4. LS2N, Université de Nantes, CNRS, 44322 Nantes, France; erwan.delage@univ-nantes.fr (E.D.); damien.eveillard@univ-nantes.fr (D.E.)
* Correspondence: Alison.murray@dri.edu (A.E.M.); pchain@lanl.gov (P.S.G.C.); bjbaker@usf.edu (B.J.B.)

Received: 16 April 2020; Accepted: 27 May 2020; Published: 2 June 2020

Abstract: Polar marine ecosystems hold the potential for bioactive compound biodiscovery, based on their untapped macro- and microorganism diversity. Characterization of polar benthic marine invertebrate-associated microbiomes is limited to few studies. This study was motivated by our interest in better understanding the microbiome structure and composition of the ascidian, *Synoicum adareanum*, in which palmerolide A (PalA), a bioactive macrolide with specificity against melanoma, was isolated. PalA bears structural resemblance to a hybrid nonribosomal peptide-polyketide that has similarities to microbially-produced macrolides. We conducted a spatial survey to assess both PalA levels and microbiome composition in *S. adareanum* in a region of the Antarctic Peninsula near Anvers Island (64°46′ S, 64°03′ W). PalA was ubiquitous and abundant across a collection of 21 ascidians (3 subsamples each) sampled from seven sites across the Anvers Island Archipelago. The microbiome composition (V3–V4 16S rRNA gene sequence variants) of these 63 samples revealed a core suite of 21 bacterial amplicon sequence variants (ASVs)—20 of which were distinct from regional bacterioplankton. ASV co-occurrence analysis across all 63 samples yielded subgroups of taxa that may be interacting biologically (interacting subsystems) and, although the levels of PalA detected were not found to correlate with specific sequence variants, the core members appeared to occur in a preferred optimum and tolerance range of PalA levels. These results, together with an analysis of the biosynthetic potential of related microbiome taxa, describe a conserved, high-latitude core microbiome with unique composition and substantial promise for natural product biosynthesis that likely influences the ecology of the holobiont.

Keywords: Antarctica; ascidian; microbiome; microbial diversity; palmerolide A; co-occurrence

1. Introduction

Microbial partners of marine invertebrates play intrinsic roles in the marine environment at both the individual (host survival) and community (species distribution) levels. Host–microbe relationships are mediated through complex interactions that can include nutrient exchange, environmental adaptation, and production of defensive metabolites. These functional interactions are tied to the structural nature (diversity, biogeography, and stability) of host and microbiome, and the ecological interactions between them. Studies of sponges, corals, and, to a lesser degree, ascidians have revealed strong trends in invertebrate host species specificity to particular groups of bacteria and archaea. These studies have documented an underlying layer of diversity (e.g., [1–3]) in which habitat and biogeography appear to have strong influences on the microbiome structure and function [4–6].

The vast majority of host–microbiome studies have been conducted at low- and mid-latitudes from coastal to deep-sea sites. High-latitude benthic marine invertebrate-associated microbiome studies are currently limited to the Antarctic, where just the tip of the iceberg has been investigated in regards to different host–microbe associations [7] and ecological understanding is sparse. Antarctic marine invertebrates tend to have a high degree of endemicity at the species level, often display circumpolar distribution, and in many cases have closest relatives associated with deep-sea fauna. Whether endemicity dominates the microbiomes of high-latitude benthic invertebrate is currently not known, nor is the extent of diversity understood within and between different host-associated microbiomes. Likewise, reports of core (conserved within a host species) microbiomes within Antarctic invertebrate species are sparse.

The few polar host-associated microbiome studies to date have documented varying trends in host species specificity, with generally low numbers of individuals surveyed. For example, low species specificity was reported in sponge microbiome compositions between different sub-Antarctic and South Shetland Island *Mycale* species [8] which shared 74% of the operational taxonomic units (OTUs), possibly representing a cross-*Mycale* core microbiome. On the contrary, high levels of microbiome–host species specificity and shared core sequences within a species was observed in five McMurdo Sound sponge species [9]. The same was found across several Antarctic continental shelf sponge species [10]. Webster and Bourne [11] also found conserved bacterial taxa dominated by microorganisms in the class Gammaproteobacteria across the soft coral, *Alcyonium antarcticum*, sampled at three sites in McMurdo Sound. Another cnidarian, the novel ice shelf burrowing sea anemone *Edwardsiella andrillae*, contained novel microbiota, though the composition across a limited set of individuals was only moderately conserved, in which some specimens were dominated by an OTU associated with the phylum Tenericutes, and others, a novel OTU in the class Alphaproteobacteria [12]. Lastly, a single representative of the Antarctic ascidian *Synoicum adareanum* revealed limited rRNA gene sequence diversity, including representatives of Actinobacteria, Bacteroidetes, Proteobacteria, Verrucomicrobia, and TM7 phyla [13], though persistence of these taxa across individuals was not studied.

Alcyonium antarcticum (formerly, *A. paessleri*) and *Synoicum adareanum* are both reported to be rich in secondary metabolites. The soft coral *A. antarcticum* produces sesquiterpenes that are unusual in bearing nitrate ester functional groups [14], while the ascidian, *S. adareanum*, is known to produce a family of macrolide polyketides, the palmerolides, which have potent activity against melanoma [15]. The role of the microbial community in contributing to host defensive chemistry, microbe–chemistry interactions and niche optimization, as well as microbe–microbe interactions, are unknown in these high-latitude environments.

Here, we have designed a study to investigate whether a core microbiome persists among *S. adareanum* holobionts that may inform our understanding of palmerolide origins. We conducted a spatial survey of *S. adareanum* in which we studied coordinated specimen-level quantitation of the major secondary metabolite, palmerolide A (PalA), along with the host-associated microbiome diversity and community structure across the Anvers Island Archipelago (64°46′ S, 64°03′ W) on the Antarctic Peninsula (Figure 1). The results point to a core suite of microbes associated with PalA-containing *S. adareanum*, distinct from the bacterioplankton, which will lead to downstream testing of the hypothesis that the PalA producer is part of the core microbiome.

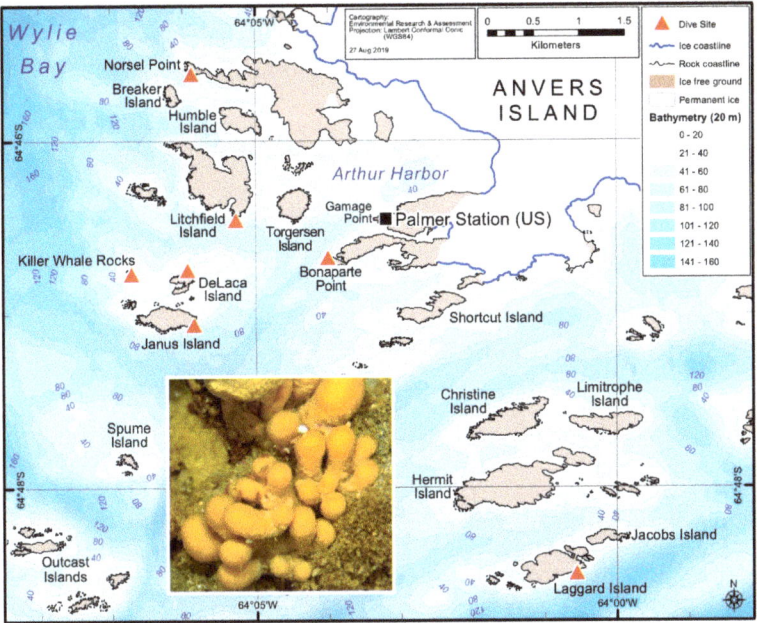

Figure 1. Bathymetric map of the study area off Anvers Island. *Synoicum adareanum* collection sites are shown with red triangles. The map was generated by Environmental Research and Assessment, Cambridge, UK, using Arthur Harbor bathymetry data from the PRIMO survey project 2004–2006 (Dr. Scott Gallagher and Dr. Vernon Asper). Inset: Colonial ascidian, *S. adareanum*, which occurs in clusters of multiple lobes connected by a peduncle which together comprise a colony on the seafloor, collected at depths ranging from 24 to 31 m.

2. Results

2.1. Variation in Holobiont PalA Levels Across Ascidian Colonies and Collection Sites

Typical procedures for natural product chemistry samples utilize bulk specimen collections for chemistry extraction (~30 individual ascidian lobes per lipophilic extraction in the case of *S. adareanum*). Prior to this study, variation in PalA content at the individual lobe or colony level (inset, Figure 1) was unknown. Our sampling design addressed within- and between-colony variation at a given sampling site, as well as between site variation. The sites were constrained to the region that was logistically accessible by Zodiac boat in the Anvers Island Archipelago off-shore of the United States Antarctic Program (USAP)-operated Palmer Station. *S. adareanum* colonies were sampled across seven dive sites (Figure 1), in which three lobes per multi-lobed colony were sampled from three colonies per dive site, totaling 63 lobes for PalA comparison. PalA stands out as the dominant peak in all LC–MS analyses of the dichloromethane:methanol soluble metabolite fraction of all samples analyzed (e.g., Figure 2a,b). The range in PalA levels varied at an order of magnitude of approximately 0.49–4.06 mg PalA x g^{-1} host dry weight across the 63 lobes surveyed. Our study design revealed lobe-to-lobe, intra-site colony level and some site-to-site differences in PalA levels ($p < 0.05$) in the archipelago (Figure 2c and Figure S1). Within a given colony, the lobe-to-lobe variation was often high and significantly different in 17 of 21 colonies surveyed. Significant differences in PalA levels between colonies were also observed within some sites (Janus Island (Jan), Bonaparte Point (Bon), Laggard Island (Lag), and Litchfield Island (Lit); see Figures 1 and 2c), in which at least one colony had significantly different levels compared to another colony or both. Despite this, we found differences between some of the sites. Namely, Bon was significantly lower than all six other sites. This site is the closest to the largest island, Anvers

Island, and Palmer Station. Samples from Killer Whale Rocks (Kil) and Lit sites were also found to have significantly higher PalA levels than Jan, Bon and Norsel Point (Nor), although these did not appear to have a particular spatial pattern or association with sample collection depth.

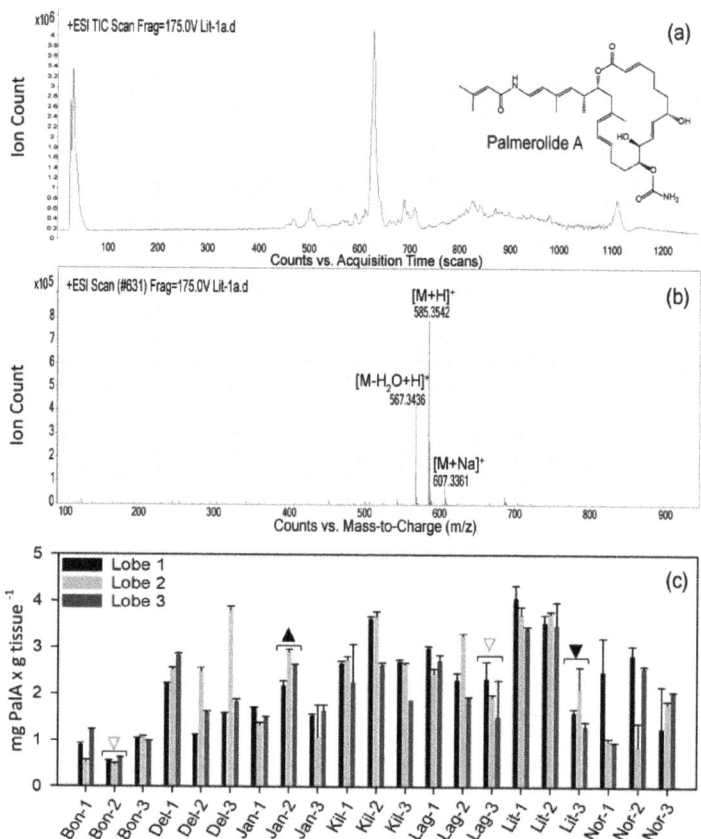

Figure 2. Palmerolide A (PalA) detection in *S. adareanum* holobionts. (**a**) Total ion chromatogram derived from sample Lit-1a. The PalA peak dominates the dichloromethane-methanol fraction of the *S. adareanum* extract. Inset: PalA structure. (**b**) Mass spectrum of PalA (sample Lit-1a) derived from peak at scan number 631 showing $[M - H_2O + H]^+$ ($C_{33}H_{47}N_2O_6$ calculated m/z 567.3429), $[M + H]^+$ ($C_{33}H_{48}N_2O_7$ calculated m/z 585.3534) and $[M + Na]^+$ ($C_{33}H_{47}N_2O_7Na$ calculated m/z 607.3359). (**c**) Levels of PalA normalized to tissue dry weight detected by mass spectrometry in *S. adareanum* holobiont tissues (three lobes per colony) surveyed in three colonies per site across the Anvers Island Archipelago. Error represents individual lobe technical replication (standard deviation). Colonies with significant differences in PalA levels within a site (e.g., Jan-1:Jan-2) are indicted with triangles, in which the direction of the point indicates a significantly higher or lower colony. Filled triangles indicate significance ($p < 0.05$) in comparison to the other two colonies, and open triangles are those that were different from only one of the two colonies. Most colonies had significant lobe-to-lobe differences in PalA concentration, and some site-level differences were observed (Figure S1).

2.2. Characterization of Host-Associated Cultivated Bacteria

Given our interest in identifying a PalA-producing microorganism [13], we executed a cultivation effort with *S. adareanum* homogenate on three different marine media formulations at 10 °C. The 16S rRNA gene sequencing revealed seven unique isolates (of 16 brought into pure culture) at a level of < 99% sequence identity. All but one of the isolates was affiliated with the class Gammaproteobacteria, including five different genera commonly isolated from marine environments (*Shewanella*, *Moritella*, *Photobacterium*, *Psychromonas* and *Pseudoalteromonas*—of which, nine were highly related). In many cases, we characterized their near neighbors as well-known marine psychrophiles, with many from polar habitats (Figure S2). The exception to this was the isolation of a cultivar associated with the Alphaproteobacteria class, *Pseudovibrio* sp. str. TunPSC04-5.I4, in which its two nearest neighbors were isolated from a temperate marine sponge and a temperate ascidian (associated with a different Ascidiacea family). This result marks the first *Pseudovibrio* sp. cultivated from high latitudes. HPLC screening results of biomass from all sixteen isolates did not reveal the presence of PalA.

2.3. Synoicum Adareanum Microbiome (SaM)

To understand the nature of conservation in the composition of the host-associated microbiome of *S. adareanum*, we identified the microbiome structure and diversity (based on the V3–V4 region of the 16S rRNA gene) with sections of the 63 samples used for holobiont PalA determinations. This effort resulted in 461 16S rRNA gene amplicon sequence variants (ASVs) distributed over 13 bacterial phyla (Table 1, Table S1). The core suite of microbes, defined as those present in > 80% of samples (referred to as the Core80), included 21 ASVs (six of which were present across all 63 samples). The Core80 ASVs represented the majority of the sequenced iTags (95% on average across all 63 samples), in which the first four ASVs dominated the sequence set (Figure 3). The ASVs present in 50%–79% of samples represented the Dynamic50 category and contained 14 ASVs, which represented only 3.3% of the data set. The remaining ASVs fell into the Variable fraction, which included 426 ASVs, representing 1.7% of the iTag sequences, yet the majority of phylogenetic richness (Table 1). Comparative statistical analyses were conducted with the complete sample set, which was subsampled to the lowest number (9987) of iTags per sample. This procedure was limited by one sample (Bon1b) that underperformed in terms of iTag sequence yield. After the elimination of this sample from the analysis, the 62-sample set had 19,003 iTags per sample with a total of 493 ASVs, the same 21 sequences in the Core80 (with seven common to all 62 samples), the same 14 Dynamic50 sequences, and a total of 458 Variable ASVs.

Table 1. Relative proportions (average +/− standard deviations, n = 63) of phyla (and class for the Proteobacteria) across the different microbiome fractions.

Phyla or Class	Whole Community	Core80	Dynamic50	Variable
Proteobacteria				
Gammaproteobacteria	71.990 ± 6.640	73.280 ± 6.330	51.300 ± 23.160	43.710 ± 23.630
Alphaproteobacteria	22.900 ± 5.390	23.830 ± 5.930		23.830 ± 19.700
Deltaproteobacteria	0.170 ± 0.100	0.160 ± 0.100		1.110 ± 2.000
Bacteroidetes	2.830 ± 2.140	0.790 ± 0.690	46.550 ± 22.910	17.40 ± 14.690
Verrucomicrobia	1.560 ± 2.800	1.590 ± 2.930		2.830 ± 3.970
Nitrospirae	0.270 ± 0.230	0.290 ± 0.240		0.020 ± 0.170
Planctomycetes	0.120 ± 0.130		2.150 ± 3.060	4.600 ± 12.840
Actinobacteria	0.100 ± 0.080	0.050 ± 0.050		3.150 ± 3.530
Patescibacteria	0.020 ± 0.090			0.840 ± 2.050
Dadabacteria	0.020 ± 0.003			1.220 ± 2.030
Uncl. Bacteria	0.009 ± 0.017			0.720 ± 1.530
Dependentiae	0.004 ± 0.018			0.340 ± 1.990
Chlamydiae	0.002 ± 0.006			0.190 ± 0.830
Acidobacteria	0.000 ± 0.003			0.020 ± 0.130
Chloroflexi	0.000 ± 0.003			0.020 ± 0.130
Epsilonbacteraeota	0.000 ± 0.001			0.010 ± 0.070

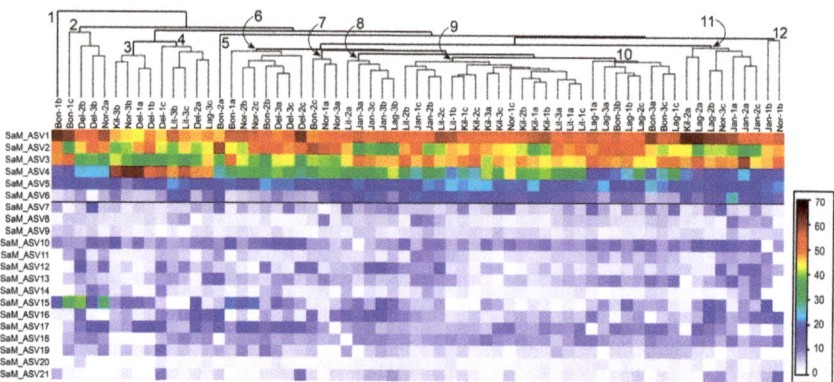

Figure 3. Heatmap of square root transformed amplicon sequence variant (ASV) occurrence data for the core microbiome. ASVs (ranked and numbered) are shown on the y-axis, and hierarchically clustered samples (63) are shown on the x-axis (site-based; square root transformed abundance data). Nodes with significant clusters are indicated from left to right ($p < 0.05$); order of clustering inside the node was not significant. The horizontal line drawn below SaM_ASV6 demarcates those ASVs that were present in all 63 samples.

The Core80 microbiome category included a relatively high degree of phylogenetic novelty, with nearly one-third of the membership having low (< 95.0%) sequence identities to nearest neighbors. At the same time, the rest of the Core80 ASVs (14) matched mostly uncultivated marine taxa from polar seas or sediments—in many cases, with identities > 97%. Several of the nearest neighboring sequences originated from marine invertebrate microbiomes. The Core80 ASVs were distributed across five phyla (Proteobacteria, Actinobacteria, Nitrospirae, Verrucomicrobia and Bacteroidetes; Table 1), in which seven highly related ASVs were associated with the Gammaproteobacteria genus *Microbulbifer*, and dominated the ASV sequences (Figure S1). Two other Gammaproteobacteria ASVs in the Core80 were affiliated with the *Endozoicomonas* genus (*SaM_ASV7*) and *Nitrosospira* (*SaM_ASV13*). There were several Alphaproteobacteria with nearest neighbors falling in *Pseudovibrio*, *Hoeflea*, *Sulfitobacter*, and *Octadecabacter*, genera. A Rhodospirillales-related sequence was only distantly related to known taxa, with an 86.6% sequence identity to its nearest neighbor. A Deltaproteobacteria *Bdellovibrio*-related ASV was also part of the Core80 microbiome (*SaM_ASV9*) that was also unique, with a sequence identity of 90.3% to its nearest neighbor. The Actinobacteria-affiliated core ASV (*SaM_ASV20*) was related to an uncultivated Solirubrobacterales sequence. ASV11 most closely matched a sequence in the Nitrospirae family from Arctic marine sediments. There were two Verrucomicrobium-affiliated sequences represented in different families (*Puniceicoccaceae*, SaM_ASV14, and *Opitutacae*, SaM_ASV15). Lastly, there were two ASVs affiliated with the phylum Bacteroidetes: one related to polar strain, *Brumimicrobium glaciale* (SaM_ASV19), and the other to a marine *Lutibacter* strain (SaM_ASV12).

Five Dynamic50 ASVs were affiliated with the marine Bacteroidetes phylum (*Cryomorphaceae* and *Flavobacteriacae*-related), in addition to six ASVs associated with the class Gammaproteobacteria (including four additional *Microbulbifer*-related sequences). There were also two additional phyla, an ASV related to a sponge-affiliated Verrucomicrobium isolate, and a Planktomycetes-related ASV (Table 1, Figure S2). Several of these ASVs were most closely related to isolates from marine sediments.

Interestingly, five sequences identified from earlier cloning and sequencing efforts with this host-associated microbiome (Figure S2; [13]) matched sequences in the Core80 and Dynamic50 data sets. Phylogenetic comparisons also revealed that the SaM isolates were distinct from the Core80 and Dynamic50 except for the *Pseudovibrio* sp. TunPSC04-5.I4 isolate, which was present in both the Core80, and the clone and sequencing study.

The hierarchical clustering of Core80 ASVs (based on Bray–Curtis similarity) across all 63 samples did not reveal strong trends in site or colony specific patterns (Figure 3). There were eight instances where two of three lobes paired as closest neighbors, and four of eight primary clusters that included three lobes derived from the same colony. Sample Bon1b clustered apart from them all. In some cases, clusters could be attributed to specific ASVs. For example, cluster 2 (Figure 3) had the highest relative levels of SaM_ASV15 (an *Opitutaceae* family-affiliated sequence), whereas cluster 3 (Figure 3) had the highest relative levels of ASV4 (affiliated with *Microbulbifer* spp.).

Overall, the community structures in the *S. adareanum* microbiomes across the 63 lobes surveyed had a high degree of similarity. Bray–Curtis pairwise similarity comparisons between lobes and colonies within each site were higher than 54% in all cases. When comparing the averages of pairwise similarity values within and between colonies, all sites, other than Lag, had higher similarity values within lobes in the same colony (ranging from 69.9% to 82.2%) compared to colonies within a site (66.5%–81.0%; Figure S3), although the differences were small, and only Bon and Jan were significantly different ($p < 0.05$). We performed a two-dimensional tmMDS analysis based on Bray–Curtis similarity to investigate the structure of the microbiome between sites (Figure 4a). The microbiomes sampled at Kil and Lit had the highest overall degree of clustering (> 75% similarity) while Kil, Lag, Lit, and Jan samples all clustered at a level of 65%. The microbiomes from DeLaca (Del) were the most dissimilar, which was supported by SIMPER analysis, in which two of the most abundant ASVs in the Core80 were lower than the average across other sites (SaM_ASV1 and 3) while others in the Core80 (SaM_ASV4, 15, and 17) were higher than the average across sites. We also performed a 2D tmMDS on the SaM fractions (Core80, Dynamic50, Variable) with and without permutational iterations, which showed similar trends although partitioning of community structures between sites was more evident with the permutations (Figure S4). Site-based clustering patterns shifted to some degree in the different SaM fractions. For the Core80 alone, Jan samples clustered apart from the others. For Dynamic50, both Jan and Kil were outliers. Finally, for the Variable fraction, Kil and Del samples clustered apart from the other sites. The Variable fraction was more homogeneous, obscuring any site-to-site variability, while the core displayed tighter data clouds that showed a modest level of dispersion.

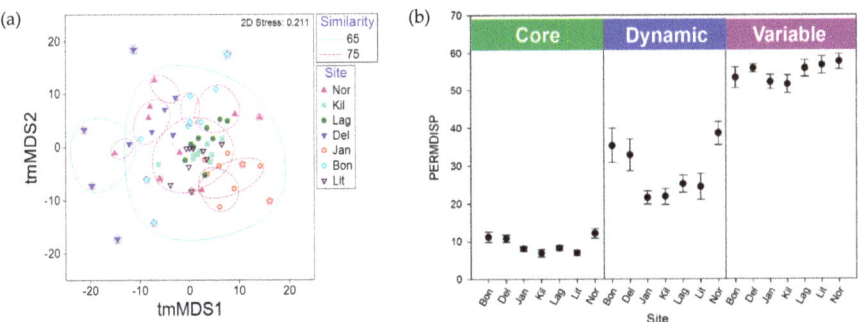

Figure 4. Similarity relationships amongst the *S. adareanum* microbiome samples in the Anvers Island Archipelago. (**a**) tmMDS of Bray–Curtis similarities of square root transformed ASV occurrence data representing the microbiome of the 63 *S. adareanum* lobe samples using the complete ASV occurrence profiles. Microbiome samples with significant levels of similarity are shown (see legend). (**b**) β-diversity across Anvers Island Archipelago sites represented by PERMDISP (9999 permutations) reveals differences between the highly persistent core, dynamic and variable portions of the *S. adareanum* microbiome (standard error shown). The degree of dispersion (variance) around the centroid changes significantly ($p < 0.0001$) for the different microbiome classifications. The lowest levels of dispersion are found in the core microbiome.

A PERMANOVA analysis investigated the drivers of variability in community structure, in which we tested the role of colony-level, site-level, and stochastic environmental variation. When evaluating the whole community (all sites and ASVs), site-to-site differences explained 25% of the variability in the microbiome (Table S2). Colony-to-colony differences explained 28%, while the remaining 47% of the variability was unexplained and is likely attributed to stochastic environmental variation. When the SaM fractions were analyzed separately, the most significant difference ($p < 0.05$) was in the Variable fraction of the microbiome, in which the site-to-site differences explained only 19.2% of the variation and the residual (stochastic) level increased to 58.4% (Table S2). Conversely, PERMDISP (Figure 4b), representing dispersion about the centroid calculated for each site (a measure of β-diversity), revealed differences in the community structures in each SaM fraction across sites, as well as differences between the microbiome fractions. The Core80 had a low level of dispersion (PERMDISP average of 9.1, range: 6.8-12.1), compared to the Dynamic50 (average 28.6, range: 24.5- 38.6), which were moderately dispersed about the centroid, and were more variable with differences between the more apparent sites; Bon, Del, and Nor had higher values compared to the other four sites. The Variable fraction had high PERMDISP values (average 54.7, range: 51.6–57.6), representing high differences in β-diversity, in which values were relatively close across the seven sites.

2.4. ASV Co-Occurrences, and Relationship to PalA

To further investigate the ascidian–microbiome ecology, we performed a network analysis of the ascidian holobiont with a particular emphasis on ASV co-occurrence and explored the relationship between ASV and PalA using direct and indirect measures. The co-occurrence network depicted a sparse graph with 102 nodes and 64 edges (average degree 1.255; diameter 15; average path length 5.81) that associated ASVs from similar SaM fractions (assortativity coefficient of 0.41), confirming the robustness of the above discrimination. Upon inspection of the co-occurrence network, a dominant connected component contained 42.1% of ASVs, in which we identified three highly connected modules (via the application of an independent network analysis WGCNA, soft threshold = 9, referred to here as subsystems; Figure 5). The network also contained several smaller systems (2–6 nodes), and 30 singletons—only one of which was in the Core80 (Gammaproteobacteria class, *Endozoicomonas*-affiliated). The three subsystems included ASVs from the Core80, Dynamic50 and Variable SaM fractions, but were unevenly distributed. Mostly driven by Core80 SaM fractions, Subsystem 1 harbored most of the highly represented ASVs, including the *Microbulbifer*-related ASVs as well as the *Pseudovibrio* ASV. Subsystem 2, interconnecting Subsystems 1 and 3, is mostly driven by Variable fraction ASVs and includes lower relative abundant Core80 *Hoeflea* and the *Opitutaceae* ASVs, as well as several *Bacteroidetes* taxa. Finally, Subsystem 3 was smaller. It included several diverse taxa dominated by Dynamic50 fraction, including *Lentimonas*, and *Cryomorphaceae*-affiliated ASVs from the Core80. The overall role of Variable ASVs in the network is surprising, as they appear to be critical nodes linking the subsystems via 13 edges that lie between Subsystems 2 and 3. Another, perhaps noteworthy smaller connected component is in the lower left of the graph, in which three Core80 ASVs, the chemoautotrophic ammonia and nitrite oxidizers, *Nitrosomonas* and *Nitrospira*, and an uncharacterized Rhodospirillales-related ASV, were linked with a Variable ASV.

To address the first-order question as to whether there was a relationship between the PalA concentration levels detected in the LC–MS analysis and the semi-quantitative ASV occurrences of *S. adareanum* ASVs, we performed three complementary analyses: correlation analysis, weighted co-occurrence networks analysis (WGCNA) and niche robust optima with PalA concentration as a variable. Pearson correlations between ASV occurrences and PalA concentrations ranged from −0.33 to 0.33 at the highest (24 of which were significant, ≤ 0.05; although none of those with a significant relationship were part of the core microbiome and were present in < 50% of the samples with the highest occurrence of 24 sequences), suggesting little relationship at the gross level of dry weight-normalized PalA and ASV relative abundance. This indicated that relative abundance of ASV is not a good predictor of PalA. A complementary WGCNA result showed no significant association between subsystem co-occurrence topology and PalA (correlations = −0.23; 0.033; −0.17 for subsystems 1, 2 and 3 respectively), pointing to the lack of relationship between microbial community structure and PalA. Finally, another aspect of the relationship between ASV occurrence and PalA levels was explored using the robust optimum method, which estimates the ecological optimum and tolerance range for ASVs about PalA. In this case, we calculated the PalA niche optimum for each ASV and ranked them based on the median (Figure S5). Core80 ASVs showed a consistent PalA niche range. Furthermore, the median optima values of the Dynamic50 ASVs lie, for the most part, in lower or higher PalA optima compared to the Core80, with a substantial niche overlap between Core80. The Variable ASVs collectively lie at the lower and higher extremes of the optimum and tolerance range. Altogether, these complementary analyses advocated for not considering an individual nor a community effect on PalA, but rather, acclimation to the high levels of PalA observed (Figure 2c) that likely rely on unknown metabolic or environmental controls.

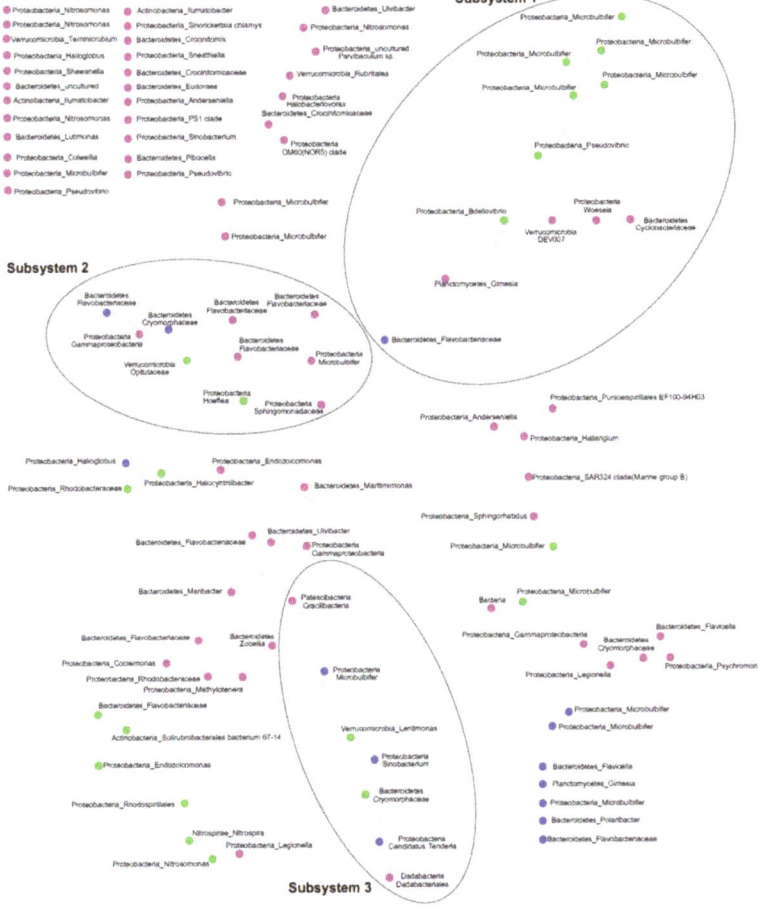

Figure 5. ASV co-occurrence network. The largest connected component of the co-occurrence network (seeded with ASVs found in at least 5 samples, 102 in total) identified three subsystems. Node colors represent the microbiome fractions (Core80, green; Dynamic50, blue; Variable, pink). Taxonomic identities of the ASVs are shown next to the nodes, with the phylum_highest level taxon identified shown.

2.5. Culture Collection: Microbiome and Bacterioplankton Comparisons

To address whether the composition of the *Synoicum adareanum*-associated bacterial cultivars was also present in the SaM or in the free-living bacterioplankton (< 2.5-µm fraction), we considered the overlap in membership between the isolate 16S rRNA gene sequences and these other two data sets. Representation of isolates in the 16S rRNA gene ASV data set was estimated by comparing the two sequence data sets, albeit different ascidian samples were used for the culture collection and the *S. adareanum* survey. Excepting *Pseudovibrio* sp. TunPSC04-5I4 that was present in the Core80 with a 100% sequence match, two other isolates also had 100% matches to sequences in the Variable SaM (BONS.1.10.24 and BOMB.9.10.19). Three other isolate 16S rRNA sequences (BOMB.3.2.14, BOMB.9.10.16, BOMB.9.10.21) were found to match sequences in the Variable microbiome at a level of 97% or higher. Only the *Pseudoalteromonas*-related isolate and the *Shewanella*-related isolate sequences were not detected with relatives at a level of at least 97% identity to the SaM ASVs; which could be explained by undersampling. The bacterioplankton composition was dominated by Gammaproteobacteria ASVs (47.35% of all ASVs; Table S3), in which six of the isolates (BOMB.9.10.21, BONS.1.10.24, BOMB.9.10.16, BOMB.3.2.20, BOMB.3.2.14, BONSW.4.10.32) matched sequences in the bacterioplankton data set at > 99.2% identity; even at a level of 95% sequence identity, the remaining ten isolates did not match sequences in the plankton, including the *Pseudovibrio* sp. str. TunPSC04-5I4 isolate.

2.6. Microbiome: Bacterioplankton Comparisons

Although at a high taxonomic level Proteobacteria and Bacteroidetes phyla dominated the microbiome and bacterioplankton (Table S3), the relative proportions varied and the taxa represented were quite different. Membership between SaM and the bacterioplankton data set indicated a low-level overlap at 100% identity, with 39 of 604 perfectly matched ASVs. At 100% ASV sequence identity, the results indicate a single, Core80 SaM ASV was a perfect match with the bacterioplankton data set—the *Microbulbifer*-associated sequence that is the most abundant across all 63 SaM data sets. Interestingly, this sequence was only identified in one bacterioplankton sample (IPY-225-9) at a low occurrence (14 of > 1.18 million tags distributed across 604 ASVs). There were three (of 14) Dynamic50 ASVs that were perfect matches with the bacterioplankton ASVs. These were affiliated with a poorly classified Bacteroidetes family Flavobacteraceae ASV (77% of SaM samples), a Gammaproteobacteria-associated *Sinobacterium* (73% of SaM samples), and a second Gammaproteobacteria-associated ASV that is associated with *Candidatus* Tenderia (71% of SaM samples). The remaining 35 perfect match ASVs between the two data sets were classified as part of the Variable microbiome. These sequences fell across four phyla and nine classes—13 of which were well distributed across the Bacterioplankton data set samples (> 50%).

At a level of 97% ASV sequence identity, there were three additional matches between the Bacterioplankton data set and the Core80. These included Alphaproteobacteria-related *Hoeflea* and *Halocynthibacter*-related sequences, and a *Nitrospira*-related sequence. There were also two other Dynamic50-related ASVs: these were both related to unclassified Flavobacteriaceae. The rest (79 ASVs) of the matches at > 97% were affiliated with the Variable fraction of the microbiome.

3. Discussion

This study reports our growing understanding of the microbiome composition of PalA-containing *S. adareanum*. To enhance our understanding of the ecology of the PalA-containing ascidian, *S. adareanum*, we investigated the ascidian colony microbiome and PalA chemistry levels at an individual lobe level, and compared the ascidian microbiome to the plankton. This comparison allowed us to address questions regarding variability in PalA content and whether a conserved core microbiome occurs across these PalA-containing Antarctic ascidians, thereby supporting the logic that if a microbial producer synthesizes PalA, the producing organism should be present in all PalA-containing *S. adareanum* samples. Before this study, however, we did not have quantitative data at the level of the individual ascidian lobe that forms the pedunculated *S. adareanum* colonies (Figure 1). This discussion focuses on the core microbiome, then takes a broader look at secondary metabolite distributions about the microbiome and in other marine invertebrates as well as the biosynthetic potential of core membership, and concludes with information gained from our initial cultivation effort.

3.1. Core Microbiome

Ascidian (host)-microbiome specificity is an active area of research. Compared to sponges and corals, for example, ascidian microbiomes have been less well characterized. To achieve a broad perspective on the microbiome composition, we also used cultivation-independent approaches. We found that the Antarctic ascidian *S. adareanum* has a persistent core microbiome across the Anvers Island Archipelago that is distinct from the plankton. This dissimilarity between ascidian host-associated microorganisms and bacterioplankton appears to be a consistent observation across the global ocean (e.g., [16–19]). The Core80 is comprised of ASVs that numerically dominate the community, as well as those representing only a fraction of a percent of the sequences surveyed. Although ascidian symbioses have not yet been systematically studied in the Antarctic, better-studied lower latitude ascidian microbiomes provide several examples for comparison. The overall trend across ascidian microbiome studies to date suggests that there is a high degree of both geographical as well as host species-level specificity of microbiome composition (e.g., [16,17,20]). The same appears to be true of *S. adareanum*. Although this study was restricted to a small geographical region, we identified a conserved core of 21 16S rRNA gene sequence types across 63 individual pedunculate lobes studied. We attribute the detection of this high degree of persistent members in part to the uniform homogenization, extraction, and sequencing methodological pipeline applied. Microbiome analysis is sensitive to sequencing depth, quality parameter choices, and algorithmic differences in data-processing pipelines (amplicon sequence variants vs. cluster-derived operational taxonomic units), which can impact direct comparisons between studies. Along these lines, the numerous highly related *Microbulbifer* ASVs would have fallen into a single OTU (97% sequence identity), resulting in a core with 14 members. These limitations aside, our findings are in line with several other ascidian microbiome studies from lower latitudes in terms of the relative size of core membership (where core definitions vary to some degree between studies). For example, *Styela plicata*, a solitary ascidian, was reported to have a core membership of 10 [21] to 16 OTUs [22]. Other solitary ascidians, including *Herdmania momus* had a core of 17 OTUs [21], while two *Ciona* species ranged from 8 to 9 OTUs [23]. Temperate colonial ascidians *Botryliodes leachi* and *Botryllus schlosseri* ranged from 10 to 11 members in their core microbiomes [20]. Further, an extensive survey of 10 different ascidian microbiomes (representing both solitary and colonial forms) conducted on the Great Barrier Reef reported core memberships ranging from 2 to 35 OTUs [16], while the numbers of individuals surveyed in each case were only 2–3. Note that a few other studies reported much higher numbers of shared OTUs ranging from 93 to 238 [18,19]; the scale of sequencing was higher in these later studies. Further, as others have reported [24], the membership of these core ascidian microbiomes is distinct, and in the case of SaM, the core microbiome diversity appears to be unique at the ASV level, although several taxa are in common with other ascidian-associated microbes at the genus level including *Microbulbifer* associated with *Cystodytes* sp. [25], *Pseudovibrio* with *Polycitor proliferus* [26] and an *Endozoicomonas*-specific clade was identified in a survey of a number of ascidians [27].

Predicted metabolic abilities of the Core80 taxa suggest aerobic heterotrophy (aerobic respiration—organic carbon is the carbon and energy source), microaerophily (growth in low oxygen conditions) and chemoautotrophy (CO_2 fixation provides carbon and reduced chemicals provide energy, e.g., NH_4^+ and NO_2^-) are themes amongst the Core80, in which the most abundant ASVs are high-molecular-weight carbon degraders. The *Microbulbifer* genus has members known to degrade cellulose [28], and perhaps noncoincidently, ascidians are the only known invertebrate capable of cellulose biosynthesis in the marine environment (e.g., [29,30]). From this, we could speculate that the *Microbulbifer* strains associated with *S. adareanum* could occupy a commensal, if not somewhat antagonistic, relationship [31]. In support of this possibility is the fact that the only overlapping sequence between the Core80 and the bacterioplankton was a *Microbulbifer* sequence, which was a rare sequence in the plankton, suggesting that it may be an opportunistic member of the *S. adareanum* microbiome. In addition, free-living and sponge-associated isolates from the *Microbulbifer* genus have been found to produce bioactive compounds including pelagiomicins [32] and parabens [33], respectively. This observation, in the least, suggests that the *Microbulbifer(s)* is/are likely well adapted to their ascidian host and might be considered a potential PalA-producing organism.

The NH_4^+-oxidizing *Nitrosopumilis*-affiliated Thaumarchaeota have been commonly detected in ascidian microbiomes [16,21,22,34], which contrasts phylogenetically, but not in terms of biogeochemical function, with the NH_4^+-oxidizing *Nitrosomonas* ASV that was part of the SaM core. The niche, however, has been reported to be different for the archaeal and bacterial NH_4^+ oxidizers, in which the archaea tend to be found in oligotrophic systems, while the bacteria (e.g., *Nitrosomonas*) can tolerate high levels of dissolved ammonia (reviewed by [35]). This result might reflect both the environment, and in situ *S. adareanum* tissue ammonia levels where it may accumulate. Several studies have reported on the high levels of oxidizing ammonia Thaumarchaeota in the coastal waters of the Anvers Island Archipelago which are numerous only in winter to early spring waters [36–38]. Our study was conducted with samples collected in Fall, when the ammonia-oxidizing Thaumarchaeota are not abundant in the coastal seawater [36], advocating for the comparisons between the SaM with bacterioplankton collected in both late summer and winter periods.

In a similar vein, although we did not intentionally conduct a temporal study, the data from samples collected in 2007 and 2011 appear to suggest that a number of the core microorganisms are stable over time. We found several ASVs in 2011 samples that matched (at 100% sequence identity) cloned sequences from samples collected in 2007 [13]. Stability of the ascidian microbiome over time has been reported in a few studies [17,24,34]. Studying the persistence of the core membership over the annual cycle would be interesting (and provide compelling evidence for stable relationships) in this high-latitude environment, where light, carbon production, and sea ice cover are highly variable.

The co-occurrence analysis indicated three subsystems of ASVs that co-occur within *S. adareanum*. A small side network included the two taxa involved with the 2-step nitrification process, including the *Nitrosomonas* ASV mentioned above and a *Nitrospira* ASV. Even though at present, the functional underpinnings of the host–microbial system have not been studied, the co-occurrence relationships provide fodder for hypothesis testing in the future. One interaction network that warrants mentioning here is the ASVs in Subsystem 1, which harbor several Core80 *Microbulbifer* ASVs, and the *Pseudovibrio* ASV are linked to a *Bdellovibrio* ASV that is also a member of the Core80. Members of the *Bdellovibrio* genus are obligate bacterial predators [39] that penetrate the outer membrane and cell wall of their prey. The linkage position in the subsystem is compelling in the sense that the *Bdellovibrio* could potentially control the abundance of the connected members of the network. Lastly, the positions of a couple of Dynamic and several the Variable ASVs in the network, as links between the subsystems, was unexpected. The central positions of these ASVs suggest that they may not be merely stochastic members of the microbiome; that they could play opportunistic, adaptive or ecological roles in the functionality of the microbiome subsystem(s) which potentially participate in different aspects of the holobiont system in particular, by promoting the switch between different ecological modes supported by different subsystems. Such roles were proposed for dynamic members of the *Styela plicata* microbiome [21].

The culturing effort succeeded in isolating a *Pseudovibrio* strain that is a crucial member of the Core80. In addition, several other Gammaproteobacteria-affiliated strains which matched sequences in the Variable SaM and the bacterioplankton were cultivated. However, the cultivated diversity using the approaches applied here reared a collection of limited diversity. It is likely that additional media types and isolation strategies could result in additional cultivated diversity as there are a number of taxa with aerobic heterotrophic lifestyles in the Core80 that have been brought into pure culture (e.g.,

Microbulbifer, Hoeflea). One challenge we experienced using the nutrient-replete media was overgrowth of plates, even at 10 °C.

3.2. Secondary Metabolite Distributions and Bioaccumulation in Marine Biota

Although the results of the archipelago spatial ascidian survey did not support a direct relationship between PalA levels and the relative abundance of microbiome ASVs, the results of the PalA niche analysis suggests that the Core80 ASVs occur in a preferred optimum and tolerance range of PalA levels. The lack of specific ASV-PalA patterns may not be entirely surprising, as secondary metabolites result from a complex combination of metabolic reactions that require a fine-tuning to environmental conditions and further metabolic modeling for the sake of understanding. Furthermore, these metabolites have been found to accumulate in the tissues in several different marine invertebrates. The Optimal Defense Theory can be applied to marine invertebrates and reflects the hypothesis that secondary metabolites are distributed in specific tissues based on exposure and anatomic susceptibility for predation [39]. For example, nudibranchs sequester toxic compounds, which have been biosynthesized by the gastropod or acquired from their prey. The toxins are concentrated in the anatomical space of their mantles, the most vulnerable portion of their soft, exposed bodies [40–42]. Bioaccumulation of secondary metabolites in invertebrates with less anatomical differentiation is also known to occur. In the phylum Porifera, different cell types and layers have been studied to determine spatial and anatomical differences in secondary metabolite concentrations [43–45]. Compounds have been found to be concentrated spatially on the surface (e.g., [46]) or apical parts of the sponge [47] in some cases. Sponges may be able to differentially bioaccumulate secondary cytotoxic metabolites based on tissues more susceptible to predation [48]. Metabolite distribution investigations that are ascidian-specific are less well documented; however, there is also evidence of ascidian secondary cytotoxic metabolite bioaccumulation. The patellazoles, marine macrolides from the ascidian *Lissoclinum patella*, bioaccumulate in the ascidian tissues to concentrations up to seven orders of magnitude higher than their cytotoxic dose in mammalian cell lines [49,50]. Additionally, there are other instances in which bioaccumulation in ascidian host tissues suggests metabolic cooperation of producer and host as well as compound translocation from producer to host [15,51,52]. Although the PalA levels were normalized to grams of dry lobe weight, tissue-specific spatial localization is a potentially confounding factor in the statistical analyses investigating the ASV:PalA relationship.

3.3. The Biosynthetic Potential of the Core

We investigated the natural product biosynthetic potential of the nine genera associated with 15 of 21 Core80 ASVs using antiSMASH (Table 2, Table S4). From this, it appears that all genera had at least one relative at the genus level with biosynthetic capacity for either polyketide or nonribosomal peptide biosynthesis or both. Even though the number of genomes available to survey were highly uneven, there is quite a disparity of biosynthetic capacity between the genera analyzed, thus, it appears that *Pseudovibrio, Nitrosomonas, Microbulbifer, Nitrospira* have the greatest capacities (in that order). Likewise, *Microbulbifer, Pseudovibrio, Hoeflea* and *Opitutaceae* might be prioritized as candidate PalA producers based solely on relative abundance ranking (Table 2; [24]). Although we did not conduct this analysis for the six ASVs that were classified at best at the family or order level, a few of these might be worth considering as potential producers considering their higher-level relationships with marine natural product producing lineages. For example, marine actinobacteria are classically associated with the production of numerous bioactive natural products (e.g., [53,54]), although speculation is difficult with actinobacteria SaM_ASV20 in the core as it is only distantly related to known natural product producers. Likewise, *Opitutaceae*-related SaM_ASV15 is ranked 7 in terms of average relative abundance and falls in the same family the ascidian-associated *Candidatus* Didemnitutus mandela, which harbors the biosynthetic gene cluster predicted to produce mandelalide, a glycosylated polyketide [55]. From this, we might prioritize the *Microbulbifer, Pseudovibrio,* and *Opitutaceae* ASVs for downstream investigation, with the lower relative abundance *Nitrosomonas* and *Nitrospira* ASVs also holding some potential given the perhaps surprising abundance of biosynthetic gene cluster content in these chemoautotrophic, and generally small genome-size taxa. Although this analysis focused on predicted pathway characterizations across genera detected, the distributions of predicted pathways varied substantially across the taxa analyzed. The potential for these new Antarctic ascidian-associated strains to harbor secondary metabolite pathways remains speculative as they are amongst the most variable component of a bacterium's genome.

Table 2. Taxonomic affiliations of core microbiome, relative abundance rank, and the potential of affiliated genus in natural product gene cluster biosynthesis. Taxonomy is shown according to genome taxonomy database (GTDB) classification and NCBI taxonomy is included (GTDB/NCBI) where they differ. Biosynthetic potential only calculated for ASVs with genus-level taxonomic assignments was based on representative genome biosynthetic gene cluster content in the same genus (See Figure S3 for list of genomes). ASVs in bold ranked in the top 10. Where more than one ASV was found per genus, the average relative abundance and standard deviations were summed. n = 63 individuals.

ASV_ID	Phylum, Highest Taxonomic Assignment	Average Relative Abundance (%)	Rank	Nearest Neighbor % Identity	NRP BGC	PKS BGC	Combined NRP-PKS
SaM_ASV1, 2, 4, 5, 10, 17, 18	**Proteobacteria, *Microbulbifer***	**77.54 ± 21.86**	**1, 2, 4, 5, 8, 9, 10**	**97.42**	**+**	**+**	**-**
SaM_ASV7	Proteobacteria, *Endozoicomonas*	0.47 ± 0.51	13	96.71	+	+	-
SaM_ASV13	Proteobacteria, *Nitrosomonas*	0.46 ± 0.35	14	99.77	+	+	+
SaM_ASV3	**Proteobacteria, *Pseudovibrio***	**19.92 ± 4.74**	**3**	**98.75**	**+**	**+**	**+**
SaM_ASV6	**Proteobacteria, *Hoeflea***	**1.59 ± 1.36**	**6**	**99.25**	**+**	**+**	**+**
SaM_ASV16	Proteobacteria, *Halocynthiibacter*	0.63 ± 0.64	11	99.75	+	-	-
SaM_ASV11	Nitrospirota/Nitrospirae, *Nitrospira*	0.27 ± 0.23	15	98.32	+	+	+
SaM_ASV12	Bacteroidota/Bacteroidetes, *Lutibacter*	0.50 ± 0.55	12	94.54	+	-	+
SaM_ASV14	Verrucomicrobiota/Verrucomicrobia, *Lentimonas*	0.16 ± 0.22	19	99.77	+	-	+
Sam_ASV21	Proteobacteria, *Rhodobacteraceae*	0.18 ± 0.26	18	98.75	-	-	-
SaM_ASV8	Proteobacteria, *Rhodospirillales*	0.22 ± 0.22	17	86.60	-	-	-
SaM_ASV9	Bdellovibrionota/Proteobacteria, *Bdellovibrionaceae*	0.15 ± 0.09	20	90.35	-	-	-
SaM_ASV19	Bacteroidetes, *Cryomorphaceae*	0.24 ± 0.23	16	89.10	-	-	-
SaM_ASV15	**Verrucomicrobiota/Verrucomicrobia, *Opitutaceae***	**1.34 ± 2.77**	**7**	**90.14**	**-**	**-**	**-**
SaM_ASV20	Actinobacteria, *Solirubrobacterales*	0.05 ± 0.05	21	91.80	-	-	-

4. Conclusions

This work has advanced our understanding of the Antarctic ascidian *S. adareanum*, PalA distributions, and microbiome in several ways. First, we found PalA to be a dominant product across all 63 samples, with some variation but no coherent trends with the site, sample, or microbiome ASV. Second, the results point to a conserved, core, microbiome represented by 21 ASVs—20 of which appear to be distinct from the Antarctic bacterioplankton. The phylogenetic distribution of these taxa was diverse and distinct from other ascidian microbiomes in which organisms with both heterotrophic and chemosynthetic lifestyles are predicted. Third, the co-occurrence analysis suggested the potential for ecologically interacting microbial networks that may improve our understanding of this ascidian–microbiome–natural product system. Likewise, based on the occurrence and likelihood of natural product biosynthesis, there are a number of taxa that may bear biosynthetic capabilities, including that of PalA. These results advance the long-term goal of palmerolide-producing *Synoicum adareanum* and host-associated microbiome research, which is compelled by the fact that by identifying the producer, genome sequencing could then provide information on PalA biosynthesis, and then lead to the development of a potential therapeutic agent to fight melanoma.

5. Materials and Methods

5.1. Cultivation-Dependent Effort

S. adareanum samples collected by SCUBA in 2004 and 2007 were used for cultivation (Table S5). The 2004 specimen were archived in 20% glycerol at −80 °C until processing by manual homogenization using sterilized mortar and pestle prior to plating a suspension onto marine agar 2216 (BD Difco™, Franklin Lakes, NJ, USA) plates in 2006. The 2007 samples were homogenized immediately following collection using sterilized mortar and pestle, and suspensions were prepared in 1X marine broth 2216 or filter-sterilized Antarctic seawater then transferred at 4 °C to DRI. Shortly after (within 1 month of collection), the 2007 isolates were cultivated on three types of media in which suspensions initially stored in marine broth 2216 were plated onto marine agar (2216), while homogenate preparations stored in seawater were plated onto VNSS agar media [56] and Antarctic seawater agar plates amended with 3 g yeast extract (BD Difco™), 5 g peptone (BD Difco™), and 0.2 g casein hydroslyate (BD Difco™) per liter. Colonies were selected from initial plates, and purified through three rounds of growth on the same media they were isolated on.

5.2. Field Sample Collections for Cultivation-Independent Efforts

Next, a spatial survey of *Synoicum adareanum* was executed in which samples were collected by SCUBA in austral fall between 23 March and 3 April 2011. Seven sampling sites (depths 24.7–31 m; Table S6) around the region accessible by Zodiac boat from Palmer Station were selected in which we sampled in a nested design where three multi-lobed colonies were selected from each site, and three lobes per colony were sampled (Figure 1). At each dive site, multi-lobed colonies were collected by hand into separate mesh collecting bags. Underwater video [57] was taken at each site, then video footage was observed to note general ecosystem characteristics (% cover of major benthic species and algae). In total, 63 *S. adareanum* lobes were sampled (9 from each site). Samples were transported to Palmer Station on ice and multi-lobed colony samples were placed in sterile Whirl-Pak®bags (Nasco, Fort Atkinson, WI, USA) and frozen at −80 °C, until processing at DRI and USF. At DRI, frozen pedunculated *S. adareanum* lobes were separated, then cut longitudinally in half for parallel processing through DNA and palmerolide detection pipelines.

Then, to address whether the composition of the SaM was distinct from the free-living bacterioplankton (< 2.5 μm fraction), we considered the overlap in membership between the SaM and bacterioplankton in the water column. To accomplish this, we used a reference seawater data set represented by samples that had been collected in the period February–March 2008 (five samples) and in the period August–September 2008 (nine samples) from LTER Station B near Anvers Island (east of the Bonaparte Point dive site), and at a few other locations in the region (Table S7). Seawater samples were collected by a submersible pump and acid washed silicone tubing at 10 m at Station B, and using a rosette equipped with 12 L Niskin bottles for the offshore samples at 10 and 500 m (2 samples each depth). The February–March seawater samples were processed using in-line filtration with a 2.5 μm filter (Polygard, MilliporeSigma, Burlington MA, USA) to screen larger organisms and bacterioplankton were concentrated using a tangential flow filtration system and the cells were harvested on 25 mm and 0.2 μm Supor filters (MilliporeSigma). The August–September seawater samples were processed using inline filtration with a 3.0 μm filter (Versapor, MilliporeSigma), and then bacterioplankton was collected onto 0.2 μm Sterivex (MilliporeSigma) filters using a multichannel peristaltic pump (Masterflex®, Cole-Parmer, Vernon Hills, IL, USA). All filters were immersed in sucrose:Tris:EDTA buffer [58] and stored frozen at −80 °C until extraction.

5.3. Palmerolide A Screening

Sixty-three frozen *S. adareanum* lobes were cut in half. Half lobes were lyophilized and then exhaustively extracted using dichloromethane for three days, followed by methanol for three days. The extracts were combined and dried on a rotary evaporator. The extracts were filtered, dried down, and reconstituted at 1.0 mg/mL to ensure the injected concentration was consistent. The residue was subjected to liquid chromatography-mass spectrometry (LC–MS) analysis using a H_2O:ACN gradient with constant 0.05% formic acid. The high-resolution mass spectra were recorded on an Agilent Technologies 6230 electrospray ionization Time-of-Flight (ESI-ToF) spectrometer. LC–MS was performed using a C-18 Kinetex analytical column (50 × 2.1 mm; Phenomenex, Torrance, CA, USA). The presence of PalA was verified using MS/MS on an Agilent Technologies 6540 UHD Accurate-Mass QTOF LC–MS.

The *S. adareanum*-associated microbial culture collection was screened for the presence of PalA. Isolates were cultivated in 30 mL volumes, and the resulting biomass was lyophilized and screened by HPLC. Each sample was analyzed in ESI-SIM mode targeting masses of 585 amu and 607 amu. The reversed-phase chromatographic analysis consisted of a 0.7 mL × min^{-1} solvent gradient from 80% H$_2$O:CH$_3$CN to 100% CH$_3$CN with constant 0.05% formic acid using the same C-18 column as above. The analysis was conducted for over 18 min. PalA had a retention time of approximately 14 min. The twenty-four sample sequence was followed by a PalA standard to confirm its analytical characteristics.

5.4. S. Adareanum-Associated Microbial Cell Preparation

The outer 1–2 mm of the ascidian tissue, which could contain surface-associated microorganisms, was removed using a sterilized scalpel before sectioning tissue subsamples (~0.2 g) of frozen (−80 °C) *S. adareanum* ($\frac{1}{2}$ lobe sections). Tissue samples were diced with a sterile scalpel before homogenization in sterile autoclaved and filtered seawater (1 mL) in 2 mL tubes. Each sample was homogenized (MiniLys, Bertin Instruments, Montigny-le-Bretonneux, France) using sterile CK28 beads (Precellys, Bertin Instruments) 3 times at 5000 rpm for 20 s, samples were placed on ice in between each homogenization. Homogenates were centrifuged at 500× *g* at 4 °C for 5 min to pellet tissue debris. The supernatant was removed to a new tube for a second spin at the same conditions. This supernatant was decanted and the cell suspension centrifuged at 12,000× *g* at 4 °C for 5 min to collect the microbial cells. Suspensions were stored on ice, then entered an extraction pipeline, in which 12 samples were processed in parallel on the QIAvac 24 Plus Manifold (Qiagen Inc., Germantown, MD, USA).

5.5. DNA Extractions

S. adareanum-associated microbial cell preparations were extracted with Powerlyzer DNEasy extraction (Qiagen Inc.) following the manufacturer's instructions starting at with the addition of the lysis solution. Samples were processed in parallel in batches of twelve at a time using the QiaVac 24 Plus Vacuum Manifold. Two rounds of lysis (5000 rpm for 60 s each with incubation on ice) were performed on the MiniLys using the 0.1 mm glass beads that come with the Powerlyzer kit. DNA concentrations of final preparations were estimated using Quant-iT Picogreen dsDNA Assay Kit (Invitrogen) fluorescence detection on a Spectramax Gemini (Molecular Devices, Mountain View, CA, USA).

DNA from bacterioplankton samples was extracted following [58], and DNA from bacterial cultures was extracted using the DNeasy Blood and Tissue kit (Qiagen Inc.) following the manufacturer's instructions. All DNA concentrations were estimated using Picogreen.

5.6. The 16S rRNA Gene Sequencing

Illumina tag sequencing for the *S. adareanum* microbiome (SaM) targeted the V3–V4 region of the 16S rRNA gene using prokaryote-targeted primers 341F (5'-CCTACGGGNBGCASCAG-3' [59]) and 806R (5'-GGACTACHVGGGTWTCTAAT-3' [60]; source: Integrated DNA Technologies). The first round of PCR amplified the V3–V4 region using HIFI HotStart Ready Mix (Kapa Biosystems, Wilmington, MA, USA). The first round of PCR used a denaturation temperature of 95 °C for 3 min, 20 cycles of 95 °C for 30 s, 55 °C for 30 s and 72 °C for 30 s and followed by an extension of 72 °C for 5 min before holding at 4 °C. The second round of PCR added Illumina-specific sequencing adapter sequences and unique indexes, permitting multiplexing, using the Nextera XT Index Kit v2 (Illumina, Inc., San Diego, CA, USA) and HIFI HotStart Ready Mix (Kapa Biosystems). The second round of PCR used a denaturation temperature of 95 °C for 3 min, 8 cycles of 95 °C for 30 s, 55 °C for 30 se and 72 °C for 30 s and followed by an extension of 72 °C for 5 min before holding at 4 °C. Amplicons were cleaned up using AMPure XP beads (Beckman Coulter, Indianapolis, IN, USA). A no-template PCR amplification control was processed but did not show a band in the V3–V4 amplicon region and was sequenced for confirmation. A Qubit dsDNA HS Assay (ThermoFisher Scientific, Waltham, MA, USA) was used for DNA concentration estimates. The average size of the library was determined by the High-Sensitivity DNA Kit (Agilent) and the Library Quantification Kit—the Illumina/Universal Kit (KAPA Biosystems) quantified the prepared libraries. The amplicon pool sequenced on Illumina MiSeq generated paired-end 301 bp reads was demultiplexed using Illumina's bcl2fastq.

The bacterioplankton samples sent to the Joint Genome Institute (JGI, Walnut Creek, CA, USA) for library preparation and paired-end (2 × 250 bp) MiSeq Illumina sequencing of the prokaryote-targeted variable region 4 (V4) using primers 515F (5'-GTGCCAGCMGCCGCGGTAA-3') and 806R (5'-GGACTACHVGGGTWTCTAAT-3' [60]; source: Integrated DNA Technologies). No-template PCR amplification controls were run as above, and were negative. Sequence processing included removal of PhiX contaminants and Illumina adapters at JGI.

The identity of the cultivated isolates was confirmed by 16S rRNA gene sequencing using Bact27F and Bact1492R primers either by directly sequencing agarose gel-purified PCR products (Qiagen Inc.), or TA cloning (Invitrogen, ThermoFisher Scientific) of PCR fragments into *E. coli* following the manufacturer's instructions, in which three clones were sequenced for each library and plasmids were purified (Qiagen Inc.) at the Nevada Genomics Center, where Sanger sequencing was conducted on an ABI3700 (Applied Biosystems, Life Technologies, Foster City, CA, USA). Sequences were trimmed and quality checked using Sequencer, v. 5.1.

5.7. Bioinformatic Analysis of 16S rRNA Gene tag Sequences

We employed a QIIME2 pipeline [61] using the DADA2 plug-in [62] to de-noise the data and generate amplicon sequence variant (ASV) occurrence matrices for the SaM and bacterioplankton samples. The rigor of ASV determination was used in this instance given the increased ability to uncover variability in the limited geographic study area, interest in uncovering patterns of host-specificity, and ultimately in identifying the conserved, core members of the microbiome—at least one of which may be capable of PalA biosynthesis. Sequence data sets were initially imported into QIIME2 working format and the quality of forward and reverse were checked. Default trimming parameters included trimming all bases after the first quality score of 2, in addition, the first 10 bases were trimmed, and reads shorter than 250 bases were discarded. Next the DADA2 algorithm was used to de-noise the reads (corrects substitution and insertion/deletion errors and infers sequence variants). After de-noising, reads were merged. The ASVs were constructed by grouping the unique full de-noised sequences (the equivalent of 100% OTUs, operational taxonomic units). The ASVs were further curated in the QIIME2-DADA2 pipeline by removing chimeras in each sample individually if they can be exactly reconstructed by combining a left segment and a right segment from two more abundant "parent" sequences. A pre-trained SILVA 132 99% 16S rRNA Naive Bayes classifier (https://data.qiime2.org/2019.1/common/silva-132-99-nb-classifier.qza) was used to perform the taxonomic classification. Compositions of the SaM and the bacterioplankton ASVs were summarized by proportion at different taxonomy levels, including genus, family, order, class, and phylum ranks. In order to retain all samples for diversity analysis, we set lowest reads frequency per sample (n = 62 samples at 19,003 reads; n = 63 samples at 9987 reads) as rarefaction depth to normalize the data for differences in sequence count. ASVs assigned to Eukarya or with unassigned taxa (suspected contaminants) were removed from the final occurrence matrix such that the final matrix read counts were slightly uneven with the lowest number of reads per sample with 9961 reads.

The SaM ASVs were binned into Core (highly persistent) if present in $\geq$ 80% of samples (Core80), Dynamic if present in 50%–79% of samples (Dynamic50) and those that comprise the naturally fluctuating microbiome, or Variable fraction, which was defined as those ASVs present in < 50% of the samples [2,3]. We used these conservative groupings of the core microbiome due to the low depth of sequencing in our study [3].

ASV identities between the SaM, the *S. adareanum* bacterial isolates and the bacterioplankton data sets were compared using CD-HIT (cd-hit-est-2d; http://cd-hit.org). The larger SaM data set which included 19,003 sequences per sample was used for these comparisons to maximize the ability to identify matches; note that this set does exclude one sample, Bon1b, which had half as many ASVs, though overall this larger data set includes nearly 200 additional sequences in the Variable fraction for comparison. ASVs with 100% and 97% identity between the pairwise comparisons were summarized in terms of their membership in the Core, Dynamic or Variable fractions of the SaM. Likewise, CD-HIT was used to dereplicate the isolate sequences at a level of 99% sequence identity, and then the dereplicated set was compared against the bacterioplankton iTag data set.

Phylogenetic analysis of the SaM ASVs, *S. adareanum* bacterial isolates, and 16S rRNA gene cloned sequences from Riesenfeld et al. [13] was conducted with respect to neighboring sequences identified in the Ribosomal Database Project and SILVA and an archaea outgroup using MEGA v.7 [63]. Two maximum likelihood trees were constructed—the first with the Core80 ASVs, and the second with both Core80 and Dynamic50 ASVs. A total of 369 aligned positions were used in both trees. A total of 1000 bootstrap replicates were run in both instances, in which the percentage ($\geq 50\%$) of trees in which the associated taxa clustered together are shown next to the branches.

5.8. Statistical Analyses

T-tests were run in Statistica (v. 13, Tibco Software, Palo Alto, CA, USA) to determine significance ($p < 0.05$) of site-to-site, within- and between-colony variation in PalA concentrations. Similarity matrix and hierarchical clustering analyses were performed using PRIMER v.7 and PERMANOVA+ (PRIMER-e, Auckland, New Zealand). Analyses were performed on the complete microbiome as well as the three microbiome fractions in most cases. The ASV occurrence data were square root transformed for all analyses. A heat map based on the Core80 ASV occurrence was generated with the transformed data, and hierarchical clustering with group average parameter was employed, which was integrated with SIMPROF confidence using 9,999 permutations and a 5% significance level. Bray–Curtis resemblance matrixes were created using ASV occurrences without the use of a dummy variable. To determine basic patterns in community structure within- vs. between-colony and site variation, the significance was determined by t-test using Statistica v. 13. To compare within- (n = 9) vs. between-colony variation (n = 27), nine between-colony pairwise similarity values were randomly sampled in order to compare equal sample sizes, checking that the homogeneity of variance was similar between them. Then threshold metric Multi-Dimensional Scaling (tmMDS) was conducted based on Kruskal fit scheme 1, including 500 iterations, and a minimum stress of 0.001. Similarity profile testing through SIMPROF was performed based on a null hypothesis that no groups would demonstrate differences in ASV occurrences. This clustering algorithm was also used to generate confidence levels on the MDS plot, which were set to 65% and 75%. In addition, 95% bootstrap regions were calculated with 43 bootstraps per group, set to ensure a minimum rho of 0.99. In order to assess the contribution of each factor to the variance of the microbial community in this nested experimental design, Site(Colony), permutational multivariate analysis of variance (PERMANOVA) was used. Site-based centroids were calculated and the PERMDISP algorithm was used to determine the degree of dispersion around the centroid for each site. Overall, site-to-site difference in dispersion was determined and pairwise comparisons were also calculated, with 9999 permutations used to determine significance (P(perm) < 0.05). Exploratory analysis of the major ASV contributors to similarity was performed using the SIMPER procedure based on sites and colonies, with a cut off for low contributions set to 70%.

Co-occurrence networks were constructed using filtered ASV occurrence data sets in which the ASV were filtered to only those that were present in at least five samples resulting in a 102 ASV data set. The 102 × 63 matrix was provided as input to FlashWeave v1.0 [64] using default parameters, and visualized in Gephi v. 0.9.2 [65]. Then to consider whether the ASVs in the Core80, Dynamic50, or Variable fractions of the SaM were affiliated with particular levels of PalA in the ascidian lobes, PalA niche robust optimum and range were computed using the occurrence and dry weight-normalized contextual data [66]. Weighted gene correlation network analysis (WGCNA package in R [67]) was used to identify modules and their correlation with PalA levels. The matrix was total-sum normalized [68], and WGCNA was used in signed mode. There were few modules detected, although they were not correlated with PalA. Modules were projected on the FlashWeave co-occurrence network and called subsystems.

5.9. Biosynthetic Gene Cluster Analysis

Subsequently, in order to predict the likelihood of Core80 ASV lineages harboring the potential for natural product biosynthesis, we designed a meta-analysis of neighboring genomes found at the Integrated Microbial Genomes (IMG) database [69]. The analysis was conducted only for ASVs in which confidence of taxonomic assignment was at the genus level. Therefore, genomes were harvested from IMG that were associated with a total of 9 genera (*Microbulbifer* (16 genomes), *Pseudovibrio* (24 genomes), *Endozoicomonas* (11 genomes), *Nitrosomonas* (19 of 68 total genomes in this genus), *Nitrospira* (14 genomes), *Hoeflea* (7 genomes), *Lutibacter* (12 genomes), *Halocynthilibacter* (2 genomes), and in the case of *Lentimonas*, since no genomes were found, we harvested 8 genomes from the *Puniciococcaceae* family). This results in 113 genomes that were submitted to antiSMASH [70] for analysis. The genomes and counts of biosynthetic gene clusters assigned to nonribosomal peptide synthase, polyketide synthase, or a hybrid of the two classes were tabulated (Table S4).

5.10. Data Availability

Synoicum adareanum microbiome Illumina sequence information and associated metadata are described under NCBI BioProject PRJNA597083 (https://www.ncbi.nlm.nih.gov/bioproject/?term=PRJNA597083), and the *S. adareanum* culture collection 16S rRNA gene sequences were deposited in GenBank under MN960541- MN960556. The bacterioplankton sequence information and associated metadata are described under NCBI BioProject PRJNA602715 (https://www.ncbi.nlm.nih.gov/bioproject/?term=PRJNA602715). Antarctic project metadata [71] and environmental metadata (data set identifiers: Synoicum_adareanum_microbiome_part1, Synoicum_adareanum_microbiome_part2, Synoicum_adareanum_microbiome_part3) are available at: POLA$_3$R (2020)—POLA$_3$R Polar Links to Antarctic, Arctic and Alpine Research. Scientific Committee on Antarctic Research, Antarctic biodiversity portal, (www.biodiversity.aq/pola3r/).

Supplementary Materials: The following are available online at http://www.mdpi.com/1660-3397/18/6/298/s1, Table S1: ASV occurrences, sequences, and taxonomic affiliations, Table S2: PERMANOVA estimators of drivers of variability, Table S3: Taxonomic distribution of bacterioplankton ASVs, Table S4: Biosynthetic gene clusters in bacterial genomes related to Core80 SaM genera, Table S5: *Synoicum adareanum* collections and preparations for microbiome cultivation, Table S6: *Synoicum adareanum* collections for palmerolide A and microbiome characterization by V3–V4 rRNA gene tag sequencing, Table S7: Bacterioplankton collections used in v4 rRNA gene tag sequencing. Figure S1: Results of pairwise t-tests of PalA levels determined by mass spectrometry, Figure S2: Maximum likelihood 16S rRNA gene phylogenetic tree, Figure S3: Average pairwise similarity within and between *S. adareanum* microbiome community structures, Figure S4: tmMDS plots representing the microbiome of the 63 *S. adareanum* samples, and Figure S5. PalA niche optimum for *S. adareanum* microbiome ASVs.

Author Contributions: This work was the result of a team effort in which the following contributions are recognized: conceptualization, A.E.M., P.S.G.C., and B.J.B. methodology and experimentation, A.E.M., N.E.A., L.B., D.E., M.L.H., S.K., C.S.R. and R.M.Y.; validation, K.W.D., M.L.H., and B.J.B. formal analysis, A.E.M., N.E.A., E.D., D.E., S.K., and C.-C.L.; data curation, M.L.H. and C.-C.L.; writing—original draft preparation, A.E.M., B.J.B., N.E.A., D.E., S.K., and C.-C.L.; writing—review and editing, A.E.M., N.E.A., B.J.B., L.B., P.S.G.C., A.E.K.D., D.E., S.K., C.S.R., and R.M.Y.; supervision, A.E.M., B.J.B., P.S.G.C., K.W.D., A.E.K.D., and C.S.R.; project administration, K.W.D.; funding acquisition, A.E.M., P.S.G.C., and B.J.B. All authors have read and agreed to the published version of the manuscript.

Funding: Support for this research was provided in part by the National Institute of Health award (CA205932) to A.E.M., B.J.B., and P.S.G.C., with additional support from National Science Foundation awards (OPP-0442857, ANT-0838776, and PLR-1341339 to B.J.B., ANT-0632389 to A.E.M. and Postdoctoral Research Fellowship award DBI-0532893 to C.S.R.). Support for the sequencing of the bacterioplankton was provided as part of the Joint Genome Institute's Community Sequencing Program (JGI-634 to A.E.M.).

Acknowledgments: The assistance of several collaborators and students is also acknowledged including Charles Amsler, Margaret Amsler, Jason Cuce, Bill Dent, Alex Dussaq, Cheryl Gleasner, Alan Maschek, Robert W. Read, Andrew Shilling, Santana Thomas, and the Palmer Station science support staff.

Conflicts of Interest: The authors declare no conflict of interest.

References

1. Taylor, M.W.; Tsai, P.; Simister, R.L.; Deines, P.; Botte, E.; Ericson, G.; Schmitt, S.; Webster, N.S. 'Sponge-specific' bacteria are widespread (but rare) in diverse marine environments. *ISME J.* **2013**, *7*, 438–443. [CrossRef] [PubMed]
2. Ainsworth, T.D.; Krause, L.; Bridge, T.; Torda, G.; Raina, J.B.; Zakrzewski, M.; Gates, R.D.; Padilla-Gamino, J.L.; Spalding, H.L.; Smith, C.; et al. The coral core microbiome identifies rare bacterial taxa as ubiquitous endosymbionts. *ISME J.* **2015**, *9*, 2261–2274. [CrossRef] [PubMed]
3. Hernandez-Agreda, A.; Leggat, W.; Bongaerts, P.; Ainsworth, T.D. The microbial signature provides insight into the mechanistic basis of coral success across reef habitats. *mBio* **2016**, *7*, e00560-16. [CrossRef] [PubMed]
4. Burgsdorf, I.; Erwin, P.M.; Lopez-Legentil, S.; Cerrano, C.; Haber, M.; Frenk, S.; Steindler, L. Biogeography rather than association with cyanobacteria structures symbiotic microbial communities in the marine sponge *Petrosia ficiformis*. *Front. Microbiol.* **2014**, *5*, 529. [CrossRef] [PubMed]
5. Kelly, L.W.; Williams, G.J.; Barott, K.L.; Carlson, C.A.; Dinsdale, E.A.; Edwards, R.A.; Haas, A.F.; Haynes, M.; Lim, Y.W.; McDole, T.; et al. Local genomic adaptation of coral reef-associated microbiomes to gradients of natural variability and anthropogenic stressors. *Proc. Natl. Acad. Sci. USA* **2014**, *111*, 10227–10232. [CrossRef]
6. Pantos, O.; Bongaerts, P.; Dennis, P.G.; Tyson, G.W.; Hoegh-Guldberg, O. Habitat-specific environmental conditions primarily control the microbiomes of the coral *Seriatopora hystrix*. *ISME J.* **2015**, *9*, 1916–1927. [CrossRef]
7. Lo Guidice, A.; Azzaro, M.; Schiaparelli, S. Microbial Symbionts of Antarctic Marine Benthic Invertebrates. In *The Ecological Role of Microorganisms in the Antarctic Environment*; Castro-Sowinski, S., Ed.; Springer Polar Sciences, Springer Nature: Basel, Switzerland, 2019; pp. 277–296.
8. Cardenas, C.A.; Gonzalez-Aravena, M.; Font, A.; Hestetun, J.T.; Hajdu, E.; Trefault, N.; Malmbergg, M.; Bongcarn-Rudloff, E. High similarity in the microbiota of cold-water sponges of the Genus *Mycale* from two different geographical areas. *PeerJ* **2018**, *6*. [CrossRef]
9. Webster, N.S.; Negri, A.P.; Munro, M.; Battershill, C.N. Diverse microbial communities inhabit Antarctic sponges. *Environ. Microbiol.* **2004**, *6*, 288–300. [CrossRef]
10. Steinert, G.; Wemheuer, B.; Janussen, D.; Erpenbeck, D.; Daniel, R.; Simon, M.; Brinkhoff, T.; Schupp, P.J. Prokaryotic diversity and community patterns in Antarctic continental shelf sponges. *Front. Mar. Sci.* **2019**, *6*, 297. [CrossRef]
11. Webster, N.S.; Bourne, D. Bacterial community structure associated with the Antarctic soft coral, *Alcyonium antarcticum*. *FEMS Microbiol. Ecol.* **2007**, *59*, 81–94. [CrossRef]
12. Murray, A.E.; Rack, F.R.; Zook, R.; Williams, M.J.M.; Higham, M.L.; Broe, M.; Kaufmann, R.S.; Daly, M. Microbiome composition and diversity of the ice-dwelling sea anemone, *Edwardsiella andrillae*. *Integr. Comp. Biol.* **2016**, *56*, 542–555. [CrossRef] [PubMed]
13. Riesenfeld, C.S.; Murray, A.E.; Baker, B.J. Characterization of the microbial community and polyketide biosynthetic potential in the Palmerolide-producing tunicate, *Synoicum adareanum*. *J. Nat. Prod.* **2008**, *71*, 1812–1818. [CrossRef] [PubMed]
14. Palermo, J.A.; Brasco, M.F.R.; Spagnuolo, C.; Seldes, A.M. Illudalane sesquiterpenoids from the soft coral *Alcyonium paessleri*: The first natural nitrate esters. *J. Org. Chem.* **2000**, *65*, 4482–4486. [CrossRef] [PubMed]
15. Diyabalanage, T.; Amsler, C.D.; McClintock, J.B.; Baker, B.J. Palmerolide A, a cytotoxic macrolide from the Antarctic tunicate *Synoicum adareanum*. *J. Am. Chem. Soc.* **2006**, *128*, 5630–5631. [CrossRef] [PubMed]
16. Erwin, P.M.; Pineda, M.C.; Webster, N.; Turon, X.; Lopez-Legentil, S. Down under the tunic: Bacterial biodiversity hotspots and widespread ammonia-oxidizing archaea in coral reef ascidians. *ISME J.* **2014**, *8*, 575–588. [CrossRef] [PubMed]
17. Lopez-Legentil, S.; Turon, X.; Espluga, R.; Erwin, P.M. Temporal stability of bacterial symbionts in a temperate ascidian. *Front. Microbiol.* **2015**, *6*, 1022. [CrossRef]
18. Evans, J.S.; Erwin, P.M.; Shenkar, N.; Lopez-Legentil, S. Introduced ascidians harbor highly diverse and host-specific symbiotic microbial assemblages. *Sci. Rep.* **2017**, *7*, 11033. [CrossRef]
19. Evans, J.S.; Erwin, P.M.; Shenkar, N.; Lopez-Legentil, S. A comparison of prokaryotic symbiont communities in nonnative and native ascidians from reef and harbor habitats. *FEMS Microbiol. Ecol.* **2018**, *94*, fiy139. [CrossRef]

20. Cahill, P.L.; Fidler, A.E.; Hopkins, G.A.; Wood, S.A. Geographically conserved microbiomes of four temperate water tunicates. *Environ. Microbiol. Rep.* **2016**, *8*, 470–478. [CrossRef]
21. Dror, H.; Novak, L.; Evans, J.S.; Lopez-Legentil, S.; Shenkar, N. Core and dynamic microbial communities of two invasive ascidians: Can host-symbiont dynamics plasticity affect invasion capacity? *Microb. Ecol.* **2019**, *78*, 170–184. [CrossRef]
22. Erwin, P.M.; Pineda, M.C.; Webster, N.; Turon, X.; Lopez-Legentil, S. Small core communities and high variability in bacteria associated with the introduced ascidian *Styela plicata*. *Symbiosis* **2013**, *59*, 35–46. [CrossRef]
23. Blasiak, L.C.; Zinder, S.H.; Buckley, D.H.; Hill, R.T. Bacterial diversity associated with the tunic of the model chordate *Ciona intestinalis*. *ISME J.* **2014**, *8*, 309–320. [CrossRef] [PubMed]
24. Tianero, M.D.B.; Kwan, J.C.; Wyche, T.P.; Presson, A.P.; Koch, M.; Barrows, L.R.; Bugni, T.S.; Schmidt, E.W. Species specificity of symbiosis and secondary metabolism in ascidians. *ISME J.* **2015**, *9*, 615–628. [CrossRef] [PubMed]
25. Peng, X.; Adachi, K.; Chen, C.Y.; Kasai, H.; Kanoh, K.; Shizuri, Y.; Misawa, N. Discovery of a marine bacterium producing 4-hydroxybenzoate and its alkyl esters, parabens. *Appl. Environ. Microbiol.* **2006**, *72*, 5556–5561. [CrossRef]
26. Fukunaga, Y.; Kurahashi, M.; Tanaka, K.; Yanagi, K.; Yokota, A.; Harayama, S. *Pseudovibrio ascidiaceicola* sp. nov., isolated from ascidians (sea squirts). *Int. J. Syst. Evol. Microbiol.* **2006**, *56*, 343–347. [CrossRef]
27. Schreiber, L.; Kjeldsen, K.U.; Funch, P.; Jensen, J.; Obst, M.; Lopez-Legentil, S.; Schramm, A. *Endozoicomonas* are specific, facultative symbionts of sea squirts. *Front. Microbiol.* **2016**, *7*, 1042. [CrossRef]
28. Gonzalez, J.M.; Mayer, F.; Moran, M.A.; Hodson, R.E.; Whitman, W.B. *Microbulbifer hydrolyticus* gen.nov., sp. nov., and *Marinobacterium georgiense* gen.nov.sp.nov., two marine bacteria from a lignin-rich pulp mill waste enrichment community. *Int. J. Syst. Evol. Microbiol.* **1997**, *47*, 369–376.
29. Schmidt, E.W.; Donia, M.S. Life in cellulose houses: Symbiotic bacterial biosynthesis of ascidian drugs and drug leads. *Curr. Opin. Biotechnol.* **2010**, *21*, 827–833. [CrossRef]
30. Dou, X.; Dong, B. Origins and bioactivities of natural compounds derived from marine ascidians and their symbionts. *Mar. Drugs* **2019**, *17*, 670. [CrossRef]
31. Little, A.E.; Robinson, C.J.; Peterson, S.B.; Raffa, K.F.; Handelsman, J. Rules of engagement: Interspecies interactions that regulate microbial communities. *Annu. Rev. Microbiol.* **2008**, *62*, 375–401. [CrossRef]
32. Imamura, N.; Nishuma, M.; Takader, T.; Adachi, K.; Sakai, M.; Sano, H. New anticancer antibiotics pelagiomicins, produced by a new marine bacterium *Pelagiobacter variabilis*. *J. Antibiot.* **1997**, *50*, 8–12. [CrossRef]
33. Quevrain, E.; Domart-Coulon, I.; Pernice, M.; Bourguet-Kondracki, M.L. Novel natural parabens produced by a *Microbulbifer* bacterium in its calcareous sponge host *Leuconia nivea*. *Environ. Microbiol.* **2009**, *11*, 1527–1539. [CrossRef]
34. Martínez-García, M.; Stief, P.; Díaz-Valdés, M.; Wanner, G.; Ramos-Esplá, A.; Dubilier, N.; Antón, J. Ammonia-oxidizing Crenarchaeota and nitrification inside the tissue of a colonial ascidian. *Environ. Microbiol.* **2008**, *10*, 2991–3001.
35. Hatzenpichler, R. Diversity, physiology, and niche differentiation of ammonia-oxidizing archaea. *Appl. Environ. Microbiol.* **2012**, *78*, 7501–7510. [CrossRef]
36. Murray, A.E.; Preston, C.M.; Massana, R.; Taylor, L.T.; Blakis, A.; Wu, K.; DeLong, E.F. Seasonal and spatial variability of bacterial and archaeal assemblages in the coastal waters off Anvers Island, Antarctica. *Appl. Environ. Microbiol.* **1998**, *64*, 2585–2595. [CrossRef]
37. Murray, A.E.; Grzymski, J.J. Diversity and genomics of Antarctic marine micro-organisms. *Phil. Trans. Roy. Soc. B Biol. Sci.* **2007**, *362*, 2259–2271. [CrossRef]
38. Grzymski, J.J.; Riesenfeld, C.S.; Williams, T.J.; Dussaq, A.M.; Ducklow, H.; Erickson, M.; Cavicchioli, R.; Murray, A.E. A metagenomic assessment of winter and summer bacterioplankton from Antarctica Peninsula coastal surface waters. *ISME J.* **2012**, *6*, 1901–1915. [CrossRef]
39. Rhoades, D. *Evolution of Plant Chemical Defense Against Herbivores. Herbivores: Their Interaction with Secondary Plant Metabolites*; Academic Press: New York, NY, USA, 1979.
40. McPhail, K.L.; Davies-Coleman, M.T.; Starmer, J. Sequestered chemistry of the Arminacean nudibranch *Leminda millecra* in Algoa Bay, South Africa. *J. Nat. Prod.* **2001**, *64*, 1183–1190. [CrossRef]

41. Carbone, M.; Gavagnin, M.; Haber, M.; Guo, Y.W.; Fontana, A.; Manzo, E.; Genta-Jouve, G.; Tsoukatou, M.; Rudman, W.B.; Cimino, G.; et al. Packaging and delivery of chemical weapons: A defensive trojan horse stratagem in chromodorid nudibranchs. *PLoS ONE* **2013**, *8*, e62075. [CrossRef]
42. Winters, A.E.; White, A.M.; Dewi, A.S.; Mudianta, I.W.; Wilson, N.G.; Forster, L.C.; Garson, M.J.; Cheney, K.L. Distribution of defensive metabolites in nudibranch molluscs. *J. Chem. Ecol.* **2018**, *44*, 384–396. [CrossRef]
43. Schupp, P.; Eder, C.; Paul, V.; Proksch, P. Distribution of secondary metabolites in the sponge *Oceanapia* sp. and its ecological implications. *Mar. Biol.* **1999**, *135*, 573–580. [CrossRef]
44. Freeman, C.J.; Gleason, D.F. Chemical defenses, nutritional quality, and structural components in three sponge species: *Ircinia felix*, *I. campana*, and *Aplysina fulva*. *Mar. Biol.* **2010**, *157*, 1083–1093. [CrossRef]
45. Roue, M.; Domart-Coulon, I.; Ereskovsky, A.; Dejediat, C.; Pererz, T.; Bourguet-Kondracki, M.-L. Cellular localization of clathridimine, an antimicrobial 2-aminoimidazole alkaloid produced by the Mediterranean calcareous sponge *Clathrina clathrus*. *J. Nat. Prod.* **2010**, *73*, 1277–1282. [CrossRef]
46. Furrow, F.B.; Amsler, C.D.; McClintock, J.B.; Baker, B.J. Surface sequestration of chemical feeding deterrents in the Antarctic sponge *Latrunculia apicalis* as an optimal defense against sea star spongivory. *Mar. Biol.* **2003**, *143*, 443–449. [CrossRef]
47. Becerro, M.A.; Paul, V.J.; Starmer, J. Intracolonial variation in chemical defenses of the sponge *Cacospongia* sp. and its consequences on generalist fish predators and the specialist nudibranch predator *Glossodoris pallida*. *Mar. Ecol. Prog. Ser.* **1998**, *168*, 187–196. [CrossRef]
48. Siriak, T.; Intaraksa, N.; Kaewsuwan, S.; Yuenyongsawad, S.; Suwanborirux, K.; Plubrukarn, A. Intracolonial allocation of tisoxazole macrolides in the sponge *Pachastrissa nux*. *Chem. Biodivers.* **2011**, *8*, 238–246.
49. Richardson, A.D.; Aalbersberg, W.; Ireland, C.M. The patellazoles inhibit protein synthesis at nanomolar concentrations in human colon tumor cells. *Anti Cancer Drugs* **2008**, *16*, 533–541. [CrossRef]
50. Kwan, J.C.; Donia, M.S.; Han, A.W.; Hirose, E.; Haygood, M.G.; Schmidt, E.W. Genome streamlining and chemical defense in a coral reef symbiosis. *Proc. Natl. Acad. Sci. USA* **2012**, *109*, 20655–20660. [CrossRef]
51. Gouiffes, D.; Juge, M.; Grimaud, N.; Welin, L.; Sauviat, M.; Barbin, Y.; Laurent, D.; Roussakis, C.; Henichart, J.; Verbist, J. Bistramide A, a new toxin from the urochordata *Lissoclinum bistratum* Sluiter: Isolation and preliminary characterization. *Toxicon* **1988**, *26*, 1129–1136. [CrossRef]
52. Schmidt, E.W. The secret to a successful relationship: Lasting chemistry between ascidians and their symbiotic bacteria. *Invertebr. Biol.* **2015**, *134*, 88–102. [CrossRef]
53. Subramani, R.; Aalbersberg, W. Culturable rare Actinomycetes: Diversity, isolation and marine natural product discovery. *Appl. Microbiol. Biotechnol.* **2013**, *97*, 9291–9321. [CrossRef]
54. Ziemert, N.; Lechner, A.; Wietz, M.; Millan-Aguinaga, N.; Chavarria, K.L.; Jensen, P.R. Diversity and evolution of secondary metabolism in the marine actinomycete genus *Salinispora*. *Proc. Natl. Acad. Sci. USA* **2014**, *111*, E1130–E1139. [CrossRef]
55. Lopera, J.; Miller, I.J.; McPhail, K.L.; Kwan, J.C. Increased biosynthetic gene dosage in a genome-reduced defensive bacterial symbiont. *mSystems* **2017**, *2*, e00096-17. [CrossRef]
56. Holmstrom, C.; James, S.; Neilan, B.A.; White, D.C.; Kjelleberg, S. *Pseudoalteromonas tunicata* sp. nov., a bacterium that produces antifouling agents. *Int. J. Syst. Bacteriol.* **1998**, *48*, 1205–1212. [CrossRef]
57. Baker, B.J.; Dent, B. *Synoicum adareanum* sampling underwater video March 2011 Palmer Station Antarctica, V3. *Dryad Dataset* **2020**. Available online: https://doi.org/10.5061/dryad.gxd2547gw (accessed on 30 May 2020).
58. Massana, R.; Murray, A.E.; Preston, C.M.; DeLong, E.F. Vertical distribution and phylogenetic characterization of marine planktonic Archaea in the Santa Barbara Channel. *Appl. Environ. Microbiol.* **1997**, *63*, 50–56. [CrossRef]
59. Takahashi, S.; Tomita, J.; Nishioka, K.; Hisada, T.; Nishijima, M. Development of a prokaryotic universal primer for simultaneous analysis of Bacteria and Archaea using next-generation sequencing. *PLoS ONE* **2014**, *9*, e105592. [CrossRef]
60. Caporaso, J.G.; Lauber, C.; Walters, W.; Berg-Lyons, D.; Lozupone, C.; Turnbaugh, P.; Fierer, N.; Knight, R. Global patterns of 16S rRNA diversity at a depth of millions of sequences per sample. *Proc. Natl. Acad. Sci. USA* **2011**, *108*, 4516–4522. [CrossRef]
61. Bolyen, E.; Rideout, J.R.; Dillon, M.R.; Bokulich, N.; Abnet, C.C.; Al-Ghalith, G.A.; Alexander, H.; Alm, E.J.; Arumugam, M.; Asnicar, F.; et al. Reproducible, interactive, scalable and extensible microbiome data science using QIIME 2. *Nat. Biotechnol.* **2019**, *37*, 852–857. [CrossRef]

62. Callahan, B.J.; McMurdie, P.J.; Rosen, M.J.; Han, A.W.; Johnson, A.J.A.; Holmes, S.P. DADA2: High-resolution sample inference from Illumina amplicon data. *Nat. Methods* **2016**, *13*, 581–583. [CrossRef]
63. Kumar, S.; Stecher, G.; Tamura, K. MEGA7: Molecular evolutionary genetics analysis version 7.0 for bigger data sets. *Mol. Biol. Evol.* **2016**, *33*, 1870–1874. [CrossRef] [PubMed]
64. Tackmann, J.; Matias Rodrigues, J.F.; von Mering, C. Rapid inference of direct interactions in large-scale ecological networks from heterogeneous microbial sequencing data. *Cell Syst.* **2019**, *9*, 286–296.e8. [CrossRef] [PubMed]
65. Bastian, M.; Heymann, S.; Jacomy, M. Gephi: An Open Source Software for Exploring and Manipulating Networks. In Proceedings of the International AAAI ICWSM Conference on weblogs and social media, San Jose, CA, USA, 17–20 May 2009.
66. Cristóbal, E.; Ayuso, S.V.; Justel, A.; Toro, M. Robust optima and tolerance ranges of biological indicators: A new method to identify sentinels of global warming. *Ecol. Res.* **2013**, *29*, 55–68. [CrossRef]
67. Langfelder, P.; Horvath, S. WGCNA: An R package for weighted correlation network analysis. *BMC Bioinform.* **2008**, *9*, 559. [CrossRef]
68. Paulson, J.N.; Stine, O.C.; Bravo, H.C.; Pop, M. Differential abundance analysis for microbial marker-gene surveys. *Nat. Methods* **2013**, *10*, 1200–1202. [CrossRef]
69. Markowitz, V.M.; Chen, I.-M.A.; Palaniappan, K.; Chu, K.; Szeto, E.; Grechkin, Y.; Ratner, A.; Jacob, B.; Huang, J.; Williams, P.; et al. IMG: The integrated microbial genomes database and comparative analysis system. *Nucleic Acids Res.* **2012**, *40*, D115–D122. [CrossRef]
70. Blin, K.; Medema, M.H.; Kottmann, R.; Lee, S.Y.; Weber, T. The antiSMASH database, a comprehensive database of microbial secondary metabolite biosynthetic gene clusters. *Nucleic Acids Res.* **2017**, *45*, D555–D559. [CrossRef]
71. Murray, A.; Baker, B. *Synoicum adareanum* Microbiome. SCAR—Microbial Antarctic Resource System Metadata Dataset. , 2020. Available online: https://doi.org/10.15468/aewoib (accessed on 30 May 2020).

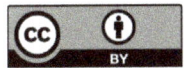

© 2020 by the authors. Licensee MDPI, Basel, Switzerland. This article is an open access article distributed under the terms and conditions of the Creative Commons Attribution (CC BY) license (http://creativecommons.org/licenses/by/4.0/).

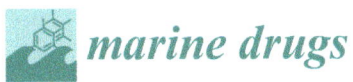

Article

Light-Mediated Toxicity of Porphyrin-Like Pigments from a Marine Polychaeta

Mariaelena D'Ambrosio [1,*], Ana Catarina Santos [1], Alfonso Alejo-Armijo [2], A. Jorge Parola [2] and Pedro M. Costa [1,*]

1. UCIBIO–Applied Molecular Biosciences Unit, Departamento de Ciências da Vida, Faculdade de Ciências e Tecnologia da Universidade Nova de Lisboa, 2829-516 Caparica, Portugal; acf.santos@campus.fct.unl.pt
2. LAQV–Associate Laboratory for Green Chemistry, Departamento de Química, Faculdade de Ciências e Tecnologia da Universidade Nova de Lisboa, 2829-516 Caparica, Portugal; aaa00010@red.ujaen.es (A.A.-A.); ajp@fct.unl.pt (A.J.P.)
* Correspondence: m.dambrosio@fct.unl.pt (M.D.); pmcosta@fct.unl.pt (P.M.C.); Tel.: +351-212-948-300 (ext. 11103) (P.M.C.)

Received: 30 March 2020; Accepted: 4 June 2020; Published: 6 June 2020

Abstract: Porphyrins and derivatives form one of the most abundant classes of biochromes. They result from the breakdown of heme and have crucial physiological functions. Bilins are well-known representatives of this group that, besides significant antioxidant and anti-mutagenic properties, are also photosensitizers for photodynamic therapies. Recently, we demonstrated that the Polychaeta *Eulalia viridis*, common in the Portuguese rocky intertidal, holds a high variety of novel greenish and yellowish porphyrinoid pigments, stored as granules in the chromocytes of several organs. On the follow-up of this study, we chemically characterized pigment extracts from the worm's skin and proboscis using HPLC and evaluated their light and dark toxicity in vivo and ex vivo using *Daphnia* and mussel gill tissue as models, respectively. The findings showed that the skin and proboscis have distinct patterns of hydrophilic or even amphiphilic porphyrinoids, with some substances in common. The combination of the two bioassays demonstrated that the extracts from the skin exert higher dark toxicity, whereas those from the proboscis rapidly exert light toxicity, then becoming exhausted. One particular yellow pigment that is highly abundant in the proboscis shows highly promising properties as a natural photosensitizer, revealing that porphyrinoids from marine invertebrates are important sources of these high-prized bioproducts.

Keywords: porphyrinoids; annelida; marine bioproducts; HPLC-DAD; toxicity; photosensitizers

---

1. Introduction

Biological pigments (biochromes) can be defined as any material from biological origin that results in color. They can have many functions, among which mimicking and communication are but a few, and are normally products of complex and varied biosynthetic pathways involving a wide span of enzymes [1]. Pigments resulting from these metabolic processes can be broadly divided in two classes: those that are directly responsible for organism colors and those that are colored secondary metabolites, which may or may not be directly involved with the organisms' primary pigmentation [2]. One of the most abundant classes of natural pigments are tetrapyrroles, considered as the "pigments of life" [3] due to their role in photosynthesis, gas transport, and redox reactions. This class includes porphyrins, which are metabolites of heme.

Arguably, the best known porphyrinoids are bilins (also termed bilichromes or bile pigments) [2,4], whose coloration can vary between yellow, green, red, and brown [5]. They are secondary metabolites devoid of metal cores and are arranged in linear (chain) structures rather than in the customary cyclic configuration of porphyrins [2]. Biliverdin and bilirubin are notorious members of this group that, despite resulting from the breakdown of heme, hold important biological functions, such as antioxidants, in humans and other animals [6]. Like many other tetrapyrroles, bilins are photosensitive, which provides them with a high interest in photodynamic therapy (PDT), since they can generate singlet oxygen when irradiated, thus triggering localized cytotoxic effects [7]. In fact, depending on their structure, porphyrinoids have a distinctive absorption spectrum in the UV-visible region, characterized by a strong band around 420 nm, named the Soret band, and a series of low-intensity absorption bands at longer wavelengths, typically between 500 and 650 nm, termed Q bands (refer to Arnaut [8] for an overview). However, photoactivation may occur when the pigments are subjected to light from the whole visible spectrum [9]. Porphyrinoids may exert light-independent toxicity, nonetheless, which renders mandatory safeguarding a high light:dark toxicity ratio to uphold a compound's value as photosensitizer [10]. Altogether, porphyrinoids are provided with a particular interest for biotechnological purposes as colorants, antimicrobial, biocides, or as biomarkers for the physiological status of animals [11–13].

Marine invertebrates, in particular, especially those of coastal environments, known for their bright and diversified coloration, seemingly have a wider span of porphyrinoids than their vertebrate counterparts. However, as for other natural products, the true diversity, nature, and function of these pigments in marine invertebrates remains largely unknown. Some of the first works on tetrapyrrole pigments from marine animals began with bonellin, a distinctive chlorin-like greenish pigment from the females of the Echiuran Polychaeta *Bonellia viridis* that is turned into a potent biocidal when photoactivated, protecting the animal from predators and biofoulants [14,15]. In turn, *Hediste* (*Nereis*) is a common intertidal worm that is known to have a diversified and seasonally changing pattern of pigments, in large part due to porphyrinoids resulting from endogenous heme breakdown [16].

Recently, we showed that an uncanny uniformly green Polychaeta, *Eulalia viridis*, an opportunistic predator of the rocky intertidal, owes its coloration to a multiplicity of endogenous porphyrin-like pigments whose abundance and distribution changes between organs [17–20]. These pigments, which seem to almost entirely replace common biochromes such as carotenoids and melanins, were found to be chiefly stored as granules allocated within unique specialized chromocytes [19,20]. The function and bio-reactivity of these pigments is not, however, fully understood. It was hypothesized that, more than mimicking the worm's surroundings, these pigments offer important protection from sunlight and that, being porphyrinoids, they may also have toxic properties modulated by light. Additionally, *E. viridis* secretes toxins that, delivered by its copious mucus secretion, are used to immobilize and partly digest prey (mostly invertebrates, especially mussels, barnacles, and other Polychaeta) before extracting a portion of flesh via suction with its jawless but highly muscular proboscis [21]. This ability also led us to hypothesize a strong investment in chemical warfare on behalf of the species that may extend to its pigmentation. On the follow-up of our preceding research, the current work aimed at a comparative screening for potential light-mediated toxicity of the novel porphyrinoid pigments extracted from *E. viridis* skin and proboscis in view of its potential biotechnological value.

2. Results

2.1. Chemical Characterization of Pigments

In accordance with Martins et al. [20], the crude extracts in cold Dulbecco's phosphate-buffered saline (PBS) from the proboscis and skin, being yellowish and greenish in color, respectively, were comprised of multiple pigments. Both extracts of skin and proboscis tissues were analyzed by HPLC-DAD and recorded at 280 and 440 nm (exemplified in Figure 1). For simplification purposes, this distinction based on visual inspection will be retained. Albeit variable among individual pigments, the absorption spectra of either extract had maxima within the UV range (ca. 280 nm), plus Soret bands between 350 and 500 nm and the characteristic Q bands (580–750 nm) of porphyrin-like pigments, which is particularly obvious for the main pigments fractionated from the skin (Figure 2). Among the main pigments in skin extracts that better fit the expected porphyrin signature, we found a yellowish pigment that was exclusive to this organ, with a retention time of 1.8 min. To this substance a greenish pigment was added with retention time 3.43 min and two yellow pigments with retention times 0.95 and 4.40 min (Figure 3). The latter, in particular, was found to be the most abundant pigment in skin extracts, as inferred from its higher absorbance (Figure 3D).

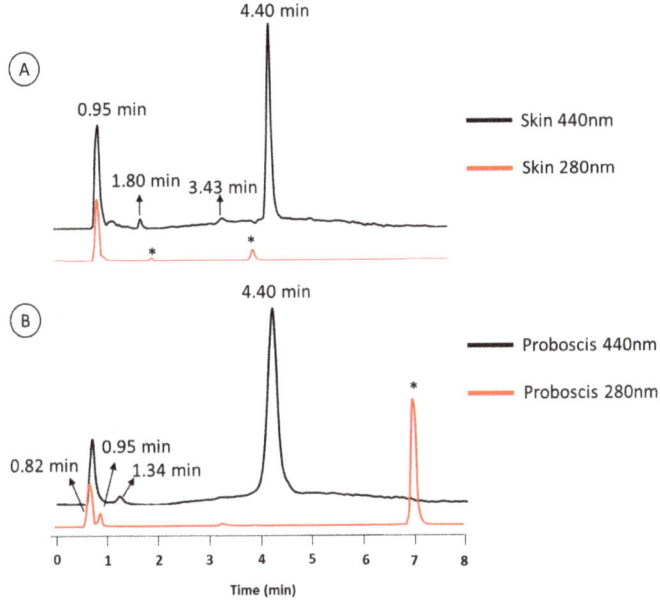

Figure 1. Representative HPLC-DAD profiles at 440 and 280 nm (black and red line, respectively). Pigments extracts from (**A**) skin, and (**B**) proboscis. Compounds with * did not present the characteristic absorption of porphyrin pigments and were not further addressed.

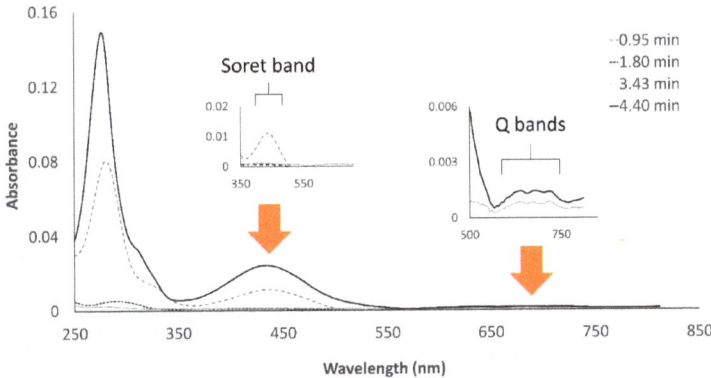

Figure 2. Absorption spectra of the four main pigments in *Eulalia viridis* skin crude pigment extracts spectra retrieved from HPLC-DAD analyses (each pigment's spectrum is identified by its retention time). The Soret (350–500 nm) and Q (580–750 nm) bands typical of porphyrinoids are highlighted.

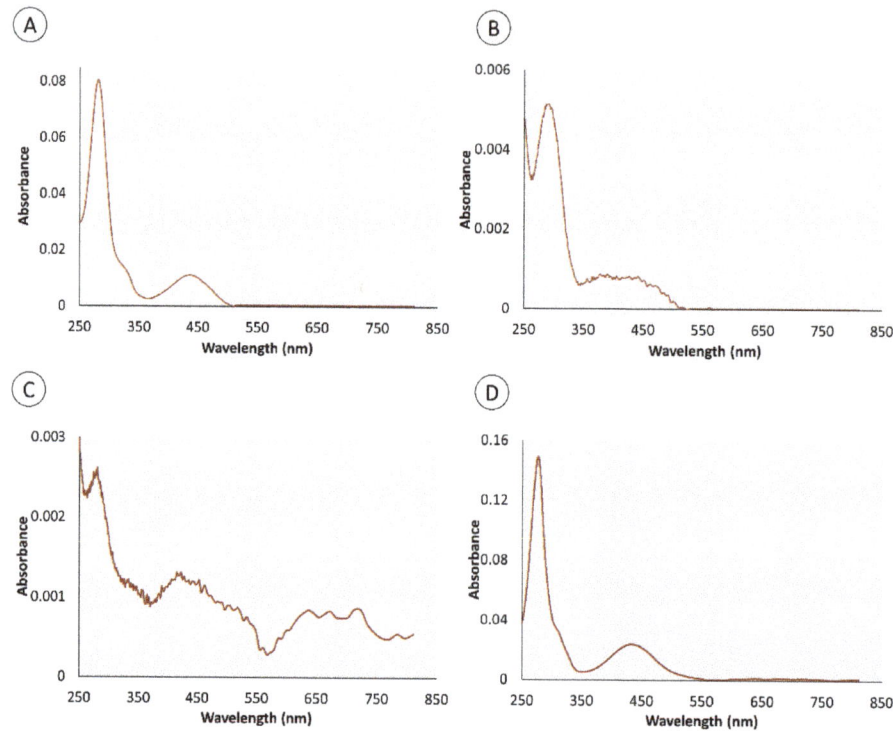

Figure 3. Spectra of the principal pigments in the crude extracts from the skin of *Eulalia viridis* fractionated by HPLC-DAD. The skin yielded mainly one greenish and three yellowish pigments. (**A**) yellow pigment (0.95 min); (**B**) yellow pigment (1.8 min); (**C**) green pigment (3.43 min); (**D**) yellow pigment (4.40 min). The pigments detected at retention times 1.80 and 3.34 min are specific to the skin.

The proboscis extract yielded two green and two yellowish main pigments with porphyrinoid signatures (Figure 4). Among the four main compounds, two yellow pigments were detected at retention times of 0.95 and 4.40 min, presenting maxima at both 282 and 286 nm, respectively. To this pigment two greenish pigments detected at retention times of 0.82 and 1.34 min were added, with absorbance maxima at 272 and 257 nm, respectively, which were exclusive to this organ (Figure 5). The yellow pigments detected in the proboscis are similar to those described earlier in the skin, judging from similar retention times (0.95 and 4.40 min) and absorbance magnitudes. As previous, the yellow pigment shown in Figure 5D with the 4.40-min retention time was most abundant, not only in extracts from the proboscis but also comparatively to the skin. Table 1 summarizes the main similarities and differences between pigment extracts from the two organs.

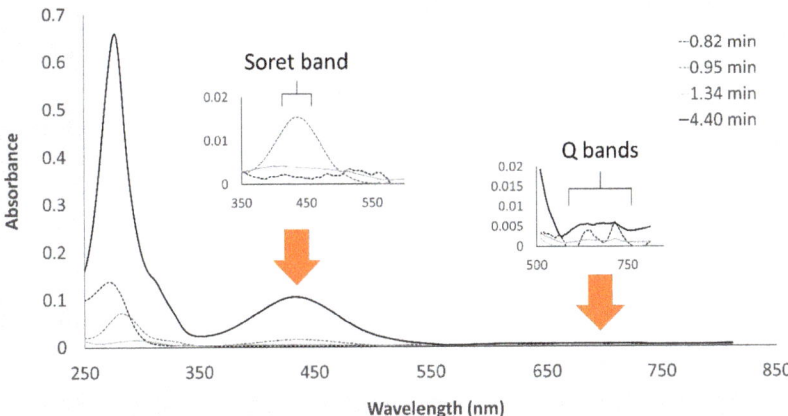

Figure 4. Absorption spectra of the four main pigments in *Eulalia viridis* proboscis crude pigment extracts spectra retrieved from HPLC-DAD analyses (each pigment's spectrum is identified by its retention time). The Soret (350–500 nm) and Q (580–750 nm) bands typical of porphyrinoids are highlighted.

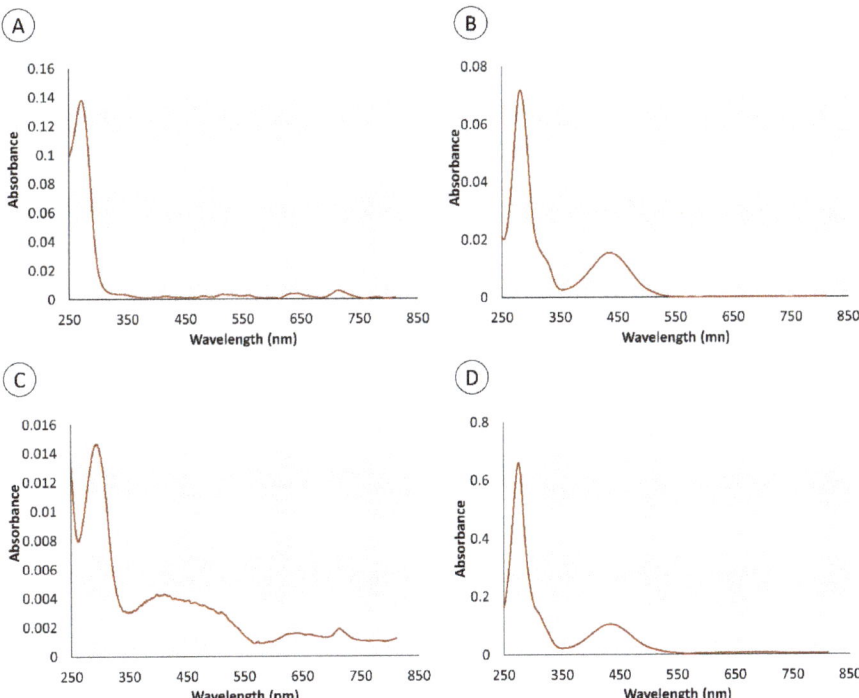

Figure 5. Spectra of the principal pigments in the crude extracts from the proboscis of *Eulalia viridis* fractionated by HPLC-DAD. The proboscis yielded mainly two yellowish and two greenish pigments. (**A**) green pigment (0.82 min); (**B**) yellow pigment (0.95 min); (**C**) green pigment (1.34 min); (**D**) yellow pigment (4.40 min). The pigments detected at retention times of 0.82 and 1.34 min are specific to the proboscis.

2.2. Comet Assay

The light/dark experimental treatment (here identified as the two-factor variable "treatment") was the only explanatory variable found to significantly modulate DNA damage (Table 2). In accordance, significant differences were found between the L (light) and D (dark) experimental conditions in gills exposed to extracts from the proboscis, albeit only for the 50% concentration (D2), attaining a maximum of ≈56% DNA in tail (Figure 6). In the case, gills exposed to the extract, in the light, revealed highest damage by ca. two-fold on average, relative to the dark condition (Figure 7). Even though pigment extracts from the skin failed to elicit significant differences between experimental conditions, regardless of dilution, the highest level of DNA damage scored in gills exposed to this extract was recorded in gills subjected to light and exposed to the highest (100%) concentration of pigments (termed D1), attaining an average of 51% DNA in tail.

Table 1. Summary of the main pigments in PBS extracts from the skin and proboscis of *Eulalia viridis*, based on data retrieved from HPLC-DAD.

Retention Time (min)	Organ		Color		Absorbance Maximum (nm)	
	Skin	Proboscis	Green	Yellow	Skin	Proboscis
0.95	•	•		•	280 nm	282 nm
4.4	•	•		•	276 nm	286 nm
0.82	–	•	•		–	272 nm
1.34	–	•	•		–	257 nm
1.8	•	–		•	288 nm	–
3.43	•	–		•	288 nm	–

[•] and [–] indicate presence or absence, respectively.

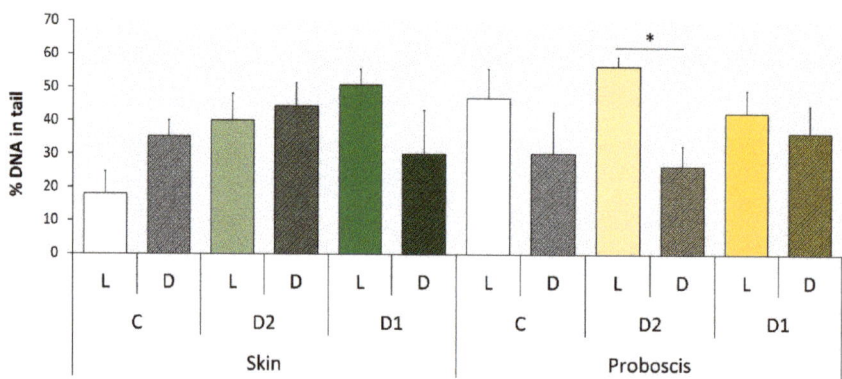

Figure 6. Comet assay results (as % DNA in tail) from the gills of *Mytilus* exposed to two dilutions of pigment extracts corresponding to the nominal concentrations of 100% (D1) and 50% (D2), plus controls, i.e., gills treated with PBS only, which was the vehicle for pigment extracts (C). Mussels were exposed to the extracts from skin and proboscis mixtures under light (L) and dark (D) conditions. The results are expressed as means + SD. [*] indicates significant differences between L and D conditions (*t*-test, $p < 0.05$).

Table 2. Results from ANOVA for GLM (based on sequential analysis of deviance) for the Comet assay on mussel gills exposed to pigments.

Variable	df	Deviance Residuals	df	Residual Deviance	p
Treatment	1	0.44403	46	5.0954	0.02629 [1]
Pigment	1	0.20322	45	4.8922	0.13280
Dilution	2	0.13029	43	4.7619	0.48465

[1] significant with $p < 0.05$.

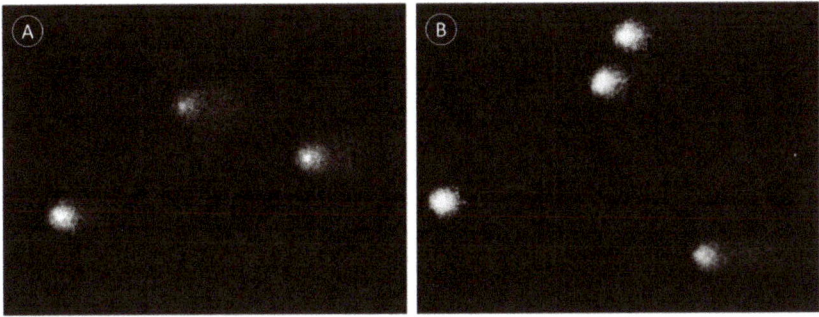

Figure 7. Exemplificative Comet fields from mussel gills treated with pigment extracts from *Eulalia* illustrating the differences between light and dark treatments. (**A**) Gills exposed to 50%-diluted extracts from the proboscis (light treatment); (**B**) same as previous but gills subjected to dark conditions, evidencing lower DNA damage, as seen by higher and lower head and tail intensities, respectively, comparatively to the previous.

2.3. Daphnia Immobilization Assay

All explanatory variables ("treatment", "exposure time", "pigment", and "dilution") were found to significantly modulate the immobilization of *Daphnia* (Table 3). Extracts from the skin were responsible for the overall highest immobilization rates, which tended to increase with concentration and total exposure time after the initial 1-h light or dark treatment (Figure 8). However, contrarily to the previous findings, exposure to pigment extracts in the dark tended to cause highest effects either at 24 (Figure 8A) or 48 h (Figure 8B), albeit the effects being more significant for assays conducted with the most concentrated extracts from the skin. Accordingly, the highest immobilization rates resulted from *Daphnia* exposed to the most concentrated (D1) skin pigment extract, followed by exposure to D2, both after 48 h, hitherto the dark treatment attaining a ca. two-fold increase relatively to the light condition. Still, after 24 h of the experiment this effect was almost three-fold higher.

Table 3. Results from ANOVA for GLM (based on sequential analysis of deviance) for the *Daphnia* immobilization assay.

Variable	df	Deviance Residuals	df	Residual Deviance	p
Treatment	1	36.461	190	862.43	1.558×10^{-9} [1]
Pigment	1	31.388	189	795.04	2.113×10^{-8} [1]
Exposure time	1	143.122	188	651.92	$<2 \times 10^{-16}$ [1]
Dilution	3	160.977	185	490.94	$<2 \times 10^{-16}$ [1]

[1] significant with $p < 0.01$.

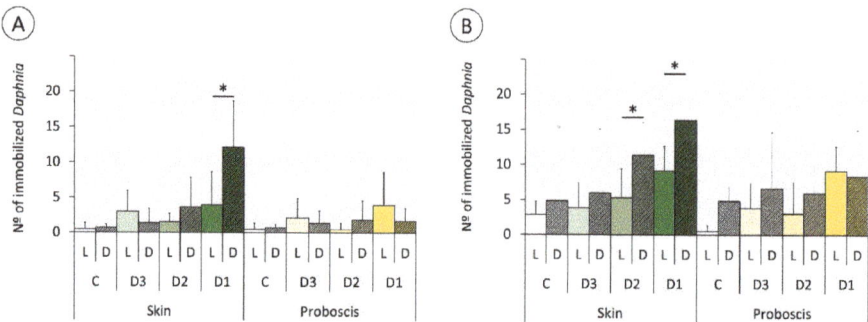

Figure 8. *Daphnia* immobilization assay after exposure to three dilutions of pigment extracts corresponding to the nominal concentrations of 100% (D1), 50% (D2), and 10% (D3), plus controls (C). *Daphnia* were exposed for 1 h to the extracts from skin and proboscis mixtures under light (L) and dark (D) conditions and analyzed after (**A**) 24 h; (**B**) 48 h. The results are expressed as mean immobilized individuals (out of 20) + SD. [*] indicates significant differences between L and D treatment conditions (t-test, $p < 0.05$).

3. Discussion

In accordance with our previous findings (Martins et al. [20]), the extracts from the "greenish" skin and the "yellowish" proboscis of *Eulalia viridis* contain multiple pigments and sustain very significant inter-organ variation. However, the extraction methods were distinct between the two works, albeit HPLC-DAD being used for fractioning in either case. Whereas we previously used HCl:acetonitrile to extract the pigments, in the present work we opted for extraction in PBS to obtain a physiologically compatible vehicle for the bioassays. The most notorious difference is the higher representativity of individual yellowish pigments in the skin found in the current work relatively to Martins et al. [20]. Nonetheless, the main pigments, in particular the yellow compound retrieved at retention time 4.40 min (Figures 3D and 5D) is seemingly present in the extracts from our preceding work. Moreover, this pigment shows the expected porphyrinoid signature. The methodological differences between the two works are likely responsible for disparities and render direct comparisons difficult, taking into account extraction efficiencies. However, it is clear from the current results that many porphyrinoid pigments in *E. viridis* are hydrophilic and compatible with PBS, which has important implications for biotechnological endeavors. It must be noted, though, that our previous paper already suggested the amphiphilic nature of porphyrinoids from *Eulalia*, similarly to what has already been described for other porphyrin-derived pigments [22]. In addition, the advantages of amphiphilic substances in therapeutics, as they can be transported through the blood stream and have facilitated crossing through the phospholipid by-layer, leads to substantial efforts to produce these compounds synthetically for the purpose of PDT (see for instance Malatesti et al. [22]). The discovery of natural bioproducts with these properties, as in the present case, is, therefore, an important biotechnological asset.

The two very distinct toxicity-testing procedures yielded divergent, albeit complementary results, in any case the presence or absence of light being a significant factor. The duration of the assays (i.e., total time of exposure) is inferred to be a key to explain the differences. Indeed, the shorter-term (1 h) assays with mussel gills revealed a trend for higher DNA-damage effects under light, whereas the *Daphnia* immobilization assay yielded the opposite tendency after 24 and 48 h of exposure following the initial 1 h treatment under light or dark conditions. Consequently, despite the differences between model and endpoint, time of exposure is seemingly a major player in the modulation of toxicity because the generation of singlet oxygen by photodynamic substances occurs swiftly after irradiation with visible light [23]. Evidently, this depends on oxygen supply, which is certainly more reduced in the test medium of *Daphnia*, especially after 48 h, even assuming minimal degradation of the pigments in the test medium or by the cladocerans' own mechanisms of porphyrinoid catabolism and elimination.

Consequently, the photodynamic effect of porphyrinoids was more evident in DNA damage determined by the standard alkaline Comet assay, which is directly sensitive to singlet oxygen radicals in the short term, with particular respect to the formation of oxidized purines [24,25]. On the other hand, after 24 and 48 h of exposure, low oxygen and photosensitizer exhaustion seemingly reduced the photodynamic effects of pigments, leaving dark toxicity of phorphyrinoids as the most evident effect. This effect has already been described for a range of porphyrin-based photosensitizers in vitro [25,26]. Even though dark toxicity for these compounds in vivo is not well understood, the results suggest significant effects in *Daphnia*. However, details on the toxicity, metabolism, and elimination of heme and its secondary metabolites are scarce (refer, for instance, to Lamkemeyer et al. [27] and references therein on *Daphnia* hemoglobin). Still, Fabris et al. [28] found *Daphnia magna* particularly sensitive to both light and dark toxicity of certain porphyrinoids after short term (1 h) and 24–48 h of incubation. It is noteworthy that the same authors employed the standard *Daphnia* immobilization assay as well. These results are thus in good alignment with the current study and show that the toxicodynamics and toxicokinetics of photosensitizers is complex as it depends on the ratio between light:dark toxicity and how it changes with time. Even though the sensitivity of our models and endpoints cannot be directly compared, the findings also demonstrate the importance of testing both immediate and longer-term effects of exposure to isolate light and dark toxicity of porphyrinoids. This subject is of particular relevance for further studies to investigate the potential of pigments in PDT, as dark toxicity can cause significant effects during the period of elimination, after the effective photodynamic capability of pigments has been exhausted.

There are also very noticeable differences between the effects caused by the two extracts that ultimately enable shortlisting the pigments with the most promising properties as photosensitizers. The findings show that the extracts from the proboscis, where the yellow pigment with 4.40 min retention time is by far more abundant than in the skin (which makes it responsible for the difference in color between the two extracts), hold higher phototoxicity. This can be ascertained from the comparison between Figures 6 and 8. Most likely, the majority of the phototoxicity causing the increment of DNA damage relatively to the dark treatment shown in Figure 6 is due to this same yellow pigment, despite inconclusive dose-response effects. On the other hand, the mixture of pigments in the skin extracts, which includes the same compounds albeit in much lower proportion, caused higher dark toxicity. Altogether, the results indicate that this yellow pigment is an interesting candidate for further research as an effective photosensitizer. It must be noted, though, that the lack of a clear dose-response is in part due to significant inter-replica variation and reduced number of concentrations tested. Nonetheless, we must emphasize that at this stage we were testing crude extracts and not the purified pigments, which also contributed to the overall variation. Further toxicity testing involving the isolation of this candidate pigment are needed, as well a complete chemical characterization. It must also be noticed that the extracts from the skin caused DNA damage and suggest a potential dose-response and light-mediated toxicity as well. However, as pointed out in our previous work, this organ holds a much wider variety of pigments than the proboscis [20], which complicates, at this stage, isolating specific substances of interest and obtaining sufficient amounts for analyses.

It can be inferred that the light toxicity of porphyrins is certain to cause deleterious effects to the worm itself. This consequence has been noted before and has, inclusively, been suggested as one of the reasons why Polychaeta are so difficult to rear in captivity [29], which explains the need to add shelter and provide dimmed light to *Eulalia* in the laboratory [18]. Considering that *Eulalia* is a diurnal forager of the rocky intertidal, its pigments likely have two important roles. First, they are either toxic or repellent to predators and parasites that cause rupture to the pigment cells where the pigments are "safely" stored in granules [19,20]. Second, they warn of excessive exposure to daylight by causing physiological stress, which can be considered a form of non-nervous sensorial arrangement. The fact that *Eulalia* uses its proboscis as the main organ for sensing and preying [19,21] explains the natural difference between the pigmentation of the skin as a major adaptive trait. These particular features, which are probably not circumscribed to *Eulalia* or even to the Order Phyllodocida, show that the Polychaeta are very promising targets for the bioprospecting of photoactive tetrapyrrolic pigments.

In conclusion, the present work revealed different porphyrin-like pigments in the body of the Polychaeta *Eulalia*, distributed differentially between the proboscis and the skin. The differential pigmentation pattern between the two organs is also reflected in distinct light:dark toxicity ratios that are influenced by time of exposure, as light-dependent toxicity occurs swiftly whereas light-independent will occur in a longer timeframe until the substances are metabolized and finally eliminated from the recipient organism. With this respect, the two bioassay procedures with mussel gills and *Daphnia* (1 and 48 h, respectively), showed the importance of performing short and longer tests to evaluate the unique toxicodynamics of photosensitizers. From the aggregate findings we were able to detect a specific pigment, yellowish in color, present in both organs albeit much more concentrated in the proboscis of the worm. This pigment, in particular, is a serious candidate as photosensitizer: (i) it is likely amphiphilic and compliant with PBS, which is an advantage for distribution during therapeutics; (ii) its light toxicity is considerably higher than its dark toxicity, and (iii) its reduced toxicity with time in vivo may be an indicator of rapid exhaustion and facilitated elimination. These highly promising results also confirm that marine invertebrates are a prolific source of natural porphyrinoids, a class of substances with high value for therapeutics and whose research is still mostly based on synthetics.

4. Materials and Methods

4.1. Animals

Adult *E. viridis* (ca. 5–10 cm length) were collected by hand in Parede Beach, an intertidal rocky beach in Western Portugal (38°41′42″ N; 09°21′36″ W), during the low tide. Organisms were then transported to the laboratory and kept in a mesocosm recreating their natural habitat consisting of dark-walled aquaria, equipped with a system providing constant aeration and water recirculation, to which natural rocks were added, with barnacles and mussels collected from the same area to provide shelter and feed to the worms, as developed by Rodrigo et al. [18]. Salinity, water temperature and photoperiod were maintained restrained at about 30, 18 °C and 16:8 h light-dark, respectively. Animals were thus acclimatized for 7–14 days until pigment extraction.

Mussels (*Mytilus* sp.) were also collected as models for the ex vivo assay. Laboratory cultures of wild-type *Daphnia pulex* were maintained in an aquarium with filtered pond water, replicating optimal environmental conditions for their reproduction (temperature: 20 ± 2 °C; pH: 7.5; photoperiod: 16 h light:8 h dark). *Daphnia* were fed with a mixture of *Arthrospira platensis* and *Saccharomyces cerevisiae*, following Pellegri et al. [30] and Santos et al. [31].

4.2. Pigment Extraction

Worms were immobilized by hypotonic shock and microdissected to collect proboscis and skin (factually the body wall containing epidermis plus underlying musculature). The organs were then homogenized separately with a pestle in cold Dulbecco's phosphate-buffered saline (PBS), pH 7.5 to extract the hydrophilic fraction of pigments. Samples were afterwards centrifuged for 5 min, 5000 g at 4 °C. The supernatant containing the pigments was collected and immediately placed on ice and in the dark. The pellet was subjected to repeated extractions until the supernatant was visibly devoid of pigments. The supernatants were then pooled. Each pooled sample contained extracts from approximately five animals.

The crude extracts of either organ were then analyzed spectrophotometrically at 440 and 700 nm, the maxima described by Martins et al. [20]. Extracts were then diluted in PBS, with the absorbance at 440 being used to normalize the dilutions until samples yielded an absorbance value of 1 (D1), corresponding to the 100% concentrated extract. This solution was necessary to overcome the absence of suitable standards for the mixtures of pigments in the extracts from either organ. Serial dilutions D1 (100%) were then produced, termed D2 and D3, corresponding to 50% and 10% of D1, respectively.

Pigment extraction was performed in a dim-lighted environment to avoid photodegradation of pigments. Exposure of worm tissues and extracts to ambient light and air was kept to the minimum. Analysis and toxicity testing involved only fresh extracts.

4.3. Chemical Characterization of Pigments

Crude extracts of the two organs (skin and proboscis) were filtered with a GHP filter before analysis. Pigments were analyzed based on the protocol for separation and quantification of human bilins developed by Woods and Simmonds [32], with many optimizations. In brief, high-performance liquid chromatography (HPLC) analyses were conducted on a Merck-Hitachi instrument equipped with a diode array detector (DAD), scan range 200–800 nm (Merck-Hitachi L-4500 Diode Array Detector, Merck, Poole, UK), operating at 20 °C, using a reversed-phase analytical column (RP-HPLC, Onix® Monolithic C18 column, 100 × 4.6 mm i.d., 13 nm and 2 µm). Samples were prepared in MeOH and the injection volume was 20 µL. Preliminary assays showed that optimal peak separation was obtained with sodium phosphate buffer 10 mM, pH 3.5 (solvent A) and pure MeOH (solvent B) at a flow rate of 2 mL/min: linear gradient from 45% to 95% B for 10 min and 95% B for 2 min. The total run time excluding equilibration was 12 min. Linear gradient from 30% to 60% B for 5 min and linear gradient from 60% to 95% B for 10 min. The total run time excluding equilibration was 15 min. Throughout analysis, the pressure was maintained at about 67 bar and the temperature column kept at environmental temperature (20 ± 2 °C).

4.4. Experimental Design

4.4.1. Assays with *Mytilus* sp. Gills

Ex vivo bioassays using *Mytilus* sp. gills were performed to investigate DNA damage resulting from exposure to pigments under light or dark conditions. For the purpose, valves of live mussels (ca. 40 mm in length) were carefully separated to retain integrity of gills and the visceral mass swiftly removed. Assays began immediately after excision. One valve being used as a test sample (pigment extract, diluted in PBS as described above) and the other as its respective control (PBS only). For both crude extracts, proboscis (P) and skin (S), the test valve was exposed to 1 mL of D1 or D2 dilutions, while the control was treated with 1 mL of PBS. Test valves and controls were subjected to either ambient light (L), i.e., indirect daylight, or dark (D) conditions for 1 h and processed immediately afterwards. All assays were made in triplicate ($n = 3$).

4.4.2. Comet Assay

Damage to DNA was evaluated using an adaptation of the alkaline single-cell gel electrophoresis (Comet) assay, developed by Singh et al. [33], adapted by Raimundo et al. [34] for molluscan solid tissue. Freshly harvested gill samples were minced with pliers in 700 mL of cold PBS and centrifuged for 1 min at 1200 rpm. The supernatant (clear cell suspension) was diluted in 1% *m/v* molten (37–40 °C) low melting point agarose (LMPA) prepared in PBS. Afterwards, two 80-µL drops of LMPA cell suspensions were placed on slides pre-coated with 1.2% *m/v* of normal melting point agarose (dried for at least 48 h) and covered with a coverslip. After LMPA solidification (15 min, 4 °C) coverslips were removed and the slides immersed in cold lysis buffer (0.45 M NaCl (*m/v*); 40 mM EDTA (*m/v*); 5 mM Tris pH 10) for 1 h. Slides were then placed in cold electrophoresis buffer (0.1 mM EDTA; 0.3 M NaOH, pH 13) for 40 min to allow DNA-unwinding and expression of alkali-labile sites. Electrophoresis was run at 25 V for 30 min at 4 °C. Then, the slides were neutralized in 0.2 M Tris-HCl, pH 7.5, and dried with methanol for archiving before analysis. Rehydrated slides were stained with GreenSafe (Nzytech, Portugal) [35] and analyzed with a DM 2500 LED microscope adapted for epifluorescence with an EL 6000-light source (Leica Microsystems). Scoring was done with CometScore 1.6 (Tritek), with 100 nucleoids being analyzed per slide. The percentage of DNA in tail was considered as a direct measure of DNA damage [36].

4.4.3. Acute Toxicity Assay with *Daphnia pulex*

Based on standard guidelines for toxicity testing with *Daphnia* sp. [37–39], daphnids with less than 24 h were selected for the assay. For the purpose, several females with mature eggs in the brood pouch were transferred to a 90-mm Petri dish containing with distilled water 12 h before the experiments. Hatched juveniles (daphnids) were afterwards collected and used for the tests. The test replicate consisted of a well of a 24-well clear bottom microplate (2-mL well) containing 20 daphnids. Each well contained 0.2 mL of extract and 1.8 mL of distilled water. Plates were then exposed under dark (D) of light (L) conditions, for 1 h, to dilutions D1, D2, or D3 of P and S pigment extracts, plus controls, which consisted of adding 0.2 mL of PBS to the test water ($n = 6$) and afterwards incubated in unchanged medium, in the dark, until analysis. The number of immobilized daphnids was evaluated after 24 and 48 h from the beginning of the exposure.

4.5. Statistical Analysis

Homoscedasticity of data was assessed by the Levene's test. After invalidation of this assumption for parametric analysis, we used generalized linear models (GLM) through a Poisson regression with a log link function, considering dilution, light/dark treatment, organ, and time (duration) of the experiment (in the case of the *Daphnia* assay) as explanatory variables. Analysis of variance based on deviance was carried out to assess the effect of independent variables on DNA damage and immobilization of *Daphnia*. Complementary comparisons were done with Student's *t*-test. All analyses were done using R [40]. Generalized linear models were computed with the package *glm2*.

Author Contributions: Conceptualization, M.D. and P.M.C.; laboratory methodology, M.D., A.C.S., A.A.-A.; data analysis, M.D., A.C.S., A.A.-A., A.J.P., P.M.C., writing—original draft preparation, M.D., P.M.C.; writing—review and editing, M.D., A.A.-A., A.J.P., P.M.C.; supervision, A.J.P., P.M.C., project administration, P.M.C. All authors have read and agreed to the published version of the manuscript.

Funding: The Portuguese Foundation for Science and Technology (FCT) funded projects GreenTech (PTDC/MAR BIO/01132014) and WormALL (PTDC/BTA-BTA/28650/2017). UCIBIO and LAQV are financed by national funds from FCT, references UID/Multi/04378/2020 and UID/QUI/50006/2020, respectively. The authors also acknowledge DPGM (the Portuguese General Directorate for Marine Policy) for funding the MARVEN project (ref. FA_05_2017_007), which includes the fellowship attributed to M.D. A.Á.-A. is grateful for the post-doctoral fellowship from Fundación Alfonso Martín Escudero.

Acknowledgments: The authors acknowledge A. Rodrigo, C. Martins, and C. Gonçalves (the SeaTox Lab at UCIBIO) for the important assistance during the work.

Conflicts of Interest: The authors declare no conflict of interest.

References

1. Diamond, J. *Concealing Coloration in Animals*; Harvard University Press: Cambridge, MA, USA, 2013; 288p. [CrossRef]
2. Needham, A.E. *The Significance of Zoochromes*; Springer: New York, NY, USA, 1974; 429p.
3. Milgrom, L.R. *The Colours of Life. An introduction to the Chemistry of Porphyrins and Related Compounds*; Oxford University Press: Oxford, UK, 1997; 256p.
4. Takemoto, J.Y.; Chang, C.T.; Chen, D.; Hinton, G. Heme-derived bilins. *Isr. J. Chem.* **2019**, *59*, 378–386. [CrossRef]
5. Bandaranayake, W.M. The nature and role of pigments of marine invertebrates. *Nat. Prod. Rep.* **2006**, *23*, 223–255. [CrossRef] [PubMed]
6. Bulmer, A.C.; Ried, K.; Blanchfield, J.T.; Wagner, K.H. The anti-mutagenic properties of bile pigments. *Mutat. Res. Rev. Mutat. Res.* **2008**, *658*, 28–41. [CrossRef] [PubMed]
7. Bonnett, R.; Berenbaum, M. Porphyrins as photosensitizers. *Ciba Found. Symp.* **1989**, *146*, 40–59. [CrossRef] [PubMed]
8. Arnaut, L.G. Design of porphyrin-based photosensitizers for photodynamic therapy. *Adv. Inorg. Chem.* **2011**, *63*, 187–233. [CrossRef]

9. Williams, T.M.; Sibrian-Vazquez, M.; Vicente, M.G.H. Design and synthesis of photosensitizer-peptide conjugates for PDT. In *Handbook of Photodynamic Therapy Updates on Recent Applications of Porphyrin-Based Compounds*; Pandey, R.K., Kessel, D., Dougherty, T.J., Eds.; World Scientific: New Jersey, NJ, USA, 2016; pp. 45–93. [CrossRef]
10. Yoo, J.-O.; Ha, K.-S. New insights into the mechanisms for photodynamic therapy-induced cancer cell death. In *International Review of Cell and Molecular Biology*; Jeon, K.W., Ed.; Academic Press: San Diego, CA, USA, 2012; Volume 295, pp. 139–174. [CrossRef]
11. Ben Amor, T.; Jori, G. Sunlight-activated insecticides: Historical background and mechanisms of phototoxic activity. *Insect Biochem. Mol. Biol.* **2000**, *30*, 915–925. [CrossRef]
12. Bozja, J.; Sherrill, J.; Michielsen, S.; Stojiljkovic, I. Porphyrin-based, light-activated antimicrobial materials. *J. Polym. Sci. Part A Polym. Chem.* **2003**, *41*, 2297–2303. [CrossRef]
13. Casini, S.; Fossi, M.C.; Leonzio, C.; Renzoni, A. Porphyrins as biomarkers for hazard assessment of bird populations: Destructive and non-destructive use. *Ecotoxicology* **2003**, *12*, 297–305. [CrossRef]
14. Schembri, P.J.; Jaccarini, V. Evidence of a chemical defence mechanism in the echiuran worm *Bonellia viridis* Rolando (Echiura: Bonelliidae). *Mar. Behav. Physiol.* **1979**, *6*, 257–267. [CrossRef]
15. Pelter, A.; Ballantine, J.A.; Ferrito, V.; Jaccariki, V.; Psaila, A.F.; Schembr, P.J. Bonellin, a most Unusual Chlorin. *J. Chem. Soc.* **1976**, 999–1000. [CrossRef]
16. Dales, R.P.; Kennedy, G.Y. On the diverse colours of *Nereis diversicolor*. *J. Mar. Biol. Ass. UK* **1954**, *33*, 699–708. [CrossRef]
17. Costa, P.M.; Carrapiço, F.; Alves de Matos, A.P.; Costa, M.H. A microscopical study of the "chlorophylloid" pigment cells of the marine polychaete *Eulalia viridis* (L.). *Microsc. Microanal.* **2013**, *19*, 15–16. [CrossRef]
18. Rodrigo, A.P.; Costa, M.H.; Alves De Matos, A.P.; Carrapiço, F.; Costa, P.M. A Study on the digestive physiology of a marine polychaete (*Eulalia viridis*) through microanatomical changes of epithelia during the digestive cycle. *Microsc. Microanal.* **2015**, *21*, 91–101. [CrossRef] [PubMed]
19. Rodrigo, A.P.; Martins, C.; Costa, M.H.; Alves de Matos, A.P.; Costa, P.M. A morphoanatomical approach to the adaptive features of the epidermis and proboscis of a marine Polychaeta: *Eulalia viridis* (Phyllodocida: Phyllodocidae). *J. Anat.* **2018**, *233*, 567–579. [CrossRef]
20. Martins, C.; Rodrigo, A.P.; Cabrita, L.; Henriques, P.; Parola, A.J.; Costa, P.M. The complexity of porphyrin-like pigments in a marine annelid sheds new light on haem metabolism in aquatic invertebrates. *Sci. Rep.* **2019**, *9*, 1–11. [CrossRef]
21. Cuevas, N.; Martins, M.; Rodrigo, A.P.; Martins, C.; Costa, P.M. Explorations on the ecological role of toxin secretion and delivery in jawless predatory Polychaeta. *Sci. Rep.* **2018**, *8*, 1–10. [CrossRef]
22. Malatesti, N.; Munitic, I.; Jurak, I. Porphyrin-based cationic amphiphilic photosensitisers as potential anticancer, antimicrobial and immunosuppressive agents. *Biophys. Rev.* **2017**, *9*, 149–168. [CrossRef]
23. Maisch, T.; Baier, J.; Franz, B.; Maier, M.; Landthaler, M.; Szeimies, R.M.; Bäumler, W. The role of singlet oxygen and oxygen concentration in photodynamic inactivation of bacteria. *PNAS* **2007**, *104*, 7223–7228. [CrossRef]
24. Ravanat, J.L.; Sauvaigo, S.; Caillat, S.; Martinez, G.R.; Medeiros, M.H.G.; Di Mascio, P.; Favier, A.; Cadet, J. Singlet oxygen-mediated damage to cellular DNA determined by the comet assay associated with DNA repair enzymes. *J. Biol. Chem.* **2004**, *385*, 17–20. [CrossRef]
25. Vicente, M.G.H.; Nurco, D.J.; Shetty, S.J.; Osterloh, J.; Ventre, E.; Hedge, V.; Deutsch, W.A. Synthesis, dark toxicity and induction of in vitro DNA photodamage by a tetra(4-nido-carboranylphenyl)porphyrin. *J. Photochem. Photobiol. B Biol.* **2002**, *68*, 123–132. [CrossRef]
26. Eckl, D.B.; Dengler, L.; Nemmert, M.; Eichner, A.; Bäumler, W.; Huber, H. A closer look at dark toxicity of the photosensitizer TMPyP in bacteria. *Photochem. Photobiol.* **2018**, *94*, 165–172. [CrossRef] [PubMed]
27. Lamkemeyer, T.; Zeis, B.; Decker, H.; Jaenicke, E.; Waschbüsch, D.; Gebauer, J.; Meissner, U.; Rousselot, M.; Zal, F.; Nicholson, G.J.; et al. Molecular mass of macromolecules and subunits and the quaternary structure of hemoglobin from the microcrustacean *Daphnia magna*. *FEBS J.* **2006**, *273*, 3393–3410. [CrossRef] [PubMed]
28. Fabris, C.; Soncin, M.; Jori, G.; Hablueetzel, A.; Lucantoni, L.; Sawadogo, S.; Guidolin, L.; Coppellotti, O. Effects of a new photoactivatable cationic porphyrin on ciliated protozoa and branchiopod crustaceans, potential components of freshwater ecosystems polluted by pathogenic agents and their vectors. *Photochem. Photobiol. Sci.* **2012**, *11*, 294–301. [CrossRef] [PubMed]

29. Mangum, C.P.; Phillips Dales, R. Products of haem synthesis in polychaetes. *Comp. Biochem. Physiol.* **1965**, *15*, 237–257. [CrossRef]
30. Pellegri, V.; Gorbi, G.; Buschini, A. Comet assay on *Daphnia magna* in eco-genotoxicity testing. *Aquat. Toxicol.* **2014**, *155*, 261–268. [CrossRef] [PubMed]
31. Santos, V.S.V.; Silveira, E.; Pereira, B.B. Ecotoxicological assessment of synthetic and biogenic surfactants using freshwater cladoceran species. *Chemosphere* **2019**, *221*, 519–525. [CrossRef]
32. Woods, J.S.; Simmonds, P.L. HPLC Methods for analysis of porphyrins in biological media. *Curr. Protoc. Toxicol.* **2001**, 1–18. [CrossRef]
33. Singh, N.P.; McCoy, M.T.; Tice, R.R.; Schneider, E.L. A simple technique for quantitation of low levels of DNA damage in individual cells. *Exp. Cell Res.* **1988**, *175*, 184–191. [CrossRef]
34. Raimundo, J.; Costa, P.M.; Vale, C.; Costa, M.H.; Moura, I. DNA damage and metal accumulation in four tissues of feral *Octopus vulgaris* from two coastal areas in Portugal. *Ecotoxicol. Environ. Saf.* **2010**, *73*, 1543–1547. [CrossRef]
35. Martins, C.; Costa, P.M. Technical updates to the Comet assay in vivo for assessing DNA damage in zebrafish embryos from fresh and frozen cell suspensions. *Zebrafish* **2020**, in press. [CrossRef]
36. Lee, R.F.; Steinert, S. Use of the single cell gel electrophoresis/comet assay for detecting DNA damage in aquatic (marine and freshwater) animals. *Mutat. Res. Rev. Mutat. Res.* **2003**, *544*, 43–64. [CrossRef]
37. Adema, D.M.M. *Daphnia magna* as a test animal in acute and chronic toxicity tests. *Hydrobiologia* **1978**, *59*, 125–134. [CrossRef]
38. Persoone, G.; Baudo, R.; Cotman, M.; Blaise, C.; Thompson, K.C.; Vollat, B.; Törökne, A.; Han, T. Review on the acute *Daphnia magna* toxicity test—Evaluation of the sensitivity and the precision of assays performed with organisms from laboratory cultures or hatched from dormant eggs. *Knowl. Managt. Aquatic Ecosyst.* **2009**, *393*, 01. [CrossRef]
39. USEPA. *Ecological Effects Test Guidelines OCSPP 850.1010: Aquatic Invertebrate Acute Toxicity Test, Freshwater Daphnids*; U.S. Environmental Protection Agency: Washington, DC, USA, 2016.
40. Ihaka, R.; Gentleman, R.R. A Language for Data Analysis and Graphics. *J. Comput. Graph. Stat.* **1996**, *5*, 299–314. [CrossRef]

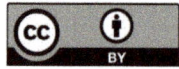

© 2020 by the authors. Licensee MDPI, Basel, Switzerland. This article is an open access article distributed under the terms and conditions of the Creative Commons Attribution (CC BY) license (http://creativecommons.org/licenses/by/4.0/).

MDPI
St. Alban-Anlage 66
4052 Basel
Switzerland
Tel. +41 61 683 77 34
Fax +41 61 302 89 18
www.mdpi.com

Marine Drugs Editorial Office
E-mail: marinedrugs@mdpi.com
www.mdpi.com/journal/marinedrugs

www.ingramcontent.com/pod-product-compliance
Lightning Source LLC
LaVergne TN
LVHW070747100526
838202LV00013B/1324

9 783036 506425